Epidemiology and the prevention of mental disorders

D1626315

Impressive strides have been made over the past 20 years in the methods for studying the occurrence of mental illness in populations. The techniques of psychiatric epidemiology are now being applied to the most pressing problems of mental ill-health in modern society: schizophrenia, major depression, suicidal behaviour, alcoholism, drug abuse, late-life dementia, and mental retardation. The contributors to this book, from a wide range of countries, discuss the incidence and distribution of these conditions in populations, and the risk factors with which they are associated.

Taking a public health approach to the prevention of mental illness, the authors report epidemiological research in psychiatry. They emphasize its importance in preventive terms, and point out that its objectives are the same in psychiatry as in other fields of medicine: to reduce the incidence of disease, to limit its course and consequences by means of early diagnosis and treatment, and to avoid whenever possible the development of disease-related chronic disability and handicap. Several contributors mark a new stage in the development of psychiatric epidemiology as a public health discipline by drawing attention to the growing concern with the implications for mental health of contemporary changes in our biological and social environment.

The Editors

Brian Cooper is Professor and Head of the Department of Epidemiological Psychiatry at the Central Institute of Mental Health, Mannheim, West Germany. Tómas Helgason is Professor and Chairman, Department of Psychiatry, University of Iceland, Reykjavik.

Published by Routledge for the World Psychiatric Association.

Epidemiology and the prevention of mental disorders

Edited by

Brian Cooper

and

Tómas Helgason

for the

World Psychiatric Association

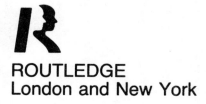

ROUTLEDGE
London and New York

First published in 1989
by Routledge
11 New Fetter Lane, London EC4P 4EE
29 West 35th Street, New York, NY 10001

© 1989 Brian Cooper and Tómas Helgason

Typeset by J&L Composition Ltd, Filey, N. Yorkshire
Printed and bound in Great Britain by
Mackays of Chatham PLC, Chatham, Kent

British Library Cataloguing in Publication Data

Epidemiology and the prevention of mental disorders.
    1. Man. Mental disorders. Epidemiology
    I. Cooper, Brian, T. II. Helgason (Tómas) III.
    World psychiatric Association
    362.2'0422

Library of Congress Cataloging in Publication Data

Epidemiology and the prevention of mental disorders / edited by Brian Cooper and
    Tómas Helgason for the World Psychiatric Association.
    p.   cm.
    Contains a selection of reports and review articles based on the ninth scientific
    symposium arranged by the World Psychiatric Association's Section of
    Epidemiology and Community Psychiatry, held in Reykjavik in September 1987
    and organized by the Department of Psychiatry, National University Hospital,
    Reykjavik.
    Includes bibliographies and index.
    1. Mental illness—Epidemiology—Congresses. 2. Mental illness-
    Prevention—Congresses. I. Cooper, Brian, 1928–   . II. Helgason,
    Tómas. III. Central Institute of Mental Health, Mannheim. IV. National
    University Hospital. Dept. of Psychiatry, Reykjavik.
    [DNLM: 1. Mental Disorders—occurrence—congresses. 2. Mental
    Disorders—prevention & control—congresses. WM 100 E637 1987]
    RC455.2.E64E655 1989
    362.2—dc19
    DNLM/DLC
    for Library of Congress   88–37105
                                      CIP

ISBN 0–415–00015–7

Contents

Contents

Tables and figures

Tables

Figures

Contributors

Anthony, James C., Ph.D., The Johns Hopkins University, School of Hygiene and Public Health, Baltimore.

Beskow, Jan, M.D., Asst. Prof., University of Göteborg, Department of Psychiatry, Göteborg.

Bickel, Dr. H., Zentralinstitut für Seelische Gesundheit, Mannheim.

Brayne, Carol, M.B., M.R.C.P., M.Sc., University of Cambridge, Department of Community Medicine, Addenbrooke's Hospital, Cambridge.

Bromet, Evelyn J., Ph.D., Prof., Department of Psychiatry and Behavioral Science, State University of New York, Stony Brook, New York.

Brook, Judith S., Ed.D., Mount Sinai School of Medicine, New York.

Brook, Drs. O. H., Geneeskundige Hoofdinspectie voor de Geestelijke Volksgezondheid, Rijswijk, The Netherlands.

Chee, Elsbeth M.L., The Johns Hopkins University, School of Hygience and Public Health, Baltimore.

Cohen, Patricia, Ph.D., Office of Mental Health, New York State Psychiatric Institute, New York.

Conover, Sarah, M.P.H., The Nathan S. Kline Institute for Psychiatric Research, Orangeburg, N.Y.

Cooper, Prof. B., Zentralinstitut für Seelische Gesundheit, Mannheim.

Dean, Laura, M.Ed., Columbia University, College of Physicians and Surgeons, Department of Psychiatry, New York.

Dilling, Prof. H., Klinik für Psychiatrie der Medizinischen Universität zu Lübeck.

Dupont, Dr. Annalise, Institute of Psychiatric Demography, Aarhus Psychiatric Hospital, Risskov, Denmark.

Eaton, W.W., Ph.D., The Johns Hopkins University, School of Hygiene and Public Health, Baltimore.

Gournas, G., M.D. University of Athens Department of Psychiatry, Community Mental Health Center, Social Psychiatry Unit, Athens.

Häfner, Prof. Heinz, Zentralinstitut für Seelische Gesundheit, Mannheim.

Harris, Tirril, MRC Department of Social Policy and Social Science, Royal Holloway & Bedford New College, London.

Helgason, Prof. Tómas, Department of Psychiatry, National University Hospital, Reykjavik.

Henderson, Dr. A.S., Social Psychiatry Research Unit, The Australian National University, Canberra.

Johnson, Jim,, Ph.D. Office of Mental Health, New York State Psychiatric Institute, New York.

King, Dr. Michael B., General Practice Research Unit, Institute of Psychiatry, London.

Kramer, Morton, Sc.D. Prof. Emeritus, The Johns Hopkins University, School of Hygiene and Public Health, Department of Mental Hygiene, Baltimore.

Leighton, Prof. A.H., Department of Community Health and Epidemiology, Dalhousie University, Halifax, Nova Scotia.

Lovell, Anne, M.S.W., New York State Psychiatric Research Institute, New York.

Madianos, Michael, G., M.D., M.P.H., University of Athens, Department of Psychiatry, Community Mental Health Center, Social Psychiatry Unit, Athens.

Madianou, D., Ph.D., University of Athens, Department of Psychiatry, Community Mental Health Center, Social Psychiatry Unit, Athens.

Magnússon, Dr. H., Department of Psychiatry, National University Hospital, Reykjavik.

Martin, J.L., Ph.D., M.P.H., Columbia University School of Public Health, New York.

Micciolo, Dr. R., Department of Medical Psychology, Institute of Psychiatry, University of Verona, Verona.

Neugebauer, Richard, Ph.D., M.P.H., The Faculty of Medicine, Columbia University, New York.

Oschinsky, Dr. A.M., Klinik für Psychiatrie der Medizinischen Universität zu Lübeck.

Parkinson, David K., M.A., B.M., B.Ch., Department of Psychiatry and Behavioral Science, State University of New York, Stony Brook, N.Y.

Rodrigo, Dr. E.K., General Practice Research Unit, Institute of Psychiatry, London.

Sartorius, Prof. N., Division of Mental Health, World Health Organization, Geneva.

Schmidtke, Dr. A., Psychiatrische Klinik u. Poliklinik, Universitäts-Nervenklinik, Würzburg.

Shapiro, S., M.D., The Johns Hopkins University, Department of Mental Hygiene, Baltimore.

Stefanis, Prof. C.N., University of Athens, Department of Psychiatry, Community Mental Health Center, Social Psychiatry Unit, Athens.

Struening, Elmer, L., Ph.D., Office of Mental Health, New York State Psychiatric Institute, New York.

Susser, E., M.D., M.P.H., The Nathan S. Kline Institute for Psychiatric Research, Orangeburg, N.Y.

Tansella, Prof. M., Department of Medical Psychology, Institute of Psychiatry, University of Verona, Verona.

Williams, Dr. P., Institute of Psychiatry, General Practice Research Unit, London.

Zimmermann-Tansella, Prof. C., Department of Medical Psychology, Institute of Psychiatry, University of Verona, Verona.

Preface

The ninth scientific symposium to be arranged by the World Psychiatric Association's Section of Epidemiology and Community Psychiatry took place in Reykjavik in September 1987, organized by the Department of Psychiatry at National University Hospital, Reykjavik. The present volume, which takes its title from the theme of the symposium, contains a selection of reports and review articles on the epidemiology of mental disorders, based on material presented on that occasion.

A number of books, derived from earlier symposia in the same series, have been published over the past twenty years (Hare and Wing 1970; Wing and Häfner 1973; Robins *et al*. 1980; Wing *et al*. 1981; Cooper 1987). Their contents reflect the progress which psychiatric epidemiology underwent during this period, from preoccupation with the construction and testing of new research tools to their increasing application in population-based investigations. The earlier meetings were largely taken up with methodological issues in data gathering and analysis, case-finding, diagnostic assessment and classification; also, to a lesser extent but increasingly, with the definition and measurement of those features of the microsocial environment thought to be implicated in the genesis of mental illness, or in determining individual susceptibility to its attack. This concentration on methods has undoubtedly paid dividends in terms of the growth of an impressive research armamentarium, as well as in changing professional attitudes within psychiatry. Operational criteria have been introduced into the major diagnostic classifications. Psychiatric case registers have been set up in many countries, and some of them at least are flourishing. Psychiatrists in all parts of the world have learned to accept the need for standardized clinical assessment and there is now an abundance of different structured or semi-structured interview procedures, a number of which are available in many languages. The opportunities thus created for international collaboration are beginning to be exploited.

The time is therefore ripe – some might say overdue – for a more systematic and intensive application of these new research techniques to the most pressing problems of mental ill-health in modern society:

schizophrenia, major depression, suicidal behaviour, alcoholism, narcotic addiction and related forms of drug abuse, late-life dementia, and mental retardation. Questions relating to the incidence and distribution of these disorders in populations, and to the risk factors with which they are associated, can and should now be addressed with the renewed vigour and confidence bestowed by methodological progress, and the increased precision which it has made possible. The present volume provides evidence that this trend is already under way.

Such a development calls for a preventive framework, since it is only in their approach to common preventive goals that the humanitarian and scientific traditions of social psychiatry can be relied upon to converge and unite. The true importance of epidemiological research, in whichever field of medicine, resides in its function as the scientific basis of preventive action. Thirty years ago, Gruenberg (1957) pointed out that an approach to the control of mental disorders calls for the same strategies to be employed as in dealing with other categories of disease and causes of death: to take the necessary steps to prevent those conditions known to be preventable (primary prevention); to terminate or arrest those which can be effectively treated (secondary prevention), and to minimize the impairments and disabilities arising from those which cannot be terminated, or which persist following illness (tertiary prevention). Success or failure in attaining these objectives is the standard by which the efficacy of health services, whether hospital or community based, must in the last analysis be judged; but it must be measured in terms of mortality and morbidity in the population as a whole, and not only among those persons who are in contact with the treatment agencies.

These arguments have been slow to gain acceptance among clinical psychiatrists and, as far as mental illness is concerned, among public health workers also. There are, however, signs that a ground-swell of change is now building up. The World Health Organization's 'Health for All 2000' campaign is gathering momentum and has served, if only fortuitously, to draw attention to an embarrassing lack of defined targets for prevention in the mental health field, and so to stimulate new activity. In 1986 the World Health Assembly adopted a resolution calling on member states to introduce measures for the prevention of mental disorders into their national health policies. The present views of WHO on this subject are summarized in this volume by Sartorius. They are now being promoted in different parts of the world by the regional offices of WHO, and the call is also being taken up by schools of public health.

That preventively oriented research is now on the upsurge in psychiatry, despite a currently unfavourable *Zeitgeist*, is suggested by the response which the Reykjavik meeting evoked: over 100 contributions, mostly reporting original research of relevance to this topic, were submitted by participants from nineteen countries. The selection included here, though it amounts to only one quarter of the total, gives some indication of the scope and variety of these reports. Two features in particular may be noted. First, while recent advances in method have been largely assimilated into this body of research, they do not themselves constitute the subject-matter: the focus of attention is fixed throughout not on the techniques but on their utilization in applied research. Second, a number of contributions – especially those from the USA – bear testimony to an increasing scientific concern with the implications for mental health of contemporary changes in man's biological and social environment. If time shows that a general trend is thus being signalized, one will be justified in regarding this book as a small but significant landmark in the development of psychiatric epidemiology as a public-health discipline.

The Editors
May 1988

References

Cooper, B. (ed.) (1987) *Psychiatric Epidemiology: Progress and Prospects*, London: Croom Helm.

Gruenberg, E.M. (1957) 'Application of control methods to mental illness', *American Journal of Public Health* 47: 944–52.

Hare, E.H. and Wing, J.K. (eds) (1970) *Psychiatric Epidemiology*, London: Oxford University Press.

Robins, L.N., Clayton, P.J., and Wing, J.K. (eds) (1980) *The Social Consequences of Psychiatric Illness*, New York: Brunner Mazel.

Wing, J.K. and Häfner, H. (eds) (1973) *Roots of Evaluation*, London: Oxford University Press.

Wing, J.K., Bebbington, P., and Robins, L.N. (eds) (1981) *What is a Case? The Problem of Definition in Psychiatric Community Surveys*, London: Grant McIntyre.

World Health Organization (1988) *Prevention of Mental, Neurological and Psychosocial Disorders*, WHO/MNH/EVA/88.1, Geneva: WHO.

Part one

Prevention in psychiatry: goals, strategies, constraints

Chapter one

Introduction: strategies of prevention

Brian Cooper

'Four cheers for prevention!' declared J.N. Morris in a memorable polemic (Morris 1974), and one might suppose that clinical psychiatrists, daily confronted in their work by evidence of the intractable nature and disastrous consequences of many cases of established mental illness, would be more than ready to endorse his opinion. Yet a cursory glance through the leading modern textbooks suffices to show that prevention remains today a grossly undervalued theme in psychiatry. The best-known American compilation, for example, devotes only three of its 2,000 pages to this topic (Kaplan and Sadock 1985), while a prestigious British handbook fails to include the word 'prevention' in the index to any of its volumes.

The reasons for this remarkable neglect do not lie primarily in any outright rejection of the idea of prevention, or even in reliance on a too-narrow biomedical model of mental illness. The roots of the problem are to be found elsewhere. To begin with, psychiatric teaching does not sufficiently emphasize the importance of secular changes in morbidity or the part that medical progress and public-health control have played together in preventing, and in some instances virtually eradicating, forms of mental disorder that were once widely prevalent. A few examples will serve to illustrate the point. Dementia paralytica, once the single most common cause of prolonged mental-hospital stay, has almost disappeared since the introduction of effective treatment of and prophylaxis against syphilis. Pellagra psychosis has been obviated with the help of improved nutrition and dietary supplements. The brain damage associated with congenital rubella is being prevented by immunization programmes, while that due to tuberculous meningitis was dramatically reduced in incidence following the introduction of streptomycin. The use of antibiotics in acute infectious disease has served incidentally to reduce the occurrence of systemic psychoses and toxic confusional states. The prevention of mental disorders, in short, is an everyday reality of modern hygiene and medical care.

Where so much has already been achieved, it is a reasonable assumption that further progress can be made. No fundamental qualitative difference is known to exist between those conditions which can, and those which as yet cannot, be prevented. But to the blinkered vision that accepts only the functional psychoses and neuroses prevalent in our own society as the legitimate sphere of psychiatric endeavour and, moreover, regards these conditions as 'endogenous' and non-communicable, the achievements of preventive medicine appear to be at best only marginally relevant.

A second, closely related cause is the identification of preventive psychiatry as a whole with those measures, based on psychodynamic theory, which are aimed at modifying human relationships, either within the nuclear family or in larger groups. Many psychiatrists still tend to think of this as being *the* preventive approach, but are highly sceptical of its value in practice. It is significant that early forays in the same direction, such as the 'mental hygiene' movement begun by Clifford Beers and Adolf Meyer (Lewis 1974), or the Child Guidance Demonstration Clinics of the 1920s (Levy 1968), were backed by philanthropic foundations and aroused greater enthusiasm among psychologists, social workers, pedagogues, and educated lay people than they did in the ranks of the medical profession. Something of the same kind could be observed in the responses to President Kennedy's 1963 Message to Congress and the Community Mental Health Centers Act which followed it. While public opinion was widely sympathetic towards a programme which placed emphasis on primary prevention through improvement of the mental health of the community as a whole, spokesmen for clinical psychiatry were dubious about the benefits and quick to point out that resources would be diverted for this purpose only at the cost of existing services for the mentally ill.

The arguments put forward on both sides in these debates express differences in underlying attitudes and contribute to an ongoing dialectic that still awaits resolution. Nevertheless, ideas about prevention are evolving slowly in the light of experience, and it seems possible that informed opinion in psychiatry and the related disciplines is now moving towards agreement with respect to a number of basic general principles, which can be stated as follows.

1. The most useful frame of reference for preventive action in psychiatry is that provided by the division into primary, secondary, and tertiary prevention, customary in other fields of preventive medicine. Such action should be concentrated on what scientific and clinical evidence has shown to be possible and aimed at preventing those conditions known to be preventable (primary level), at terminating or arresting those which are amenable to treatment (secondary level), and at minimizing the disability and handicap caused by those which cannot yet be effectively treated, or whose consequences persist after the illness (tertiary level).

2. It follows that, in a balanced preventive programme, secondary and tertiary measures directed at diagnosed cases of mental illness will play an

important part; they may indeed merit higher priority than primary prevention at the current stage of knowledge.

3. In order to undertake such measures, services for the mentally ill and handicapped should be organized for defined populations, and their clinical and preventive functions should be demarcated and co-ordinated in this population-based frame of reference.

4. Prevention at each level may call for the participation of a number of different medical and social agencies. Primary prevention will depend largely on action taken outside the sphere of psychiatry; for example, in maternal and child health care, environmental control, or political legislation. Secondary prevention will result from early case detection, treatment, and referral by community-based services. Tertiary prevention implies co-operation with social welfare agencies in avoiding the need for prolonged hospital stay and in improving facilities for rehabilitation and resettlement.

5. Any systematic approach to prevention must give high priority to epidemiological and health services research. Advances in knowledge of the risk factors of mental disorders is essential for reducing their incidence; studies of services in action are necessary to assess and improve their effectiveness; progress towards preventive goals must be monitored with the aid of health information systems. No theoretical framework can compensate for the lack of an adequate research component.

Acceptance of these postulates would establish some common ground and help to ensure that future preventive programmes evoke a more balanced, constructively critical response than did their predecessors. It would also ensure their development within the mainstream of health care, rather than as a highly specialized form of provision, organized independently from, or even in competition with, the established clinical services.

The subject is a topical one, since the debate about preventive measures and their relative importance in psychiatry seems destined to flare up again as the 'Health for All 2000' campaign gathers momentum and its relevance for mental health care begins to be examined (Cooper 1988). It is therefore encouraging that the World Health Organization has recently come to grips with this issue and has produced a useful report (WHO 1988), which sets out in concise summary the magnitude and extent of the problems to be tackled, proposals for action to be taken in dealing with them, and, if only briefly and in very general terms, some suggestions for establishing research priorities.

The report concludes, on the basis of the evidence reviewed, that preventive programmes making use of currently available methods could effect a substantial reduction in the burdens due to mental disorders and that they should be directed at both the biological and the social causes of these conditions. The various public health and social actions required for the purpose are grouped together into the following categories:

5

– measures aimed at promoting child health and development, including programmes of prenatal and perinatal care, nutrition, immunization, family planning, and accident prevention;
  – measures to reduce the risk of cognitive and social maldevelopment, including educational programmes for parenthood, health education in schools, and improved day care facilities for children;
  – provision of crisis intervention facilities in the context of primary health care;
  – avoidance of iatrogenic damage due to faulty or excessive prescribing of medication or to unnecessary hospital admission and treatment;
  – measures to minimize chronic impairment and disability, including treatment of hypertension and CNS infections, control of epilepsy, and avoidance of chronic social breakdown in psychotic patients.

Finally, the report emphasizes the need for a commitment at governmental level to preventive principles, proposes that there should be explicit reference to mental health measures in statements of national health and development policy, and recommends that inter-sectoral co-ordinating bodies should be set up in each country to promote and monitor national progress towards preventive goals.
  The limitations of a document of this kind are obvious enough and easy to criticize. A list of proposals couched in such general terms is neither comprehensive nor specific enough to serve as a blueprint for national planning. It also does not mention the formidable barriers, discussed by Kramer in this volume, which will have to be overcome before preventive goals are attained. To advocate, for example, steps to reduce alcoholism, accidents, and violence without making explicit reference to alcohol taxation and licensing laws, highway speed limits, or control of the sale of firearms is to run the risk of not being taken seriously. Reform in these areas cannot succeed without encountering massive opposition, and this fact needs to be recognized and stated at the outset. Nevertheless, the report is valuable in demonstrating that a systematic approach to prevention in the mental health field is possible with the knowledge already available, and that it should take account of physical, biological, and psychosocial risk factors. Promulgation of this concept by the World Health Organization represents a significant step forward.
  The present publication, like the symposium on which it is based, focuses on the contributions that epidemiological and health services research can make to preventive psychiatry. There are a number of ways to classify and order material of this kind. The one adopted here, which is very simple, is derived from Morris's analogy of preventive action with a campaign against disease, in which vulnerable points are selected for attack and appropriate strategies employed against them (Morris 1974).
  The logical first stage is to find out which persons in a population develop

a particular type of illness, and when and under what circumstances this occurs. The information can be applied in two principal ways. First, it can be used to provide the statistics for computing incidence rates, both for the population as a whole and for more homogeneous sub-groups within it, and these data in turn can help to establish which biological and environmental variables are risk factors, at least in the predictive sense of being positively associated with onset of the disorder in question. Second, it helps to set those cases known to treatment agencies in the wider perspective of morbidity in the population and to suggest how systems of early detection, referral, and treatment could be introduced or improved.

The next stage will then be to set up preventive programmes based on the epidemiological findings, and here a number of possibilities present themselves. One major strategy, which presupposes a knowledge of the risk factors involved, is to identify those individuals or sub-groups within a population with a high illness expectancy and to find ways of protecting them. A second is to modify the structure and mode of operation of diagnostic and treatment agencies, so as to increase their potential for secondary and tertiary prevention. Each of these approaches can be explored by extending the functions of existing health-care and social agencies, and each can be tested in the context of a local area population.

A third strategy is to promote general preventive measures by means of public-health policy at national level. This approach differs from the others in that it does not usually depend for its implementation on the specialist services; also, because legislation, fiscal measures, or other aspects of economic and social policy may be involved, it is less readily subjected to trial testing on local communities.

These various lines of attack, each of which is represented among the following contributions, has already demonstrated its relevance to preventive psychiatry. Some have been widely employed, others only in isolated experiments. All, without exception, pose unresolved problems of research method.

Case-finding and early detection

Incidence rates must be calculated from the frequency of occurrence of new cases in defined populations. Since continuous case monitoring of a whole population or representative sample is seldom feasible, investigators must in practice fall back on one or other of two expedients: either to monitor all first contacts with the relevant health-care agencies which serve the population at risk or else to make a retrospective estimate of frequency on the basis of repeated cross-sectional surveys of the same population, allowing a sufficient time-interval to elapse between them.

The former method can yield an acceptable approximation to the true incidence of those conditions, such as acute psychotic episodes, which are severe and conspicuous enough to result in contact with treatment agencies in the great majority of cases. It is represented here by the WHO-sponsored collaborative study of schizophrenia in ten countries, reported by Sartorius, which was designed to provide maximum coverage by including primary health care, social services, and other 'helping agencies' in the screening network, as well as psychiatric departments and practices. Although the service structures vary widely from country to country, the range of variation in the computed incidence rates for schizophrenia lay only between seven and fourteen per 100,000 annually.

The latter method seems more appropriate in studying disorders which tend to be insidious in onset and which may not at any stage result in acute behavioural disturbance or crisis situations. The paradigm in our society is late-life dementia, since field-study findings in a number of countries have demonstrated that the large majority of affected persons remain in the community, without psychiatric support, until a late stage of the illness or until death. Incidence rates for severe or moderately severe chronic brain syndrome in the elderly, obtained by means of this type of enquiry, are reported here by Bickel and Cooper. Again, the range of variation is limited, the annual incidence rates from studies in a number of European countries lying between eleven and eighteen per 1,000 at risk. The case material in all these surveys is, however, heterogeneous; reliable incidence rates for relatively specific diagnostic categories such as senile dementia of Alzheimer type and multi-infarct dementia are not yet available. More-over, this report underlines the point that the boundary between mild cognitive decline and clinical dementia in old age is still far from clear-cut, and hence that more precise diagnostic criteria will have to be laid down before the findings of field studies carried out on different populations can be safely comparable. It also emphasizes the difficulties that are involved in diagnosing the onset of dementing illness retrospectively in persons who have died by the time a follow-up study or second wave of interviewing is undertaken.

Despite these problems, dementing illness conforms to a fairly simple model in that it has a single point of onset (even if this cannot be recognized at the time) and usually runs a progressive course thereafter. These are favourable conditions for computing rates of incidence, though not for the clinical prognosis. Fortunately for humankind, most psychiatric disorders do not behave in this way, but manifest great variability in course and outcome. They may recover completely after a single episode, remit and relapse repeatedly, or persist for years without definite remission, but with no clear evidence of long-term deterioration either. The difficulties that can ensue in trying to compute reliable incidence rates are demon-strated here by Eaton and his co-workers, on the basis of data from the US Epidemiologic Catchment Areas survey. By examining in detail the findings at second-wave interviews, they are able to show that about half of all persons who had had a positive history of psychiatric disturbance recorded in the first interviewing wave now did not report any previous psychiatric abnormality. This source of bias could result in a gross over-estimate in incidence rates, many apparently new cases being in fact simply a result of measurement error. Retrospective 'lifetime prevalence' data are evidently of limited value in trying to establish which members of a population should be considered to be at risk for a new illness-onset. There is a strong need to distinguish clearly between 'first ever' cases and new episodes in the course of remittent illness, and hence in causal investigation to decide whether the focus of enquiry is fixed on aetiology in the narrow sense or on the provoking and precipitating factors of individual illness episodes.

Early case-detection by the application of screening techniques in communities is an approach which has a good deal in common with the investigation of disease incidence, but also differs from it in certain important respects. It is usually selective, concentrating for the sake of economy and efficiency on sub-groups of the population which, at the time they are screened, are believed to carry an increased risk for the illness in question. It normally assumes a two-stage procedure in which the initial screening can be followed, in all suspect cases, by a more detailed diagnostic examination. This kind of procedure may or may not be indicated in epidemiological field studies, depending on practical considerations. Finally, screening surveys, unlike field studies, tend to be opportunistic, in that they take advantage of situations in which the persons at high risk are most readily accessible to investigation.

The study reported here by Dilling and Oschinsky, of alcohol abuse among patients admitted to the departments of a general teaching hospital, provides a good example of this approach. The findings indicate a case frequency of 30.6 per cent among psychiatric admissions, 13.8 per cent on internal medical wards, and 7.3 per cent among surgical patients. Systematic screening of general-hospital admissions, using a rapid, economic method, can thus over a period of time serve to identify a high proportion of the alcohol-dependent members of a community, many of whom would not participate, or would not be diagnosed, in a general population survey.

At the same time, this report also highlights the problem of unreliability that can arise with screening techniques that are at least partly dependent upon the help of physicians as key informants. The scoring system for the 'MALT' screening for alcoholism prescribes that each item assessed by the physician (F-score) receives a weighting of four points, whereas each response given by the patient (S-score) receives only one point. Since, however, the surgeons who took part in the study were much less aware of alcohol abuse among their patients than were the internists and psychiatrists, the sensitivity of the screening instrument varied according to the hospital department in which it was used. This is a particularly clear example of a source of error which is commonly present in the screening of medical-agency populations and which points to an outstanding need for further methodological research.

Identifying and assessing risk factors

Numerous social and ecological variables have been proposed over the years as risk factors of mental illness, including poverty, low socio-economic status, unemployment, migration, social mobility, social isolation, overcrowding, urbanization, status incongruence, and residence in anomic urban areas (Ødegaard 1975). Some at least of these variables continue to occupy a central position in sociological theories of mental disorder. On the whole, however, their investigation and empirical testing as concomitant factors, in the setting of population-based research, has proved to have little heuristic value. In recent years, such studies have been increasingly augmented or replaced by more sophisticated approaches, which reveal methodological progress in a number of ways. Variables now tend to be selected on the basis of stated hypotheses, rather than simply because they are available in the form of ready-to-hand census data. More emphasis is being placed on features of the microsocial environment, such as life events, whose occurrence can be related in time to the onset and subsequent course of illness. New attention is being given to those positive, health-promoting features of the individual's lifestyle and social situation which appear to be protective against the onset of mental disorder or to improve the clinical and social prognosis when it does occur. Descriptive surveys, finally, are giving way more and more to case-control designs.

All these trends can be discerned in the group of contributions on psychiatric risk factors included in this volume. Once again, however, the overall impression is of a field of research in transition, characterized by unresolved methodological problems. Thus, Henderson's review of epidemiological knowledge on the risk factors of Alzheimer-type dementia clearly demonstrates that the most challenging findings to emerge in recent years have come from a handful of case-control studies, in which the exposure to certain putative risk factors of individuals suffering from this condition has been compared with that of otherwise comparable elderly persons who are free from the disease. This research has provided tentative evidence of associations – for example, with a history of head injury, thyroid disease, viral infection, and exposure to domestic animals – which call in the first instance for replication studies. But the findings have been inconsistent and, apart from the need for larger samples (notably by means of multi-centre collaborative studies), it seems clear that methods must be developed to improve both representativity and the quality of anamnestic data. The index groups have been selected mainly from among patients of presenile age under treatment in neurological departments. Research findings have varied according to whether controls are selected from among other hospital patients or from the ranks of elderly persons living in the local community. The need to ascertain and quantify the individual's exposure, often much earlier in the lifespan, to risk factors which, in themselves, would not necessarily have led to hospital admission and treatment poses a methodological problem of great complexity.

In this general context, it may also be important to preserve a clear distinction between the factors that determine risk and those which influence prognosis. The findings of the recent international study of schizophrenia, summarized here by Sartorius, provide strong support for this argument. His data show no evidence that the incidence of new cases of schizophrenia differs either significantly or consistently as between industrial developed countries, on the one hand, and developing Third World countries, on the other. Yet the pattern of course and outcome of the disorder appears to differ markedly as between the two types of society. The proportion of affected persons who manifest a definitely favourable course and outcome is nearly twice as high in the developing as in the developed countries, whereas this ratio is reversed with respect to the proportion of those affected who suffer from chronically impaired social functioning. While the specific factors responsible for these large differences have still to be isolated, the lesson for epidemiological research is already clear.

Protecting the vulnerable individual

This is still an imprecise concept and calls for clearer definition. What, to begin with, should be taken as evidence of vulnerability in psychiatric terms? Morris has rightly emphasized that whole sub-sections of the population are in distress to an extent that endangers their health:

> Every society creates its own casualties, consigns some of its people, individuals and families, to a life under very special stress; by design or acquiescence, apathy or denial, imposes its own deprivations, frustration and indignities on particular minority groups, denying their human needs and social rights. In our society, they often overlap: the chronic poor in the cities, the abandoned aged, the children who are 'finished before they are five', jobless (coloured) youngsters, the hundreds of thousands in substandard housing, the homeless, the middle-aged disabled thrown on the scrapheap, the patients in some long-stay hospitals, the coloured ghettoes, men in and out of the local prisons, the deviants we harass ... the catalogue of waste and misery could readily be lengthened. (Morris 1974: 281)

Undoubtedly, a significant proportion of the mentally ill is drawn from among these handicapped and socially disadvantaged groups. So long as our society continues to manufacture waste and misery on this scale, a large part of the task of psychiatrists will consist, in effect, of trying to ameliorate the effects on individuals and families. Thus, the consequences for mental health of the current massive increase in long-term unemployment in industrial countries are incalculable. A related problem is posed by the rapidly growing population of homeless persons, especially in the big cities, whose overlap with the psychiatric population and immediate relevance for mental health policy are documented in the review by Susser, Lovell, and Conover.

But this is only part of the story. The different categories of psychiatric disorder have been shown repeatedly to have their own characteristic distributions in the general population. Their causal factors, predisposing or provoking, must be to some extent specific in nature and are not always directly linked with distress in Morris's sense of the term. The social origins of depression in women constitute one case in point (Brown and Harris 1978). The risk of occurrence of a depressive illness appears to be partly determined by socio-economic status. Nevertheless, the research evidence, summarized here by Harris, has led these workers to focus, not on socio-economic variables such as income or quality of housing, but on the significance that an intimate, confiding relationship carries in protecting against illness onset, and hence to stress the potential importance for secondary prevention of volunteer befrienders and of local community agencies that can promote and organize this form of social support.

A distinction has to be made between vulnerability as an aspect of predisposition to illness – i.e., a long-term or even permanent characteristic of an individual – and vulnerability as the temporary effect of a life crisis, transitional period, or concatenation of stressful events. Cohen and her co-workers, for example, in their study of family changes of home as a psychological risk factor, point to this as one cause of a temporary emotional vulnerability among children. Neugebauer, reporting an intriguing instance of serendipity in research, highlights both the increased risk of depression in women following a miscarriage and the beneficial effect that a supportive interview shortly after this kind of stressful life event may have. All these contributions tend to suggest that current notions of crisis intervention may provide the foundations for a broader concept of crisis prevention in the primary care setting. Clearly, however, research is so far only touching the edges of this field of preventive endeavour.

Preventive action in health services

Research undertaken in the 1960s demonstrated a connection between the quality of psychiatric hospital care and the severity of chronic mental impairment found among schizophrenic in-patients (Wing and Brown 1970). This work seemed to open up a most promising line of investigation into the scope, within these institutions, for secondary and tertiary prevention: an impression strengthened by the growth during that period of 'industrial therapy' and other programmes of rehabilitation for the chronically mentally ill. Over the past three decades, however, there has been a major shift in the locus of psychiatric care, from mental hospital to community, and this has been matched by a corresponding change in research priorities. The assumption is now widely held that psychiatric services fulfil a preventive function only in so far as they provide out-patient, day care, and complementary facilities, and succeed in avoiding the necessity for prolonged in-patient stay.

The study in Athens reported by Madianos and his colleagues provides confirmation that a community-based extramural service can indeed exercise important preventive functions: notably a reduction in psychiatric emergencies and in relapse rates among schizophrenic patients. This ambitious project, which exemplifies the recent impressive progress of social psychiatric research in southern European countries, made use of a control design and epidemiological measures to test the impact of such a service on the local area population. In aims and design, it must be regarded as paradigmatic for a type of evaluative research that is still unusual in most parts of the world.

Brook's critique of mental health policy in the Netherlands sets different accents. On the basis of current statistical trends, he suggests that the era of diminishing psychiatric bed numbers is now at an end, and that an increasing population of 'new long-stay' patients will have to be reckoned with in the years ahead. This projection, combined with an awareness of the limitations that economic recession and demands for cost-containment must be expected to impose, leads him to question the realism of an official policy which, he believes, relies too heavily on extramural care and preventive concepts. His arguments, though expressed in national terms, are essentially a contribution to the ongoing international debate on this topic, and will awaken interest outside his own country. This study serves incidentally to remind one, as does also Beskow's account of in-patient suicides in Sweden, that the psychiatric hospital itself remains an important subject for scientific inquiry and that there are still unanswered questions concerning the essential nature of both therapeutic and harmful aspects of the institutional environment and their implications for prevention.

One other facet of psychiatric care considered in this section is the danger of iatrogenic damage resulting from faulty prescribing of benzo-diazepines and other tranquillizers. Williams and his co-workers compute that in the UK alone between 800,000 and 1,600,000 patients have taken tranquillizers regularly for twelve months or more, despite a growing consensus of informed medical opinion that prolonged prescribing of these substances should be avoided. At least one-third of long-term users appear to develop pharmocological dependence, which can result in severe withdrawal symptoms. This scale of prescribing, which is equalled or surpassed in many other countries, underlines the conclusion that continuous monitoring of psychopharmacological prescribing patterns and their consequences should be seen as an indispensable part of the task of mental health information systems.

Promoting healthier public policies

Increasing attention is now being paid to the possibility of improving mental health standards in populations by means of general preventive measures, deliberately incorporated into public-health and social policies. In the synopsis which Sartorius gives here of this issue, the promotion of mental health takes its place alongside more traditional preventive strategies aimed at the reduction of mortality and morbidity. This approach is wholly consistent with the public-health philosophy embodied in the targets of the 'Health for All' programme (WHO 1985).

The contributions to the final section of this book touch upon three main aspects of public policy. First, public action is necessary to set up, maintain, and make available appropriate types of service for the treatment and prevention of mental disorders. Epidemiological research can provide the basic descriptive information on the extent and distribution of morbidity in the population required in planning these services. Action of this kind involves questions raised in the preceding section, concerning, for example, government policy on the development of community-based extramural services, or improvement of the quality of care provided in hospitals. It may also extend, as the review by Bromet and Parkinson makes clear, to the provision of preventive care in the work-place, and hence to the influence on mental health protection of both private and nationalized industries, the trade unions, and other interested groups. Bromet and Parkinson are careful to emphasize that the most fundamental and important part of prevention in this context is the identification of workplace exposures which may lead to illness and that the first and foremost priority of physicians engaged in the industrial setting must be the health of the employees. This point is crucial in establishing the ethical basis for epidemiological or other forms of research into mental health in industry.

Second, public-health action is necessary to reduce the population's exposure to known risk factors of mental disorder. Epidemiological methods may be applied both in identifying specific risk factors and in testing the efficacy of preventive measures introduced to deal with them. The type of strategy invoked can range from investigation of small, localized outbreaks ('clinical' epidemiology) to large-scale statistical surveys.

Dupont supplies a number of telling examples, drawn from the field of mental retardation research. The prevention and control of iodine-deficiency disorders, to which at present some 800 million people living in iodine-deficient areas of the world are exposed, could have a major impact on the mental health of affected populations. The frequency of lead encephalopathy in children could be reduced by means of screening programmes and prohibition of lead-containing cosmetics. Training programmes for primary care workers could serve both to promote the early diagnosis and treatment of disorders that can result in brain damage in childhood and to foster public awareness of the risk factors involved.

The need for greater public awareness is not confined to developing Third World countries. Dupont points out that few European countries have so far developed national screening programmes for inborn errors of metabolism, as recommended by the Council of Europe in 1981. Dilling and Oschinsky deplore the comparative neglect of alcoholism research and prevention in their country. Häfner and Schmidtke, taking advantage of an 'experiment of opportunity', demonstrate convincingly the influence of a television programme in provoking suicidal acts among young people, and by so doing underline the need to achieve agreement on codes of conduct for the communications industry that pay regard to research findings and to the importance of modelling and imitation for suicide, violence, drug taking, and delinquency in the younger generation. A disturbing comment on contemporary social mores is provided by the hard opposition which projects of this type now encounter from data-protection authorities and populist groups, who apparently see in them only a violation of individual rights and a breach of confidentiality.

Finally, public policy may be called upon to enhance the mental health of populations by improving the human environment and promoting healthy lifestyles. Sartorius sees the key issue here as 'change of the abominably low place which mental life and health occupy on the scales of value of most societies', and suggests that it will prove both the most important and the most difficult task of mental health programmes in the future. Leighton also considers mental health promotion to be potentially a major component of preventive efforts, but adds cautiously that we do not yet know what effects general measures may have on the occurrence of mental illness, and that simple analogies drawn from organic medicine could be misleading.

It can be safely predicted that research in psychiatric epidemiology will continue for the forseeable future to rely mainly on indices of illness, impairment, and disability, both for description of populations and as outcome variables when trying to assess the effects of preventive programmes. Changes in such measures could certainly be employed as one way to judge the efficacy of public policies directed towards lifestyles or the quality of life. There are also grounds for arguing that data on morbidity should at times be augmented by measurement of the attitudes of physicians and other health professionals, as well as of family members and the local community, towards mental illness and mentally impaired persons. This is one important area in which psychiatric epidemiology can usefully contribute to a change for the better in societal values, and with which future symposia of the kind reported here may display an increasing concern.

References

Brown, G.W. and Harris, T. (1978) *Social Origins of Depression: a study of psychiatric disorder in women*, London: Tavistock.

Cooper, B. (1988) 'Psychiatry in the era of "Health for All"', *Social Psychiatry and Psychiatric Epidemiology* 23: 2–5.

Kaplan, H.I. and Sadock, B.J. (eds) (1985) *Comprehensive Textbook of Psychiatry*, fourth edition, Baltimore, MD: Williams & Wilkins.

Levy, D.M. (1968) 'Beginnings of the child guidance movement', *American Journal of Orthopsychiatry* 38: 799–804.

Lewis, N.D.C. (1974) 'American psychiatry from its beginnings to World War II', in S. Arieti (ed.) *American Handbook of Psychiatry (second edition), vol. 1: The Foundations of Psychiatry*, New York: Basic Books, pp. 28–42.

Morris, J.N. (1974) 'Four cheers for prevention', in J.N. Morris *Uses of Epidemiology*, third edition, Edinburgh: Churchill Livingstone, pp. 270–83.

Ødegaard, Ø. (1975) 'Social and emotional factors in the aetiology, outcome, treatment and prevention of mental disorders', in K.P. Kisker, J. –E. Meyer, C. Muller, and E. Strömgren (eds) *Psychiatrie der Gegenwart III*. 2. Auflage, Berlin: Springer.

Wing, J.K. and Brown, G.W. (1970) *Institutionalism and Schizophrenia*, Cambridge: Cambridge University Press.

World Health Organization (1985) *Targets for Health for All*, Copenhagen: WHO Regional Office for Europe.

World Health Organization (1988) *Prevention of Mental, Neurological and Psychosocial Disorders*, WHO/MNH/EVA/88.1, Geneva: WHO.

Chapter two

Global and specific approaches to prevention

Alexander H. Leighton

Introduction

I should like to begin by offering a map that shows the position of prevention in the total spectrum of the efforts society makes in order to control mental illnesses. After this review of prevention in context, I shall turn to the question of its content. This will open the way for introducing some ideas derived from epidemiological considerations and for discussion of the meaning of 'global' and the meaning of 'specific'. At the end, on the basis of the material brought forward, there will be suggestions for the construction of a new map.

The effort spectrum

Let us begin with the first map, shown in Figure 2.1.

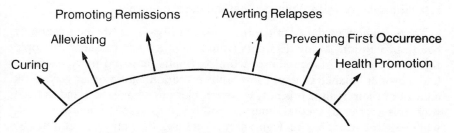

Figure 2.1   The effort spectrum in mental health

The map assumes that, although there are a great many different kinds of effort across the spectrum, they may be grouped and labelled in six major sets, each represented by an arrow. The base curve with the arrows perpendicular is intended to give the eye a sense of efforts on numerous frontiers, each of which looks in a somewhat different direction. As a consequence, the segments of the spectrum tend to strive forward like a battle-front, with a degree of independence and lack of co-ordination that can at times be wasteful and counter-productive.

1. *Curing* refers to the complete removal of a pathological process. Except for a few disorders with a mainly organic aetiology, it is, alas, exceedingly rare in our field.

2. *Alleviating* refers to reducing disability, to shortening the duration of episodes and to diminishing symptoms. This is the part of the spectrum in which advances have occurred, especially in recent years. The methods include psychodynamic therapy, chemotherapy, cognitive-behavioural intervention, group treatment, rehabilitation, manipulation of psychosocial variables, etc. Although much work still remains to be done to assure the effectiveness of these interventions, it seems safe to say that in the main they are able to reduce disabilities and improve adaptive capacities in a way that is exceedingly important to persons with mental illness, to their families, and to society.

3. *Promoting remissions* hinges on the assumption that every individual has self-healing powers to a greater or lesser degree. Although little is known about the process, it is thought to be an important aid in most treatment endeavours and to appear in certain cases as 'spontaneous recovery'.

4. *Averting relapse* refers to preventing a return to disability by a patient who has reached a greatly improved level of alleviation.

5. *Preventing first occurrence* is sometimes all and sometimes a part of what is meant by primary prevention. We shall return to this presently.

6. *Health promotion* puts emphasis on general improvement in well-being through changes in lifestyle. It seeks to fortify and further develop normal health, and it assumes that a reduction in illness rates and illness-related disability will follow as a natural consequence.

There is much evidence in the territories of organic medicine to support health promotion. Many disorders would be much less frequent if people refrained from substance abuse, wore seat belts, enjoyed more exercise, had a proper balance of work, rest, and recreation and in other ways took control of their health. It is not, however, clear to what extent and in what ways this applies to mental illnesses, and it is important to be aware that, while in some instances analogies may be helpful, they may also at times be misleading.

Preventing first occurrence

Let us return to the segment of the map that is concerned with preventing first occurrences. This goal has been strongly and recurrently advocated in psychiatry since the days of Robert Burton, but has always run into problems over whether or not it is feasible. Evidence is elusive and consequently often replaced by faith. This is again in contrast to many biomedical disorders, regarding which it is plain that primary prevention can be made to occur. Granting, however, the uncertainty which at present surrounds the primary prevention of mental illnesses, let us also note that there are some leads and some cogent theories that strongly suggest the possibility, at least for certain kinds of disorder.

The processes commonly thought about in relation to the prevention of first occurrences may be grouped in four bundles of variables, as shown in Table 2.1.

Table 2.1. Prevention variables

1. Reduction of extraordinary environmental hazards
2. Increase of environmental resources
3. Reduction of personality liabilities
4. Increase in personality assets

The first variable – 'Reduction of extraordinary environmental hazards' – rests on a complex of loosely related aetiological ideas regarding the capacities of both social and physical environments to impose pathogenic strains on human beings. I am calling these capacities 'hazards' rather than stresses, in order to avoid confusing them with the feelings of stress which they induce among individuals. I am also adding the modifier 'extra-ordinary' to indicate that it is not a question of everyday 'slings and arrows', but of those which through duration or intensity have an impact that exceeds the tolerance characteristic of our species.

Aetiologic theories of this general type are both ancient and modern and are embedded in an extensive literature. Scientific study probably goes back at least to the First World War and the investigations of Rivers (1917, 1918) and others regarding what was then called 'shell shock'. The Second World War produced Sargant and Slater's report (1940) on the retreat from Dunkirk and Grinker and Spiegel's book *Men under Stress* (1945). A major event in theory development was Lindemann's (1944) analysis based in part on the now-famous fire in the Coconut Grove nightclub in Boston. Later on came the comprehensive Lewis and Engle (1954) edited volume on war-time experiences.

There is in addition a literature on the long- and short-term effects of concentration camp living, as well as a growing list of publications on the effects of torture and on the experiences of boat people and other forced migrants.

Also to be mentioned are the studies, such as those conducted by Tyhurst (1951), focused on natural and man-made disasters. Recent work has included the effects of the dam burst at Buffalo Creek (Church 1974; Erickson 1977; Glescer *et al.* 1984), the busload of children held at

Chowchilla in California (Terr 1981, 1983, 1984), the toxic oil syndrome in Spain (Lopez-Ibor *et al*. 1985), the Three Mile Island nuclear leak (Davidson and Baum 1985; Gatchel *et al*. 1985) and James Shore's investigation of the Mt St Helens eruption (Shore *et al*. 1986). The list of such studies is now quite long.

Investigations of hazards by my colleagues and myself began with Navaho families during the great economic depression of the late 1930s (Leighton and Leighton 1944; Kluckhohn and Leighton 1946), followed by interviews with survivors of the atomic bomb in Hiroshima (Leighton 1949) and then, during the early 1970s, study of the effects of war on civilian populations in Vietnam (Murphy 1977). In the course of our long-term Stirling County study we have also given attention to observing relationships between mental illness rates and the hazards of poverty and social disintegration (Leighton *et al*. 1963). To clarify a little more what I mean by hazards, Table 2.2 may be helpful.

Table 2.2 Types of hazards

1. Threats or actuality of physical injury, as in war and social disintegration
2. Deprivation in physiological needs for food, sleep, exercise, etc.
3. Deprivation in affective needs, such as giving and receiving love
4. Deprivation in cognitive needs such as pursuing interests and solving problems
5. Deprivation of social interaction as in forced isolation

Research on hazards has led virtually everyone to the same overwhelming conclusion: that the pathogenic impact of hazards is not due to hazards alone, but also to the presence or absence of multiple other factors. Of these a major set may be called environmental resources, and is listed as item 2 in Table 2.1.

Environmental resources consist in factors which lend themselves to removing environmental hazards or to buffering the stresses which the hazards generate. Thus, individuals can draw to their aid, in this regard, religion, material goods, money, job opportunities, friends, intimate confiding relationships, social networks, social supports, and so on. There is a large consensus in the literature today that impact largely depends on the mix of hazards and resources.

Hazards and resources as characteristics of the environment are necessarily governed by the kind of societal systems that are present and how they function. Approaches with this orientation have, therefore, been called 'systems level strategy' by Cowen (1986), one of today's major researchers in prevention. Such a strategy puts emphasis on altering societal systems so as to reduce hazards and increase resources, and is, therefore, basically *global* in its orientation.

Turning now to items 3 and 4 in Table 2.1 – 'Reduction of personality liabilities' and 'Increase in personality assets' – we arrive at what Cowen has called the 'person-centred strategy' of prevention. Here again we have two sets of factors capable of balancing, and which in net effect may be termed the 'coping ability' of the individual.

Personality assets as seen in the prevention literature comprise all those capacities that are helpful to an individual in his or her struggle against hazards. Some assets are cognitive, such as the ability to search out, analyse, store, and utilize information. Some are affective, as, for instance, the ability to maintain self-respect, to be emotionally controlled, and to be able to postpone gratification. Some involve social competencies such as the capacity to get along with people, to participate in social networks, and to develop strong relationships in family, work-place, and community.

The *liabilities of personality* are to a large extent the obverse of the assets. They are generally conceived to be in part constitutional and in part the product of conditioning by life experiences. Either way, they are seen as to some extent modifiable through education and training.

'Person-centred' strategies aimed at the improvement of coping belong for the most part in the category of specific approaches to prevention. People thought to be at risk for a particular kind of disorder are selected and offered a specific intervention aimed at the improvement of coping. Nowadays such programmes appear to be largely based on cognitive-behavioural and social theories.

To illustrate, Lewinsohn (1987) in Oregon has experimented with a didactic course on how to cope with depressed feelings. The course lasts eight weeks and there are twelve two-hour sessions. Such topics as the relationship of tension to depression are covered and there is training in relaxation methods. It also includes opportunity to practise constructive rather than negative thinking together with practice in how to improve one's social skills.

Vega and his colleagues (1987) in Los Angeles have taken poor Hispanic women as a high-risk group, and have developed ways of teaching them stress reduction and stress management, together with asset acquisition through learning how to gather and utilize information that is relevant to their concerns. Emphasis is placed on enabling these women to build up positive self-images.

The interactive, process relationships of all four preventive variables are shown diagrammatically in Figure 2.2.

The personality circle at the centre of the diagram represents an individual engaged in the business of continuous adaptation to life. Going on within the personality is the process of adjusting and balancing assets and liabilities designated as coping. This is directed at the exploitation of resources in order to change, neutralize, or otherwise avoid hazards and their damaging consequences.

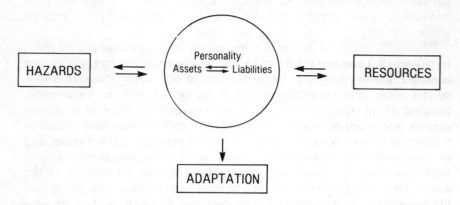

Figure 2.2 The interactive process relationships of four preventive variables

Prevention variables and the rest of the effort spectrum

I shall come back to both global and specific approaches later, but at this point I should like to draw attention once more to Figure 2.1, the map of the effort spectrum, and reconsider it in the light of these four prevention variables. A noteworthy conclusion that may be drawn is that the variables are not only relevant to prevention, but apply widely across the whole spectrum.

So far as *curing* is concerned, there is not much to say, but *alleviating* is quite another matter. It appears highly probable that the impact of the four variables is of major importance here. For many patients it seems likely that it would be helpful were it possible to change their social environment so as to lower hazards and increase resources. At the same time, the improvement of the patient's own cognitive, affective, and social coping through education and training opportunities could have an equally positive effect. There would be, of course, important questions of timing in relation to the stage of illness; but in principle, therapy and methods of strengthening personality by the management of assets would seem to have a potential for multiplying each other's benefits.

Similar points can be made with regard to *promoting remissions*, and even more so in regard to *preventing relapss*. In sum, it appears that reducing hazards and developing resources in the social environment and reducing liabilities and developing assets in personalities have about as much bearing on the clinical portion of the effort spectrum as they do on the prevention segment.

When one looks at the *health promotion* segment, the relevance is equally strong. Indeed, much of what is being advocated in health promotion is a combination of Cowan's systems level strategies and his person-centred strategies.

Some contributions from epidemiology

Let us now hold on one side the social system and personality variables and consider certain epidemiologic data that have relevance to these matters. At this point, in order to keep from wandering into unwarranted generalizations, I will narrow the focus to depression and anxiety, although I suspect that much of what I shall say applies to other disorders as well.

The first item for attention is that cases of depression and/or anxiety tend to have long durations. In our study of Stirling County, a sixteen-year follow-up of a population sample indicated a mean duration of over ten years with a range that extended from a few months to a large portion of life (Murphy *et al.* 1986). From these data we also estimate that about a quarter of the people included in the case-prevalence at any particular time are long-standing chronic cases.

This picture of chronicity in population surveys is also shown by follow-up studies of psychiatric patients. For example, Keller *et al.* (1982), working in the NIMH Psychobiology of Depression Study, report that 50 per cent of the patients with depression recovered within one year, but that the remaining 50 per cent had a much more protracted course. The probability of recovery among those remaining ill in the second year was found to be only 28 per cent and by the fourth year was down to 18 per cent of the remainder. Such a curve is in keeping with the notion that some cases never recover.

These findings suggest that the 'averting relapse' part of the effort spectrum is an area of considerable importance. We have found that the incidence rate in the Stirling County sample is about ten per 1,000 per year for depression and anxiety disorders combined (Murphy *et al.* 1988). It is difficult to calculate relapse rates so as to make a direct comparison with incidence rates, but there is more than a little to suggest that relapses may be a heavy contributor to prevalence. We estimate, for example, that another quarter of the cases in our prevalence estimate are due to relapses. If this finding stands up in other longitudinal studies it will indicate that preventing relapses could have a major impact on prevalence.

Global and specific approaches

I would like now to return to the words 'global' and 'specific' and consider them in the light of what I am supposing is a fact, namely that the kinds of activities thought about as prevention have a high degree of relevance across the entire effort spectrum from clinical treatment to health promotion.

As we have seen, global approaches are largely based on the notion of altering society so as to reduce hazards and promote resources. This leads to advocating very large-scale aims such as the elimination of poverty, racism, and war and the promotion of vastly better programmes than presently exist in health, welfare, and education. Although such ambitions offer very few opportunities for scientific assessment, their proponents are apt to regard anything less as a 'band-aid' offered where major surgery is needed. Opponents, while often accepting the ideals, see the global approach as both over-expansive and simplistic, as for instance in the 'empowerment' advocacy which came to the fore in the 1970s (Rappaport 1984). If scientific investigation is to play a part, goals that are much smaller in scope and more clearly defined must be formulated.

Because of this, the more narrowly defined person-centred approaches aimed at helping high-risk individuals improve their coping abilities has greater appeal to many investigators. Such work seems more open to action research and the measurement of effects. To some extent, however, this is illusory, because of the very serious problems in such matters as sample and control selection, the extended time periods involved and the drop-out rates of subjects, researchers, and funding. When change is found, furthermore, it is very difficult to be sure that the intervention was a significant factor. Nevertheless, there is the possibility that with continuing effort a dependable knowledge-base and methodology may gradually be developed.

Meanwhile, I should like to suggest that the concept of a global approach should not be avoided. Rather, let it be divested for the time being of its over-expansive meaning and brought to a focus on populations of limited size and on the four major variables we have been discussing: hazards and resources in the environment and assets and liabilities in persons. In other words, a global approach would be one that is applied to a population clearly defined in time and space and that utilizes both systems-level and person-centred strategies.

As is evident, this definition implies that a global approach must contain within it specific approaches, and this I think is as it should be. On the other hand, it does not imply that all specific approaches must lie within a global approach.

When one mentions a population as a target, there is some tendency to think in terms of a geographically defined group. It is perhaps worth mentioning therefore that trade unions, industrial plants, military units, and branches of civil government are non-geographically defined populations that have been usefully studied.

Geographically defined populations remain, however, for many reasons particularly interesting. They tend to have ecological characteristics that are helpful in understanding both the systems-level and the individual-level processes – and their interactions. One variant that is particularly close to us professionally is the population to which care is given by a mental health service or, in other words, its catchment area. Here we see a possible site for a global approach to a geographically defined population served by a comprehensive mental health centre.

Visualize a mental health centre surrounded by the population for whose care it is responsible and consider its potentialities in relation to the total effort spectrum and the four major variables: hazards, resources, liabilities, and assets. Such a centre, if typical, would be taken up with the treatment task of trying to reduce those particular intra-person liabilities we call mental illnesses. This is most likely to be successful in persons who aside from these illnesses are well endowed with assets, are not greatly exposed to extraordinary hazards, and who have reasonable access to resources. On the other hand, for a person who does not have these advantages, reducing intra-person liabilities alone is apt to have little permanence. Instead, to the extent that extraordinary hazards, few resources, and failures in coping are determinants, that person is apt to lead a life of recurrent or chronic illness.

Most communities, however, do contain numerous systems focused on hazard-reduction, resource-building, and coping-improvement. These are, in fact, main component processes in all cultures and go by a host of specific names which vary from time to time and place to place. In Stirling County they take shape in formal and informal programmes directed at educational opportunity, recreational activities, health promotion, child welfare, youth opportunity, care of the elderly, the fostering of religious life, and so on.

One opportunity for a community mental health centre, therefore, is to promote co-ordination of these activities with each other and with its own in such a way as to make them more accessible and effective for those in need of the opportunities offered. As has been observed frequently, patients, ex-patients, and those who seem to be on their way to becoming patients are often out of touch, even alienated, in relation to the societal processes that could be helpful to them and in which they could in turn be helpful.

In addition to promoting the more effective engagement of resources that already exist, a community mental health centre also has a potential for identifying major needs that are not being met at all by the social systems of the population, for drawing attention to these gaps, and for catalysing the formation of appropriate organizations to fill them.

If this seems a tall order for a community centre, it is. It is not likely to be done by clinics as they currently exist. Two bodies of knowledge and technical skill would have to be added to their capacities or else co-ordinated with them. One consists in the social and behavioural scientific competence necessary for investigating, describing, and analysing the social and cultural systems of a catchment area and thus arriving at a diagnosis of its needs from the perspective of hazards, resources, and coping abilities.

The other consists in the technical skills of *community development*. By this term I refer to a professional field with roots in rural sociology, applied anthropology, economics, and systems theory (Cardoza *et al.* 1975; Coombs and Manzoor 1974; Gow and Van Sant 1981; Holdcroft 1978; Inter-American Development Bank 1966; Johnston and Clark 1982; Meister 1972; Ruttan 1984; Spicer 1952). There is controversy as to whether community development is capable of inducing social change in large populations such as a developing country, but there is wide agreement that it can be very effective in more local populations. Hundreds of successes have been reported widely from all over the world. The changes this technique aims at accomplishing are precisely those we have been discussing: hazard-reduction, resource-building, and the improvement of coping. I should like to suggest, therefore, that its application to the population of a catchment area would be one way of seeing whether global changes could be brought about and whether these would have a beneficial effect on prevalence rates.

Space does not allow my describing this experimental idea further, nor discussing what I see as the pros and cons. I should, however, like to note that as part of the Stirling County study, colleagues and I did apply social science diagnosis and community development methods to the population of a catchment area over a period of ten years and some reflection of this may be found in Cardoza *et al.* (1975). The experience taught us much that was daunting and something that was encouraging. It is the latter that leads me to think that this kind of global approach deserves further attention, one in which measuring effects would be a major feature.

The spectrum re-drawn

I should like to conclude by showing in Figure 2.3 a re-drawn effort spectrum as it would look if some of the ideas I have been presenting were given implementation.

This shows prevalence as the enemy and its reduction as the common goal. The segments of the spectrum are the same as before. The curve of the arc is reversed in order to give the eye a sense of convergence towards the common goal. The broken arrows represent the linking and co-ordination of efforts, with particular reference to actions involving the social-systems level and the person-centred level. This representation is of something that is not a single-minded emphasis on therapy, or prevention, or health promotion, but rather a co-ordinated all-out attack on prevalence rates across the whole effort spectrum.

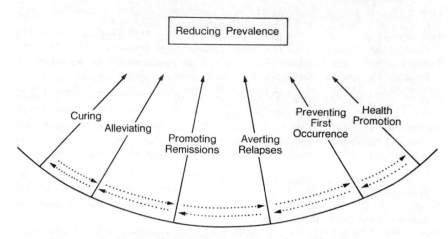

Figure 2.3 Spectrum of effort in mental health and mental illness

Acknowledgement

The preparation of this paper was supported by Dalhousie University. Grateful acknowledgement is also made to J.M. Murphy for review and suggestions, to Hemali Ostbye and James Roeber for assistance in library research and Jocelyn LeClerc for preparation of the manuscript.

References

Cardoza, V.C., Ackerly, W.C., and Leighton, A.H. (1975) 'Improving mental health through community action', *Community Mental Health* 11: 215–27.

Church, J.S. (1974) 'Buffalo Creek disaster – extent and range of emotional and/or behavioural problems', *Omega* 5: 61–3.

Coombs, P.H. and Manzoor, A. (1974) *Attacking Rural Poverty*, Baltimore, MD: Johns Hopkins Press.

Cowen, E.L. (1986) 'Primary prevention in mental health, ten years of retrospect and ten years of prospect', in M. Kessler and S.E. Goldston (eds) *A Decade of Progress in Primary Prevention*, Vermont: University Press of New England.

Davidson, L.M. and Baum, A. (1985) 'Physiological symptoms of post-traumatic stress at Three Mile Island', *Psychosomatic Medicine*, 47: 80–1.

Erickson, K.T. (1977) *Everything in its Path – the Destruction of Community at Buffalo Creek*, New York: Simon & Schuster.

Gatchel, R.J., Schaeffer, M.A., and Baum, A. (1985) 'A psychophysiological field study of stress at Three Mile Island', *Psychophysiology* 22: 175–81.

Glescer, G.C., Green, B.L., and Winget, C. (1984) *Prolonged Psychosocial Effects of Disaster – a study of Buffalo Creek*, New York: Academic Press.

Gow, D.P. and Van Sant, J. (1981) 'Beyond the rhetoric of rural development participation: how can it be done?', Integrated Rural Development Working Paper No.9., Washington, DC: Development Alternatives, Inc.

Grinker, R.R. and Spiegel, J.P. (1945) *Men under Stress*, New York: Blakiston (McGraw Hill).

Holdcroft, L.E. (1978) *The Rise and Fall of Community Development in Developing Countries, 1950–65*, Lansing MI: Michigan State University Press.

Inter-American Development Bank (1966) *Community Development: Theory and Practice*, Mexico City: Inter-American Development Bank.

Johnston, B.F. and Clark, W.C. (1982) *Redesigning Rural Development: A Strategic Perspective*, Baltimore, MD: Johns Hopkins Press.

Keller, M.B., Shapiro, R.W., Lavori, P.W., and Wolfe, N. (1982) 'Recovery in major depressive disorder – analysis with the life-table and regression models', *Archives of General Psychiatry* 39: 905–10.

Kluckhohn, C. and Leighton, D.C. (1946) *The Navaho*, Cambridge, Mass: Harvard University Press.

Leighton, A.H. (1949) *Human Relations in a Changing World*, New York: E.P. Dutton.

Leighton, A.H. and Leighton, D.C. (1944) *The Navaho Door*, Cambridge, Mass: Harvard University Press.

Leighton, D.C., Harding, J.S., Macklin, D.B., et al. (1963) *The Character of Danger*, New York: Basic Books.

Lewinsohn, P.M. (1987) 'The coping-with-depression course', in R.F. Munoz (ed.) *Prevention: Research Directions*, Washington, DC: Hemisphere.

Lewis, D.C. and Engle, B. (eds) (1954) *Wartime Psychiatry*, New York: Oxford University Press.

Lifton, R.J. and Olson, E. (1976) 'Human experience of total disaster – Buffalo Creek experience', *Psychiatry* 39: 1–18.

Lindemann, E. (1944) 'Symptomatology and management of acute grief', *American Journal of Psychiatry* 101: 141.

Lopez-Ibor, J.J., Soria, J., Canas, F., and Rodriquez, M. (1985) 'Psychopathological aspects of the toxic oil syndrome catastrophe', *British Journal of Psychiatry* 147: 352–65.

Meister, A. (1972) 'Characteristics of community development and rural animation in Africa', *Community Development* 27/28: 75–132.

Murphy, J.M. (1977) 'War stress and civilian Vietnamese: a study of psychological effects', *Acta Psychiatrica Scandinavica* 56: 92–108.

Murphy, J.M., Olivier, D.C., Sobol, A.M., Monson, R.R., et al. (1986) 'Diagnosis and outcome: depression and anxiety in a general population', *Psychological Medicine* 16: 117–26.

Murphy, J.M., Olivier, D.C., Monson, R.R., et al. (1988) 'Incidence of depression and anxiety: the Stirling Co. Study', *The American Journal of Public Health* 78: 534–40.

Rappaport, J. (1984) 'Studies in empowerment: introduction to the issue', *Prevention in Human Services* 3: 1–7.

Rivers, W.H.R. (1917) 'Freud's psychology of the unconscious (evidence afforded by the war)', *Lancet* 1: 912–14.

Rivers, W.H.R. (1918) 'The repression of war experience', *Lancet* 1: 173–7.

Ruttan, V.W. (1984) 'Integrated rural development programmes: a historical perspective', *World Development* 12: 393–401.

Sargant, W. and Slater, E. (1940) 'Acute war neuroses', *Lancet* 2: 1–2.

Shore, J.H., Tatum, E.L., and Vollmer, W.M. (1986) 'Psychiatric reactions to disaster – the Mount Saint Helens experience', *American Journal of Psychiatry* 143: 590–4.

Spicer, E.H. (1952) *Human Problems in Technological Change*, New York: Russell Sage Foundation / Wiley.

Terr, L.C. (1981) 'Psychic trauma in children – observations following the Chowchilla school bus kidnapping', *American Journal of Psychiatry* 138: 14–19.

Terr, L.C. (1983) 'Chowchilla revisited – the effects of psychic trauma four years after a school bus kidnapping', *American Journal of Psychiatry* 140: 1543–50.

Terr, L.C. (1984) 'Flaws found in Chowchilla study – reply' (letter), *American Journal of Psychiatry* 141: 1645.

Tyhurst, J.S. (1951) 'Individual reactions to community disaster; natural history of psychiatric phenomena', *American Journal of Psychiatry*, 107: 764–9.

Vega, W.A., Valle, R., Kolody, B., and Hough, R. (1987) 'The Hispanic social network prevention intervention study: a community-based randomized trial', in R. Munoz (ed.) *Depression Prevention: Research Directions*, Washington, DC: Hemisphere.

Chapter three

Barriers to prevention

Morton Kramer

Introduction

The 39th World Health Assembly in May 1986 adopted a resolution calling on all member states to apply the preventive measures identified in the report of WHO's Director General on the *Prevention of Mental, Neurological and Psychosocial Disorders* and to include these activities in their strategies to achieve health for all by the year 2000 (WHO 1987a).

The report referred to in this resolution summarized the magnitude of the world-wide public health burden resulting from the following mental, neurological and psychosocial disorders and problems (WHO 1986a, 1986d):

- Mental retardation
- Acquired lesions of the central nervous system
- Peripheral neuropathy
- Psychosis
- Epilepsy
- Emotional and conduct disorders
- Psychoactive substance abuse
- Conditions of life that lead to disease
- Violence
- Excessive risk-taking behaviours among youth
- Family breakdown

I will not go into the details of the epidemiologic data on the incidence and prevalence of these disorders and the burdens they create for individuals affected by one or more of these conditions, their families, friends, and the communities in which they live. For the purposes of this chapter it is sufficient to say that the above-named disorders and problems – to be referred to as MNP disorders – take a heavy toll in each period of the lifespan. What I will dwell on are phenomena that I perceive to be major barriers to carrying out preventive activities, indeed, to applying knowledge which could prevent certain mental disorders from occurring, particularly those of organic aetiology (e.g., chronic brain syndromes associated with syphilis, pellagra, poisonings, accidents) and knowledge which, in other instances, could reduce considerably the disabling conditions resulting from disorders of unknown aetiology that as yet cannot be prevented from occurring (e.g., schizophrenia, depressive disorders, Alzheimer's disease).

I will direct my comments principally to barriers to primary prevention. However, in my illustrations I will be using prevalence data to illustrate points I wish to make since the types of incidence data I need for my illustrations are hard to come by. Since prevalence varies as the product of incidence and duration, the reduction of prevalence can be accomplished by reducing either incidence or duration or both. Where I use prevalence data I will direct my remarks accordingly.

Population growth

By regions of the world

A major barrier to prevention is the rate of growth of the world's population. The rapid rate of total population growth will be adding large numbers of persons to populations already experiencing high prevalence rates of specific MNP disorders. These additions contain many persons with biological, social, and economic characteristics that place them at high risk of developing at least one MNP disorder. This means that the prevalence of these disorders will increase more rapidly than society can prevent their occurrence. This will happen *unless* programmes are instituted rapidly, with sufficient manpower and resources, to prevent from occurring specific disorders that can be prevented, to terminate disorders that respond to specific treatments, and to reduce the duration of the disabling effects of those disorders that cannot be terminated or prevented.

The following data will illustrate these points. As of 1985 the population of the world was estimated to be 4.8 billion persons. In May 1987 the population reached the 5 billion mark and by the year 2000 it is projected to be 6.1 billion (medium variant). The 2000-year estimate is 27 per cent higher than that in 1985. The corresponding estimates for the more developed regions are 1.2 billion in 1985 increasing to 1.3 billion in 2000, an increase of 8 per cent, and for the less developed regions, 3.7 billion in 1985 increasing to 4.9 billion in 2000, an increase of 32 per cent (United Nations 1986a).

Although the annual rates of population growth of the more and less developed regions of the world have been decreasing steadily (Figure 3.1), the number of persons being added annually is and will continue to be considerable. To illustrate, between 1985 and 2000 the average annual increment to the population of the world (medium variant) is expected to be about 85.7 million, with the annual increment in the more developed

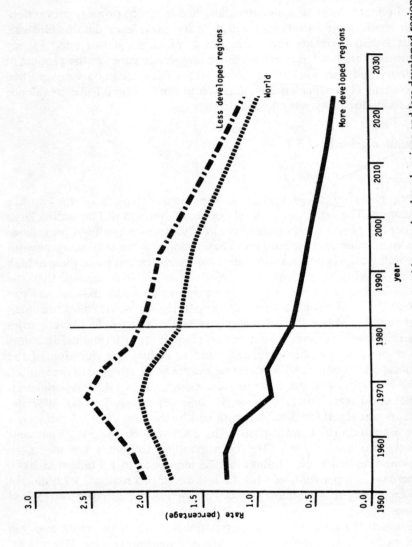

Figure 3.1 Average annual rate of population growth for the world, more developed regions and less developed regions, medium variant, 1950–2025 (United Nations 1985)

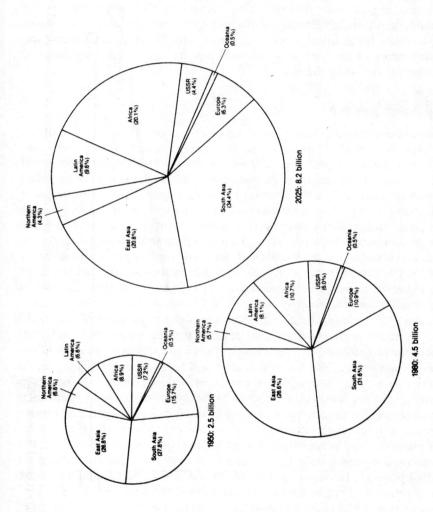

Figure 3.2 Percentage distribution of population by region, medium variant, 1950, 1980 and 2025 (United Nations 1985)

regions accounting for 6.9 million or 8 per cent of this total and that for the less developed regions accounting for 78.8 million or 92 per cent.

Figure 3.2 shows the projected increase in the population of the world and the percentage distribution by regions for the years 1950, 1980, and 2025. The population increased from 2.5 billion to 4.5 billion between 1950 and 1980 (80 per cent) and is projected to increase to 8.2 billion by 2025, 82 per cent higher than in 1980. The changes in the proportion of the population in the different regions are quite striking and have major implications for political, economic, social, and health policies facing the governments of the various states in these regions and for international collaboration among them.

Population growth by age and sex

If we assume a world-wide prevalence of all mental disorders to be of the order of at least 15–20 per cent and that no change in this prevalence rate will occur between 1985 and 2000 we can obtain a very crude estimate of the increase in the number of persons who will have some type of disorder. However, since each MNP disorder has its own age and sex distribution, it is important to go beyond the estimates of the total populations given in the preceding section and to determine the extent to which each age and sex group contributes to the total. To accomplish this requires data on the numerical size of the populations of the world and its regions by age and sex for 1985 and for the year 2000. This information is essential to obtain the expected numerical and percentage change in the number of cases in the specific age-sex groups.

Table 3.1 presents the age distribution of the population of the world and its more and less developed regions for the years 1985 and 2000 (medium variant) and the percentage change in number of persons in the specific age groups. For the world, there will be a considerable increase in every age group, the lowest percentage increase being in the age group under 15 (14 per cent) and the highest in the age group 35–44 (55 per cent). The age specific percentage increases in the more developed regions are considerably lower than those in the less developed regions (Figure 3.3). To illustrate, the percentage increase in the age group under 15 in the developed regions is only 1.9 per cent while that in the developing regions is 16.4 per cent. In the age groups 15–24 and 25–34, the populations in the more developed regions will *decrease* by 6.4 per cent and 4.7 per cent respectively, while in the less developed regions the corresponding populations will *increase* by 17 per cent and 47 per cent, respectively. The percentage increases expected in each of the other age groups in the less developed regions will *exceed* by considerable amounts the corresponding increases in the more developed regions.

Table 3.1 Estimated population of the world (medium variant) 1985 and 2000 and numerical and percentage change in world population 1985–2000 for more and less developed regions of the world by age[1]

Age years		1985			2000	
	Total	More developed regions[2]	Less developed regions[3]	Total	More developed regions	Less developed regions
			Population in 000s			
Total	4,842,048	1,172,863	3,669,185	6,127,120	1,275,656	4,851,464
<15	1,631,768	260,062	1,371,706	1,862,195	265,089	1,597,106
15–24	940,368	185,947	754,421	1,061,520	173,990	887,530
25–34	744,317	186,227	558,090	1,000,595	177,495	823,100
35–44	519,537	152,318	367,219	805,056	190,974	614,082
45–54	418,179	137,691	280,488	590,501	169,355	421,146
55–64	310,491	119,991	190,500	402,287	130,441	271,846
65–74	183,465	78,158	105,307	271,096	104,023	167,073
75+	93,923	52,469	41,454	133,870	64,289	69,581
	Change in number of persons in 000s, 1985–2000			Percentage change in number of persons 1985–2000		
Total	1,285,072	102,793	1,182,279	26.54	8.76	32.22
<15	230,427	5,027	225,400	14.12	1.93	16.43
15–24	121,152	−11,957	133,109	12.88	−6.43	17.64
25–34	256,278	− 8,732	265,010	34.43	−4.69	47.49
35–44	285,519	38,656	246,863	54.96	25.38	67.23
45–54	172,322	31,664	140,658	41.21	23.00	50.15
55–64	91,796	10,450	81,346	29.56	8.71	42.70
65–74	87,631	25,865	61,766	47.76	33.09	58.65
75+	39,947	11,820	28,127	42.53	22.52	67.85

[1] Source: United Nations (1985).
[2] More developed regions include: Northern America, Japan, all regions of Europe, Australia-New Zealand and Union of Soviet Socialist Republics.
[3] Less developed regions include: all regions of Africa, all regions of Latin America, China, other east Asia, all regions of south Asia, Melanesia and Micronesia-Polynesia.

There are differential growth rates of the population by sex which are reflected in changes expected between 1985 and 2000 in the age-specific sex ratios (males per 100 females) of the developed and developing regions of the world. There are also differential rates of population growth by region of the world as shown in Figure 3.2. In addition there are differential rates of growth of countries within regions and among different ethnic/racial groups in these countries. This is illustrated by the striking differences in the projected rates of growth of the White, Black and Hispanic populations of the United States between 1985 and 2000 (Table 3.2). The expected percentage increases in every age group for the Hispanic population

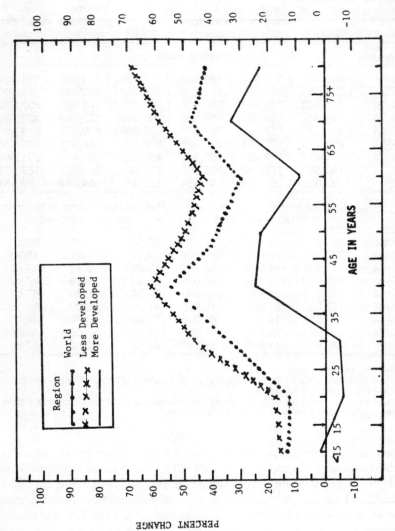

Figure 3.3 Projected percentage change in population of the world, more developed and less developed regions (medium variant) by age – 1985–2000

exceed by a considerable amount those for the Black population and those for the Black population exceed those for the White (US Bureau of the Census 1984, 1986d).

Table 3.2 Estimated population (in 000s) – Whites, Blacks, and persons of Spanish origin – in USA 1985–2000

Age (years)	Year 1985	Year 2000	Change in no. persons 1985–2000	Percentage change
		White		
Total	203,111	222,654	19,543	9.62
<15	42,123	44,314	2,191	5.20
15–24	32,883	29,002	−3,881	−11.80
25–34	35,323	29,590	−5,733	−16.25
35–44	27,620	36,355	8,735	31.63
45–54	19,529	31,662	12,133	62.13
55–64	19,759	20,605	846	4.28
65–74	15,188	15,589	401	2.64
75+	10,686	15,537	4,851	45.40
		Black		
Total	29,078	35,754	6,676	22.97
<15	8,061	9,500	1,439	17,85
15–24	5,732	5,672	−60	−1.05
25–34	5,212	5,316	104	2.00
35–44	3,404	5,811	2,407	70.71
45–54	2,336	4,124	1,788	76.54
55–64	2,003	2,355	352	17.57
65–74	1,410	1,589	179	12.70
75+	920	1,387	467	50.76
		Spanish origin		
Total	17,287	25,224	7,937	45.91
<15	5,317	7,344	2,027	38.12
15–24	3,311	4,124	813	24.55
25–34	3,254	3,804	550	16.90
35–44	2,129	3,803	1,674	78.63
45–54	1,376	2,811	1,435	104.29
55–64	1,015	1,619	604	59.51
65–74	553	1,041	488	88.25
75+	332	678	346	104.22

Source: US Bureau of the Census 1986d.

Effect of population growth on prevalence

I will give an example to illustrate how the age-specific increases in population affect the total prevalence of a specific disorder in an area. Let us assume for the moment that the one month age-specific prevalence rates for schizophrenia and schizophreniform disorders for the US as determined from the five-site Epidemiologic Catchment Area surveys in the US (Regier *et al.* 1988), applied to the population of the more developed and less developed areas of the world in 1985 and 2000 for persons 18 years of age and over (Table 3.3). Let us assume that there would be no change in these rates during this interval of time. The relative increase in the number of cases specific for age would be the same as the relative increase in the population in each age group. These rates would generate a total of 6.2 million cases in the more developed areas of the world in 1985 and 6.7 million cases in 2000, an increase of about 8 per cent. The number of cases that would occur in the less developed areas would be 16.7 millions in 1985 and 24.4 milions in 2000, an increase of 46.1 per cent. Notice also that world-wide the age group 25–44, with the highest prevalence rate (11 per 1,000) and the highest percentage increase in population (43 per cent), accounts for about two-thirds of all the cases. In this instance a large population increase is occurring in an age group with a high prevalence rate.

Table 3.3 Expected number of cases of schizophrenia and schizophreniform disorders[1] for the more[2] and less developed[3] regions of the world by age: 1985–2000

Age (years)	Rate[4] per 1,000	Population (000s) 1985	2000	Percentage change	Expected cases total number 1985	2000	Percentage change
			More developed regions				
18–24	8	132,940	120,814	−9.12	1,063,520	966,512	−9.12
25–44	11	338,545	368,469	8.84	3,723,995	4,053,159	8.84
45–64	5	257,682	299,796	16.34	1,288,410	1,498,980	16.34
65+	1	130,627	168,312	28.85	130,627	168,312	28.85
Total 18+		859,794	957,391	11.35	6,206,552	6,686,963	7.58
			Less developed regions				
18–24	8	501,157	608,689	21.46	4,009,256	4,869,512	21.46
25–44	11	925,309	1,437,182	55.32	10,178,399	15,809,002	55.32
45–64	5	470,988	692,992	47.14	2,354,940	3,464,960	47.14
65+	1	146,761	237,654	61.93	146,761	237,654	61.93
Total 18+		2,044,215	2,976,517	45.61	16,689,356	24,381,128	46.09
			World				
18–24	8	634,097	729,503	15.05	5,072,776	5,836,024	15.05
25–44	11	1,263,854	1,805,651	42.87	13,902,394	19,862,161	42.87
45–64	5	728,670	992,788	36.25	3,643,350	4,963,940	36.25
65+	1	277,388	405,966	46.35	277,388	405,966	46.35
Total 18+		2,904,009	3,933,908	35.46	22,895,908	31,068,091	35.69

[1] Source: United Nations 1985.
[2,3] See Table 3.1.
[4] Based on one month prevalence rates for DIS/DSM–III schizophrenia and schizophreniform disorders, Regier 1988.

It should be noted that the prevalence rates used in this example are quite low, the maximum being about 1 per cent in the age group 25–44 and the lowest 0.1 per cent in the age group 65+. Although these rates are from US surveys based on DIS diagnoses – and there will undoubtedly be questions raised about the propriety of applying them to the populations of other countries – they are used here simply to illustrate the consequences of rates of this magnitude for the number of cases of a disorder in an area. The prevalence rates for schizophrenia are quite low in relation to those reported for affective disorders (posssibly five times as high), anxiety disorders (possibly seven times as high), alcohol and drug use, epilepsy, and, in older age groups, dementias of all types (Alzheimer's, multi-infarct, etc.) (Mortimer *et al*. 1981; WHO 1986b; Folstein *et al*. 1985).

The frequencies of different disorders will vary by country, sex, socio-economic status, etc. As has been emphasized over and over again, the size of the problems that exist currently and those that are predicted to occur by virtue of population growth will outdistance by far our current capabilities of dealing with them.

Urbanization

The other demographic phenomenon that is producing a barrier to prevention – and will continue to do so – is the increasing urbanization of the world's population. As stated in the UN *Report on the World Social Situation* (1986a):

> Urbanization, largely a result of a long transformation in the structure of the economy and technology, brings about changes which are often synonymous with the transition of society from the traditional to the modern, with its accompanying tensions, problems and opportunities. The process of urbanization, or the concentration of a large population in a relatively small area, performing a diverse set of economic and social functions, implies a changing living and working environment, new life styles, aspirations and social institutions.

The percentage of the world's population living in urban areas has increased from about 37 per cent in 1970 to 42 per cent in 1985. It is projected to increase to about 48 per cent in 2000 and to 63 per cent in the year 2025 (United Nations 1985).

Between 1985 and the year 2000 the percentage of the population living in urban areas in the developed regions will have increased from 72 per cent to 78 per cent and that in the less developed regions from 32 per cent to 40 per cent (Table 3.4). This means that by the year 2000 the urban population of the developed regions will be over 992 million and of the developing regions over 1,959 million.

A disturbing feature of this trend is the proliferation of slums and

Table 3.4 Distribution of population of the world[1], its more[2] and less[3] developed regions, by urban and rural areas (numbers in 000s) and percentage change 1985–2000

Years	Total	Urban areas	Rural areas	Percentage urban
		World		
1985	4,842,048	2,013,324	2,828,724	41.6
2000	6,127,117	2,951,633	3,175,485	48.2
% Increase	26.5	46.6	12.3	15.9
		More developed regions		
1985	1,172,863	849,061	323,802	72.4
2000	1,275,655	992,148	283,507	77.8
% Increase	8.8	16.9	−12.4	7.5
		Less developed regions		
1985	3,669,185	1,164,264	2,504,922	31.7
2000	4,851,462	1,959,485	2,891,976	40.4
% Increase	32.2	68.3	15.5	27.4

[1] Source: United Nations 1985.
[2,3] See Table 3.1.

squatter settlements in the developing countries. Between a quarter and a half of the urban population in many of these countries live under appalling conditions, lacking the minimum infrastructure and basic amenities of life. The population of such settlements is expected to rise to over a billion by the year 2000. The World Health Organization has commented on the consequences of this unplanned and unchecked urban growth in *The Social Dimensions of Mental Health* (WHO 1981a):

> Overcrowded slums are the most glaring result of unplanned and unchecked urban growth. Tens of millions live in such slums in un-developing countries with disastrous effects on the quality of life. Psychological tension, alcohol abuse and its related problems, traffic accidents, drug dependence, educational failure, violence and crime are rampant within.

Impact of urbanization on rural areas

As a result of the rapid increase in the urbanization of the less developed regions, the percentage of the population living in rural areas is *decreasing*, but the number of persons living in these areas is *increasing* (Table 3.4). Between 1985 and 2000 the rural population of the less developed regions will increase by about 16 per cent, from 2.5 billion to 2.9 billion. In many countries unemployment of the young has swelled the migration from rural to urban areas where, as indicated above, increasing numbers of young people living in overcrowded conditions are exposed to unhealthy influences (e.g., drug abuse, alcoholism, smoking, and violence) and the consequent social tensions (WHO 1986a, 1986c, 1987b).

This pattern of migration – from rural to urban areas – produces a residual population in the rural areas that is weighted heavily with persons suffering from physical, mental, social, and economic problems that need attention. As in the urban slums, absolute poverty is rampant in the rural areas where nearly '1000 million people are trapped in the vicious circle of poverty, malnutrition and disease and despair that saps their energy, reduces their work capacity and limits their ability to plan for the future' (WHO 1981b). Lack of human, material, and financial resources, along with poor transport and communications in rural areas are major obstacles to the delivery of health services.

As stated by the *WHO Study Group on Mental Health Care in Developing Countries* (WHO 1984):

> The vast majority of the population of the developing world does not have access to mental health care. Most of those suffering from epilepsy receive no treatment despite the fact that, for many of them, such treatment is cheap, simple and effective. In some developing countries alcohol abuse is a major public health problem and in others drug dependence has assumed alarming proportions.

Thus, the conditions in rural areas and in slums of the urban areas of the developing countries exacerbate the 'vicious circle of poverty, malnutrition and disease and despair'.

Changing household and family structure and living arrangements

As stated in the *Social Dimensions of Mental Health* (WHO 1981a):

> In contrast to the teeming slums of developing countries, a problem in many developed countries is that up to one third of urban households contain only one person, and small family units that find it difficult to look after a disabled member are much more common than large households which are usually able to buffer stress.

The increase in numbers of persons living alone is only one aspect of a major demographic trend, one that is of considerable importance to mental health and other public health and social programmes. This phenomenon is the change in household and family structure and living arrangements of the populations of the developed world and also of the developing world. International demographic data on these trends are difficult to find so I will use data from the US to illustrate barriers that the changing household and family structure of the US is presenting to mental health.

Between 1950 and 1985 married couple families increased by 48 per cent, male householder families without spouse by 91 per cent, female householder families without spouse by 182 per cent, and non-family households by 411 per cent. About 85 per cent of the non-family households consist of persons living alone (one-person households). The number of one-person households increased by 421 per cent during this period. The trends for the number of households per 1,000 population by type highlight the gradual decline in the number of married couple families per 1,000 population and accentuate the striking increases occurring in the ratios of the other types of family and non-family households (Kramer *et al*. 1987; US Bureau of the Census 1985a, 1985b, 1986c).

Several factors have brought about these changes in household and family structure: the increase in divorce rates; increase in the number of widows and widowers; migration of workers to areas of the country with opportunities for employment, and trends in behaviour, lifestyle, value systems, and aspirations of the various social-class strata of our society.

It is well known that persons who are separated, divorced, widowed, or never married, persons living alone or in non-family households and children living with one parent are at relatively high risk for developing a mental disorder. The US Census Bureau (1986a) has recently published data on the living arrangements of several of these groups: divorced men and women, children under 18 living with one parent by marital status of parent, and the non-institutional living arrangements of the elderly. The latter are shown in Figures 3.4 and 3.5. These charts portray quite dramatically the different configurations of the living arrangements of children and old people.

Another characteristic of the female householder family with children is that a very large proportion of these families (about 35 per cent) live below the poverty level, another variable known to be a risk factor for mental disorder (Moynihan 1985).

As a result of the continuing emphasis on community care, it is important to learn more about the living arrangements of persons in these high-risk groups – who among them has a mental disorder, the role of this person in the household (i.e., head of household, spouse of head, child, or other relative), the impact of the persons with a disorder on the other persons in the household and vice versa – and to gather additional information about the familial aggregation of mental disorders (Downes and Simon 1954; Kellam and Ensminger 1980; Kellam *et al*. 1982; Rutter and Quinton 1984; WHO 1976). Indeed, more knowledge is needed about the family-household aggregation of mental and physical disorders in an era when the importance of primary health care and family-based preventive care is being increasingly emphasized.

The Eastern Baltimore Mental Health Survey provided a unique opportunity to collect data in a way that made it possible to allocate persons with

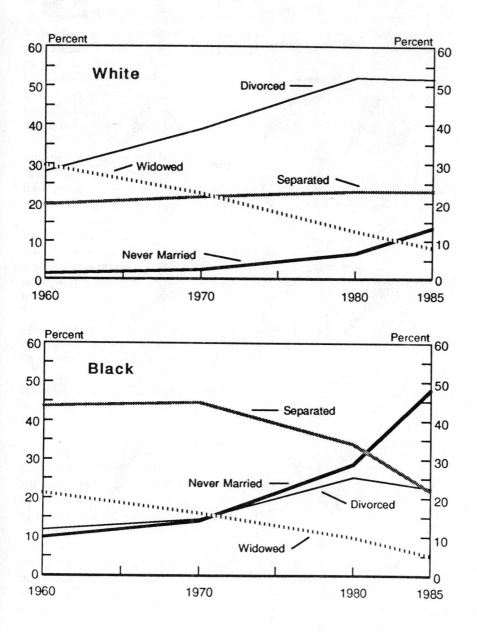

Figure 3.4 Children under 18 years living with one parent, by marital status of parent: 1985, 1980, 1970, and 1960 (US Bureau of the Census, 1986a)

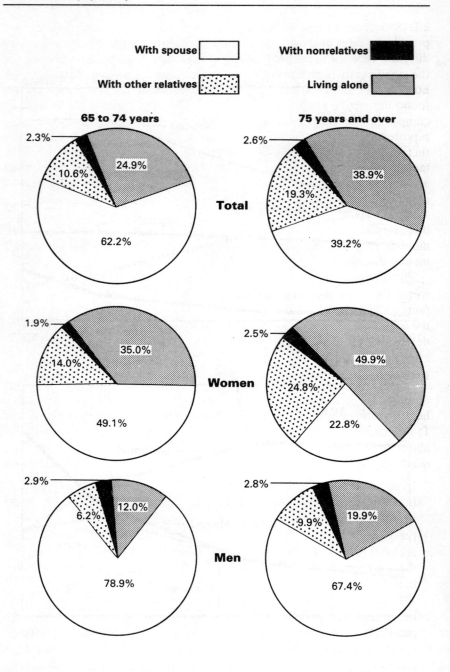

Figure 3.5 Noninstitutional living arrangements of the elderly: 1985 (percentage distribution) (US Bureau of the Census 1986a)

a DIS disorder to type of household in which they lived and to determine prevalence rates of specific DIS/DSM-III disorders among persons living in different types of households (Kramer *et al.* 1987). These data underscore the significantly higher prevalence of mental disorders in male and female householder families and non-family households, as compared to that found in married couple families. As a result of changes in the household composition of the US during the past thirty years, results similar to those reported for Eastern Baltimore are likely to be quite general throughout the US and probably in other developed countries. This follows from the fact that female and male householder families and non-family households are heavily weighted with persons at high risk for mental disorder. As a result of the expected increases in the number of such households between 1985 and 2000, shown in Table 3.5, and the high prevalence of mental disorders in these households, a marked increase can be expected in the number of US households in which one or more members will have a mental disorder.

The situation in poor developing countries is of course incomparably worse than this. For example, over 80 million children live without any family and growing numbers of children are left to fend for themselves in the cities of developing countries as economic and social conditions deteriorate (WHO 1987b).

Refugees and the homeless

Another group of persons at high risk for MNP disorders and many other health problems are refugees. It is estimated that there are between 10 and 15 million refugees in the world, that their number is increasing at a rate of about 3,000 per day and that half of them are children (WHO 1987b). To quote this WHO report:

Events have once again demonstrated the magnitude and complexity of the refugee problem, which in the final analysis is a reflection of the troubled conditions of today's world. Concentrations and movement of refugees, often sizable, have been reported in almost all geographical areas. It is estimated that there are between 10 and 15 million refugees in the world, their number increasing at a rate of about 3000 per day, and half of them children.

In Africa alone there are five million refugees, approximately one in every hundred people. The efforts required merely to care for and protect such numbers, not to mention the human suffering, are vast. The steady increase in the number of persons in holding centers in several countries could have serious implications, since no durable solution by resettlement, repatriation or local integration has yet been found. Physical safety in some of the refugee settlements has become very precarious. The long-term solutions to this growing problem lie in national and international sociopolitical and economic policies that are concerned above all with human development.

Table 3.5   Type of households and family units USA 1985–2000[1]

Type of household and family	1985	2000	Percentage change
Number 000s			
Total	86,789	105,933	22.1
Family households	62,707	72,277	15.3
Married couple	50,350	56,294	11.8
Other, male householder	2,228	3,282	47.3
Other, female householder	10,129	12,701	25.4
Non-family households	24,082	33,656	39.8
Male householder	10,114	15,452	52.8
Female householder	13,968	18,204	30.3
Living alone	20,602	28,944	40.5
Two or more persons	3,480	4,712	35.4
Percentage of Total			
Total	100.0	100.0	
Family households	72.3	68.2	−5.7
Married couple	58.0	53.1	−8.5
Other, male householder	2.6	3.1	19.2
Other, female householder	11.7	12.0	2.6
Non-family households	27.7	31.8	14.8
Male householder	11.7	14.6	24.8
Female householder	16.1	17.2	6.8
Living alone	23.7	27.3	15.2
Two or more persons	4.0	4.5	12.5
No. of households per 1,000 population			
Total	363.7	395.3	8.7
Family households	262.8	269.7	2.6
Married couple	211.0	210.1	−0.4
Other, male householder	9.3	12.2	31.2
Other, female householder	42.4	47.4	11.8
Non-family households	100.9	125.6	24.5
Male householder	42.4	57.7	36.1
Female householder	58.5	67.9	16.1
Living alone	86.3	108.0	25.1
Two or more persons	14.6	17.6	20.5
Population US (000s)	238,631	267,956	12.3

[1] Source: US Bureau of the Census (1986c)

A problem which bears some semblance to that of refugees and other homeless persons in the developing world is that of the homeless of the developed world. The refugee problems in the developing areas of the world have been created by international sociopolitical and economic policies of nations that have deprived persons and their families of a permanent residence. Almost all arise for socio-economic reasons, particularly the migration of large numbers of persons from rural to urban areas to find better economic opportunity. In the US some persons have become homeless for the same reasons but some for other reasons, including loss of employment resulting from major changes in industry, agriculture, and other segments of the economy; migration to other sections of the country to seek employment opportunities; government policy that has promoted deinstitutionalization of large numbers of patients from state mental institutions into communities without adequate housing or services; severe alcohol and drug abuse problems that have caused family breakdown; loss of friends, loss of finances, loss of job, and affiliative relationships; and desire on the part of some individuals to escape from a society that is too complicated and stressful for them (Fischer and Breakey 1987). Whatever the reasons, there are in the US an estimated 250,000 homeless on any given night and as many as three million who experience some type of homelessness during a year (Roper and Boyer 1987).

Homelessness is a complex medical, social, psychological, and economic problem. Detecting high-risk individuals and preventing them from entering into the state of homelessness is a difficult, sometimes thankless task. Once individuals are in this state there are many barriers that must be overcome to prevent them from deteriorating and to motivate them to seek and to use the help needed to return them to an appropriate niche in the community. Some of the barriers relate to personal characteristics, such as geographical instability; others are societal, such as lack of funds for programmes that provide relevant services and personnel to implement them (Breakey 1987).

Poverty

In the preceding sections mention has been made of the extensive poverty that exists in the developing areas of the world. WHO has underscored the dramatic increase in poverty in the developing countries: 'Absolute poverty traps almost one thousand million people, 90% of whom live in rural areas; more than 50% are small farmers and almost 25% are laborers without land' (WHO 1987b).

There is also evidence that growing numbers of elderly persons in the developed countries live in poverty, particularly among the elderly who live alone, and, as already indicated, the same is true among the increasing number of one-parent families (Commonwealth Fund Commission 1987; US Senate Special Committee 1986).

Many epidemiologic surveys of mental disorders have demonstrated the inverse relationship between socio-economic status and the prevalence of specific MNP disorders (Eaton 1986; Roman and Harrison 1967). The effect of poverty on disease is well summarized in the WHO statement (1987b): 'The risk of disease and disablement is much greater for the poverty-stricken, threatening families with further demands on their limited resources and thus even deeper poverty.'

Other barriers to prevention

The preceding sections have provided a review of demographic factors that are barriers to prevention of MNP disorders. There are many other health, social, cultural, and economic factors that place major obstacles in the way of preventing these disorders and their disabling consequences, which can only be touched on here. Among these are: hunger, malnutrition and nutritional deficiencies; inadequate prenatal and perinatal care; acquired lesions of the central nervous system; lack of shelter and ancillary services; illiteracy; lack of programmes and trained manpower, particularly in developing countries; natural disasters; discrimination against girls and women; racism and apartheid; torture; ongoing military actions and conflicts; and deterioration and pollution of the environment.

A detailed exposition is given in the *Seventh Report on the World Health Situation* (WHO 1987b) and possible preventive strategies are summarized in the Report of the Director-General (WHO 1986a).

Confusion about what we are trying to prevent

Another major barrier to prevention results from problems created by the proliferation of diagnostic instruments used to identify persons with a specific mental disorder. In the US, we now have the following diagnostic instruments: SADS, SADS–L, DIS, PSE, SPE, PERI, SCID, CIDI, and SADD (Weissman *et al.* 1986). Each one incorporates a specific interpretation of criteria for a specific diagnosis, includes questions that attempt to operationalize these criteria, and provides procedures for eliciting responses from persons to determine whether they meet the criteria for a specific diagnosis. Several of these instruments have been translated into many different languages, which further complicates the situation.

A question remains as to whether persons allocated to a given diagnostic category by each procedure have the same or different symptom profiles. For example, persons assigned to 'schizophrenia' on the basis of DIS criteria and procedures may have symptom profiles that differ from those assigned to that diagnosis on the basis of PSE criteria and procedures. As a result of differences in diagnostic assignment that may result from the other diagnostic instruments, the risk factors associated with DIS/DSM–III schizophrenia may also differ from those found for a diagnosis of schizophrenia based on SADS and CIDI procedures. A similar problem can be formulated for persons assigned a diagnosis of major depressive disorder as well as other disorders.

Data from the Eastern Baltimore Mental Health Survey illustrate this point. A probability sample of subjects evaluated by the DIS procedure was examined by psychiatrists using a procedure for assigning DSM–III diagnoses modelled on the PSE. The prevalence rate of schizophrenia, based on the clinical reappraisal examination, was not significantly different from that based on the DIS but the individuals in numerators of the rates were to a large extent different subjects. With regard to major depressive disorders the prevalence rates were significantly different and the individuals in the numerators of each of these rates were also quite different subjects (Anthony *et al.* 1985).

There may also be differences in response to treatment with a given psychotropic drug between patients with the same diagnosis but derived from a different diagnostic procedure. For example, the responses of patients with a DIS/DSM–III diagnosis of major depressive disorder may differ from the responses of patients with the same diagnosis derived from SADS, PSE, CIDI, or SADD diagnostic procedures. The same may be true for the outcome of prevention trials to be carried out in the community. It is also possible that there may be genetic differences among patients with a diagnosis of schizophrenia obtained from the different interview procedures.

Accordingly, it is important to initiate research to determine whether risk factors, outcome of treatment, results of preventive trials, and genetic factors differ among persons with the same diagnostic label but derived from different diagnostic interview methods. The results of such investigations will help define more clearly the disorders we are trying to prevent and provide improved guidelines for the design of research for their prevention and control.

Inadequate information support for planning programmes for prevention of MNP disorders

There is still another barrier to the prevention of MNP disorders: the lack of epidemiological, demographic, and health services information needed for sound planning of programmes to accomplish this. In its evaluation of progress being made by member states in their formulation of national strategies for achieving the goals of Health for All by the year 2000, WHO found that practically all reported that inadequate information support was the main constraint to the development of these strategies (WHO 1987b).

With respect to MNP disorders the lack of essential information is particularly critical. Only a few countries have the trained manpower and resources needed to collect systematic data about the prevalence of these disorders in the various demographic and geographic sub-groups of their populations and to monitor trends of these rates. There is a similar problem with respect to the collection of data on the utilization of health, mental health, and related human services by persons with MNP disorders and of the additional data needed to evaluate the effectiveness of these services.

The lack of these essential data is a very serious problem for most of the countries of the developing areas of the world. But it is also a problem in many countries of the more developed areas. To illustrate, Freeman *et al.* (1985) carried out a study of the impact of WHO's long-term programmes on mental health for Europe and, in particular, its effect on mental health policies, principles, and practices at both national and regional levels. One of the major conclusions of the study was: 'Because of deficiencies in information submitted to WHO, very few meaningful comparisons could be made between the situations in 1972 and 1982 in the region as a whole.'

Thus, considerable effort is needed to assist member states of WHO in developing information systems that will facilitate the planning and implementation of programmes for the prevention and control of MNP disorders and evaluation of their effectiveness.

Implications of the rising pandemic of AIDS for MNP prevention programmes

This paper would not be complete without mentioning the implications of the rising pandemic of acquired immune deficiency virus (HIV) syndrome for programmes for the prevention and control of MNP disorders.

The transmission of the virus results from behaviour and actions of persons who manifest certain MNP problems: homosexual and bisexual men and intravenous drug users. They account for the largest number and proportion of reported cases. To illustrate, these groups account for almost 90 per cent of the 39,594 cases reported to the surveillance programme of the Centers for Disease Control of the US Public Health Service between January 1981 and 3 August 1987 (Centers for Disease Control 1987a). The remaining 10 per cent of the cases consisted of blood transfusion recipients, haemophiliacs, children of infected mothers, and heterosexual partners of infected persons.

One of the conditions associated with AIDS is HIV encephalopathy giving rise to dementia. For surveillance purposes the Centres for Disease Control recommend the following definitive diagnostic method for this disorder (Centers for Disease Control 1987b):

HIV encephalopathy (dementia): clinical findings of disabling cognitive and/or motor dysfunction interfering with occupation or activities of daily living, or loss of behavioral developmental milestones in a child, progressing over weeks to months, in the absence of a concurrent illness or condition other than HIV infection that could explain the findings. Methods to rule out such concurrent illnesses and conditions must include cerebrospinal fluid examination and either brain imaging (computer tomography or magnetic resonance) or autopsy.

About 90 per cent of the cumulative number of cases reported to the CDC between 1 January 1981 and 3 August 1987 (39,594) were among persons in the age range 20–49. Thus, AIDS can produce a type of dementia in persons in the middle years of the lifespan, an age group in which currently the incidence of dementia is very low.

The Director of the WHO Special Programme on AIDS has commented on this problem as follows (Mann 1987):

During a five-year period, 10–30% of all HIV-infected persons can be expected to develop AIDS. An additional 25–50% will develop AIDS-related illnesses. The proportion of infected persons who will develop HIV neurological-disease (particularly dementia) is unknown, but an epidemic of progressive neurological disease among HIV-infected persons must be considered a possibility.

As a result, from the 5–10 million persons already infected with HIV worldwide, between 500,000 and 3 million AIDS cases are likely to emerge during the next five years, along with 1–5 million cases of AIDS-related illnesses and an unknown number of neurological illnesses.

Mann also stresses the considerable social and economic costs of the HIV epidemic (1987):

The personal, social and economic costs of the HIV epidemic are very high. Uncertainties regarding prognosis, along with fears and realities of exposure and ostracism, lead HIV-infected but asymptomatic persons to experience higher levels of stress than AIDS patients themselves. The family structure and function is threatened both by infection and the loss of mothers and fathers. The social and economic fabric is seriously affected by the epidemic of illness and death among productive 20–40 year olds, which is typical of AIDS epidemiology in industrialized and developing countries. In Africa, social and economic development may be threatened by the loss of a substantial proportion of 20–40-year-old persons, particularly among the urban elites. The direct economic costs of AIDS are also enormous. For example, in the United States, it is estimated that the total cost of direct medical care for AIDS patients in 1991 will reach U.S. $16 billion. In some central African hospitals, 20–50% of adult patients on medical wards have AIDS or other HIV-related conditions, placing an additional burden upon already limited health care systems. The combined impact of the HIV pandemic, of AIDS, AIDS-related diseases and neurological disease upon health care, insurance and legal systems, economic and social development and indeed entire cultures and populations is already extraordinary and will become increasingly profound.

In summary, the HIV epidemic presents an unprecedented challenge to biomedical research and to public health and mental health: to biomedical research, the development of vaccines to protect persons against HIV infection and therapies to treat persons with AIDS and AIDS-related illnesses; to public health, the development of effective prevention and control programmes to reduce morbidity and mortality from these illnesses and to ease the socio-economic burdens and stress they cause the community.

Conclusion

This review has dealt with what the author perceives to be major barriers to prevention of MNP disorders and associated disabling conditions in the developed and developing countries of the world. Many of these problems are due to the behaviour of people living in these areas. Others are the result of actions of governments, some of whom have enacted policies and laws intended to improve the mental, physical, and social well-being of the populations under their jurisdictions, while others have conducted policies that maintain the status quo of conditions known to result in MNP problems and still others have actively increased world tensions which are a threat to the physical and mental health of their populations and their state of well-being.

It is quite clear that much more research will be needed on the bio-psycho-social factors that determine the differential incidence of MNP disorders and their outcome and the organizational, human, and financial resources needed to apply the results of these research efforts. However, it must be emphasized that progress in achieving the goals of prevention is very much dependent on social progress and much remains to be done to remove the obstacles that are preventing this progress (UN 1986a). To quote from WHO's *Seventh Report on the World Health Situation* (1987b):

The Global Strategy for Health for All by the Year 2000 stresses the close and complex links that exist between health and socioeconomic development. Health not only results from genuine socioeconomic development as distinct from mere growth, it is also an essential investment in such development. The economic development of a country is clearly limited when one out of five children dies before completing one year of life, when a high proportion of children suffer from stunted growth due to malnutrition, when a lifetime can be shortened by as much as a tenth by disease, or when a person is beset by disability and disease at what is potentially the most productive age.

Achievement of health goals is determined to a large extent by policies that lie outside the health sector and in particular by policies, whatever their nature, aimed at assuring universal access to the means to earn an acceptable income. But a mere increase in income is no guarantee of health. Health authorities will have to be vigilant in identifying those aspects of development that can threaten health and in introducing the elements that are essential to health development in national, regional and global socioeconomic development plans.

It is my hope that the World Psychiatric Association, WHO, professional and non-governmental organizations, and the people themselves will continue to put pressure on our governments and institutions to remove the social, economic, psychological, and political barriers that continue to thwart our efforts to prevent mental, neurological, and psychosocial disorders and their disabling effects and other health and social problems that currently affect such a large portion of the world's population.

References

Anthony, J.C., Folstein, M., Romanoski, A.J., *et al*. (1985) 'Comparison of the Lay Diagnostic Interview Schedule and a Standardized Psychiatric Diagnosis', *Archives of General Psychiatry* 42: 667–75.

Breakey, W.R. (1987) 'Treating the homeless', *Alcohol* 11: 42–6.

Centers for Disease Control (1987a) 'AIDS weekly surveillance report', United States AIDS Program, 3 August 1987, Atlanta, Georgia: CDC.

Centers for Disease Control (1987b) *Draft of the Revision of AIDS Case Definition for Surveillance Purposes*, Atlanta, Georgia: CDC.

Commonwealth Fund Commission on Elderly People Living Alone (1987) *Old, Alone, and Poor*, a plan for reducing poverty among elderly people living alone. Baltimore, MD: Commonwealth Fund Commission.

Downes, J. and Simon K. (1954) 'Characteristics of psychoneurotic patients and their families as revealed in a general morbidity study', *Milbank Memorial Fund Quarterly* 32: 42–64.

Eaton, W.W. (1986) *The Sociology of Mental Disorders*, second edition, New York: Praeger.

Fischer, P.J. and Breakey, W.R. (1987) 'Profile of the Baltimore homeless with alcohol problems', *Alcohol* 11: 36–7.

Folstein, M., Anthony, J.C., Parhad, I., Duffy, B., and Gruenberg, E.M. (1985) 'The meaning of cognitive impairment in the elderly', *Journal of the American Geriatric Society* 33: 228–35.

Freeman, H.L., Fryers, T., and Henderson, J.H. (1985) *Mental Health Services in Europe: 10 Years on. Public Health in Europe 25*, Copenhagen: WHO Regional Office for Europe.

Kellam, S.G. and Ensminger, M.E. (1980) 'Theory and method in child psychiatric epidemiology in studies of children', in F. Earls (ed.) *Monographs in Psychological Epidemiology*, New York: Prodist.

Kellam, S.G., Adams, R.G., Brown, C.H., and Ensminger, M.E. (1982) 'Long-term evolution of the family structure of teenage and older mothers', *Journal of Marriage and the Family* August: 539–54.

Kramer, M., Brown, H., Skinner, A., *et al.* (1987) 'Changing living arrangements in the population and their potential effect on the prevalence of mental disorder: findings of the Eastern Baltimore Mental Health Survey', in B. Cooper (ed.) *Psychiatric Epidemiology: Progress and Prospects*, London: Croom Helm.

Mann, J.M. (1987) 'The global AIDS situation', *World Health Statistics Quarterly* 40: 185–92.

Mortimer, J.A., Schuman, L.M., and French, L.R. (1981) 'Epidemiology of dementing illness', in J.A. Mortimer and Schuman, L.M. (eds) *Epidemiology of Dementia*, New York: Oxford University Press, pp. 3–23.

Moynihan, D.P. (1985) 'Family and nation: the Godkin Lectures', Harvard University, 8–9 April 1985.

Reiger, D.A., Boyd, J.H., Burke, J.D., *et al.* (1988) 'One-month prevalence of mental disorders in the U.S. – based on Five Epidemiologic Catchment Area Sites', *Archives of General Psychiatry* 45: 977–86.

Roman, P. and Harrison, M.T. (1967) *Schizophrenia and the Poor*, Ithaca, NY: New York State School of Industrial and Labor Relations.

Roper, H.R. and Boyer, R. (1987) 'Homelessness as a health risk', *Alcohol* 48: 38–41.

Rutter, M. and Quinton, D. (1984) 'Parental psychiatric disorder: effects on children', *Psychological Medicine* 41: 853–80.

United Nations (1985) *World Population Prospects: Estimates and Projections as Assessed in 1982*, Department of International Economic and Social Affairs; Population Studies No. 86 ST/ESA/SER.a/86, New York: UN.

United Nations (1986a) *1985 Report on the World Social Situation*, Department of International Economic and Social Affairs, ST/ESA/165. E/CN–5/1985, Revision 1, New York: UN.

United Nations (1986b) *Living Conditions in Developing Countries in the Mid 1980's*, Supplement to the 1985 Report on the World Social Situation, Department of Economic and Social Affairs/ESA/165 Add 1, New York: UN.

United Nations (1986c) *World Population Prospects: Estimates and Projections as Assessed in 1984*, Departmental of International and Economic and Social Affairs, Populations Studies No. 98, New York: UN.

US Bureau of the Census (1984) *Projections of the Population of the United States by Age, Sex, and Race, 1983 to 2080*, Current Population Reports, Series P–25, No. 952, Washington DC: US Government Printing Office.

US Bureau of the Census (1985a) *Households, Families, Marital Status and Living Arrangements March 1985 (Advance Report)*, Series P–20 No. 402, Washington DC: US Government Printing Office.

US Bureau of the Census (1985b) *Marital Status and Living Arrangements, March 1984*, Series P–20 No. 399, Washington, DC: US Government Printing Office.

US Bureau of the Census (1986a) *Marital Status and Living Arrangements, March 1985*, Series P–20, No. 410, Washington, DC: US Government Printing Office.

US Bureau of the Census (1986b) *Households, Families, Marital Status and Living Arrangements, March 1986 (Advance Report)*, Series P–20, No. 412, Washington, DC: US Government Printing Office.

US Bureau of the Census (1986c) *Projections of the Number of Households and Families, 1986–2000*, Series P–25, No. 986, Washington, DC: US Government Printing Office.

US Bureau of the Census, Gregory Spencer (1986d) *Projections of the Hispanic Population, 1983 to 2080*, Current Population Reports, Series P–25, No. 995, Washington, DC: US Government Printing Office.

US Senate Special Committee on Aging with the American Association of Retired

Persons, the Federal Council on Aging and the Administration on Aging (1986) *Aging America, Trends, and Projections*, 1985–86 Edition, PF, 3377 (1085), Washington, DC: US Government Printing Office.

Weissman, M.M., Myers, J.K., and Ross, C.E. (eds) (1986) *Community Surveys of Psychiatric Disorders*, New Brunswick, NJ: Rutgers University Press.

World Health Organization (1976) *Statistical Indices of Family Health*, Report of a WHO Study Group, Technical Report Series No. 587, Geneva: WHO.

World Health Organization (1981a) *The Social Dimensions of Mental Health*, Geneva: WHO.

World Health Organization (1981b) *Global Strategy for Health for All by the Year 2000*, 'Health for All' Series, No. 3, Geneva: WHO.

World Health Organization (1984) *Report of the WHO Study Group on Mental Health Care in Developing Countries: A Critical Appraisal of Research Findings*, Technical Report Series 698, Geneva: WHO.

World Health Organization (1986a) *Prevention of Mental, Neurological, and Psychosocial Disorders*, Report by the Director-General, A 39/9, 25 February 1986, Geneva: WHO.

World Health Organization (1986b) *Dementia in Later Life: Research and Action*, Report of a WHO Scientific Group on Senile Dementia, Technical Report Series 730, Geneva: WHO.

World Health Organization (1986c) 'Smoking, Alcohol and Drugs', *World Health*, June 1–31.

World Health Organization (1986d) *World Health Statistics Annual*, Geneva: WHO, (a) global overview: mental, neurologic, and psychosocial disorders, pp. 24–8; other problems, pp. 3–23; 22–30; (b) evaluation of the global strategy for health for all, pp. 33–46.

World Health Organization (1987a) *Handbook of Resolutions and Decisions of the World Health Assembly and the Executive Board III*, first edition (1985–86), Geneva: WHO, p. 28.

World Health Organization (1987b) *Evaluation of the Strategy for Health for All by the Year 2000: Seventh Report on the World Situation 1, Global Review*, Geneva: WHO.

Part two

Towards earlier detection: case-finding and diagnosis

Chapter four

Incidence of dementing illness among persons aged over 65 years in an urban population

Horst Bickel and Brian Cooper

Introduction

The incidence rate of any given disease – i.e., the number of new cases which occur in a defined population unit during a specified time period – is of importance in the epidemiological search for causes, since this requires the frequency of illness-onset to be established in relation to the population's exposure to putative aetiological or risk factors. Because the occurrence of new cases, especially of chronic forms of disease, may be difficult to monitor directly, epidemiologists often have recourse to indirect measures, such as the numbers of new cases notified from medical practice, or of hospital first admissions. Data of this kind, however, will be subject to variability arising from diagnostic inconsistency, differences in the level of medical-care provision, and other extraneous influences.

In the case of late-life dementia, reliance on hospital admission figures or other treatment statistics seems in general to lead to a serious underestimation of the true extent of the problem. While rates of 'treated incidence', derived from hospital and case-register statistics, have been of the order of two to three per 1,000 for men and two to four per 1,000 for women over the age of 60, field survey findings from a number of countries suggest that the total incidence is much higher than this (Bergmann and Cooper 1986). Thus, on the basis of a two-and-a-half to four year follow-up of their Newcastle samples, Bergmann et al. (1971) estimated an annual rate of fifteen per 1,000 for the age range above 60 years. The 'Lundby' study in southern Sweden (Hagnell et al. 1981) yielded a rate of 16.3 per 1,000 for the decade 1947–57, though this fell to 10.7 per 1,000 over the following fifteen years. A survey on the Danish island of Samsø in the years 1972–7, making use of second-hand data from the local medical and social agencies, provided an estimate of twelve per 1,000 annually for persons aged over 60 (Nielsen et al. 1982). On average, therefore, field-study estimates have been about four times as high as those derived from hospital censuses or psychiatric case registers (Cooper 1989).

A disparity of this order – which, incidentally, is consistent with the repeated finding in cross-sectional surveys that far more dementing old people are to be found living in the community than in hospital care – casts doubt on the representativity of hospital-based samples and underlines the need to draw unselected case samples from the elderly population as a whole.

In order to carry out population-based studies, a number of outstanding problems of method must be tackled. To begin with, because dementing illnesses often have a slow, insidious onset and continuous population monitoring is seldom feasible, the appearance of new cases cannot usually be recorded at the time. In practice, investigators have relied upon the replication of cross-sectional surveys at fairly long intervals, and on computing the number of newly identified cases against the time period since the previous survey wave (see, for example, Hagnell et al. 1981; Nilsson 1984). This approach requires that diagnostic judgements be made in retrospect about those individuals in the sample or cohort who have died meanwhile.

Second, since dementing processes usually develop slowly, some specification of clinical severity or degree of functional impairment is called for in defining a case. According to current diagnostic classifications, milder degrees of cognitive decline in the elderly should not be designated as cases of dementia, although their subsequent course and outcome may make this necessary later on (Cooper 1988). Hence, each mild or borderline case of cognitive impairment or decline must be compared with a glossary description, or with prescribed diagnostic guidelines, in order to decide whether or not it fulfils the case criteria.

Third, the relatively high mortality which is found in the highest age groups of the population can lead to serious errors when denominators for epidemiological rates are being computed. To overcome this difficulty, incidence can be calculated as the hazard rate, or 'force of morbidity', for which the index used as denominator is not the number of persons at risk but, instead, the product of population and time at risk, i.e., the number of 'person-years' of exposure for the sample under enquiry (Last 1983).

Finally, the fact that late-life dementia is not a single disease entity, but rather a heterogenous grouping in terms of the underlying pathology and, in all probability, the causal agents involved means that attention must be paid to the question of differential diagnosis. Although a specific diagnosis cannot as a rule be confirmed under field survey conditions, broad criteria are now available which make it possible to assign cases, with a fair degree of probability, to a major diagnostic category such as dementia of Alzheimer type (DAT), multi-infarct dementia (MID), or secondary dementia (McKhann et al. 1984; Roth et al. 1986).

Each of these methodological problems was taken into account in the design and method of a recently completed longitudinal study of a sample of old people in the industrial city of Mannheim.

Research aims and method

The aims of the study were as follows:

1. To establish the rate of incidence of dementing illness in a representative sample of persons aged over 65 years, living in the community, and to examine any variation observed in relation to medical and social characteristics.

2. To ascertain the frequency of new cases of dementia among the elderly residents of geriatric and old people's homes, drawn from the same background population, and to compare it with that found among the community residents.

3. To assess the prospects for predicting the onset of dementia in this elderly population on the basis of the observed distribution and the association with personal characteristics of the sample members ('probands').

Mannheim has a total population of just over 300,000 of whom some 50,000 (16.4 per cent) are aged over 65 years. For the original cross-sectional survey, seven districts with contrasting features were selected which together contained one-fifth of the population and were broadly representative for the city as a whole. In each of these districts a 5 per cent random sample was drawn from the current residents' lists of persons aged over 65 living in private households (Cooper and Sosna 1983). In addition, a separate sample was drawn of persons in this age range who were living in geriatric or old people's homes and had been admitted from addresses in the seven survey districts (Cooper et al. 1984).

Two interviews were conducted with the members of these samples: one focused on the physical and mental health status and the other on the family and social situation. The mental health status was assessed with the aid of a German translation of the standardized Clinical Psychiatric Interview, modified for use with the elderly (Cooper and Schwarz 1982). This interview provided the basis for a profile of psychiatric symptoms and an over-all rating of clinical severity. In addition, a psychiatric diagnosis was recorded whenever appropriate, according to the International Classification of Diseases, Chapter V and the six-category system used by the Newcastle group (Kay et al. 1964).

The modified version of the interview includes a short 'dementia scale', similar in form and content to most such instruments. It consists of fourteen simple questions dealing with orientation for time and place and general knowledge, the responses being given a score of 0, 1, or 2 points each, so that the total (unweighted) score ranges from 0 to a maximum of 28 points.

The initial community survey began in 1978 and was completed in 1980; the survey of home residents was then undertaken in the period 1981–2. The follow-up study was conducted in the years 1986–7, the community sample again being contacted first and the home residents and staff afterwards. This meant in practice that the follow-up interval was from seven to nine years (on average 7.8 years) for the community sample and five to six years (on average 5.6 years) for the old people living in homes.

At this stage, the standardized psychiatric interview was repeated whenever possible, the interviewer having no knowledge of the earlier findings or diagnostic assessment. If the old person was too confused or mentally inaccessible for a structured procedure, a free interview was carried out, with simple questions to try to establish the state of their memory and orientation, and other relevant information was obtained from the nearest relative or care-giver.

In the case of each proband who had died, contact was made with relatives or former care-givers who could act as informants. Again, interviews were carried out and systematic inquiry made about the proband's mental condition, any hospital or other institutional admissions and the events preceding death. Evidence of cognitive impairment, confusion, or disorientation was assessed and rated on a scale of severity (Hughes *et al.* 1982), provided this had persisted for at least six months prior to death. Mental deterioration commencing within six months of death was not accepted as evidence of a dementing illness. An independent check of the date of death was made by a search in the municipal register office.

A retrospective diagnostic assessment of each new case of dementia was made on the basis of all the available information. The authors scrutinized the case material and made independent diagnostic judgements, using predetermined guidelines (Roth *et al.* 1986). They also in each instance made an independent rating of the severity of each new illness, on the basis of the operational criteria.

In order to test for possible risk factors of dementia, the incidence of new cases during the follow-up period was examined in relation to a large series of variables derived from the findings of the original psychiatric and social interviews. These were intended to represent the following types of characteristic of the sample members and their situation: demographic; social (in particular, socio-economic status, housing conditions, and social integration or isolation); physical health status and functional ability; mental health status.

Since the risk of a dementing condition is known to be related to age within the senium, and this variable in turn is associated with a number of other potentially important risk factors, techniques of multivariate analysis are essential in a study of this kind. For the purposes of the present report, only one such technique requires mention: the Cox proportional hazards regression model, which confers the important advantage that the occurrence of new cases of illness can be analysed in relation to various individual characteristics, regardless of variation in the follow-up interval and the presence of 'censored' data (Allgulander and Fisher 1986).

Research findings

Contact and response rates

Complete data were obtained for 343 of a total of 418 persons included in the original survey sample (81.2 per cent) and on 146 of the 167 persons in the sample of home residents (87.4 per cent). The remaining individuals either refused to participate or could not be contacted after repeated attempts.

At follow-up, eight years later, 198 members of the community sample (57.7 per cent) were still alive and 145 (42.3 per cent) had died. An interview was completed either with the proband or, in the case of a deceased person, with an informant in 312 instances, and partial information was obtained on the remainder. In all, the presence or absence of a dementing condition, up to the time of death or follow-up, could be ascertained for 331 probands, representing a successful follow-up rate of 96.5 per cent.

The mortality rate among the home residents was, as expected, much higher than that for the community sample. At follow-up, 45 (30.8 per cent) of the 'homes' sample were still alive and 101 (69.2 per cent) had died in the interim. Information could be obtained at interview with the proband, alone or together with relatives, or, in the case of deceased home residents, from the matron or warden of the establishment in 144 instances (98.6 per cent). The mental status at follow-up was ascertained for all home residents, without exception, who had not shown evidence of a dementing condition at the time of first interview, and hence were at risk for a new illness.

Incidence of dementing illness in the community sample

In the initial survey, seventeen persons had been diagnosed as cases of severe or moderately severe organic mental disorder, and were therefore considered to be no longer at risk for a new illness. Persons with mild, non-psychotic degrees of cognitive impairment (corresponding to category 310 in the current, ninth revision of the ICD), of whom there were a further nineteen in the sample, were included as being at risk. By computing the period of survival from the first interview until the date of death or disease onset, or until the follow-up interval, a total was obtained for the person-years of exposure to risk, and this was then used as the denominator when estimating incidence rates.

At follow-up, thirty-four new cases of clinically manifest dementia were identified in the community sample. This total, distributed over 1,911 person-years of survival, corresponds to a mean rate of 17.8 per 1,000 annually. The nine male cases, occurring in 640 person-years of survival, correspond to a mean rate of 14.1 per 1,000 annually and the twenty-five

Table 4.1 Incidence of organic mental disorder (severe or moderately severe) in the elderly population, reported from area field surveys. Annual age-specific rates per 1,000 population

Author(s)	Survey area & period	Sample size[1] (persons aged over 60)	Age group			
			60–69	70–79	80+	Total (60+)
Bergmann et al. 1971	Newcastle, UK (a) 1960–4; (b) 1964–7	760 (2,000)	–	–	–	15.0
Hagnell et al. 1981	'Lundby', Sweden, 1947–57	655 (4,224)	5.1	18.8	57.3	16.3
	dto. 1957–72	696 (7,959)	2.9	14.8	33.7	10.7
Nielsen et al. 1982	Samsø Island, Denmark 1972–7	1,564 (6,580)	2.8	22.7	34.6	12.0
Nilsson 1984	Gothenburg, Sweden 1971–81	364 (2,655)	–	16.2	–	–
Bickel and Cooper present study	Mannheim, F.R.G. 1978–86[2]	314 (1,912)	4.8	12.2	34.1	17.8[3]

[1] Figures in brackets refer to numbers of 'person-years' at risk.
[2] Age groups 65–69; 70–79; 80+.
[3] Total for age group 65+.

female cases, occurring in 1,271 person-years of survival, to a mean rate of 19.7 per 1,000 annually. Allocation of the new cases to broad diagnostic categories indicated an incidence rate of 9.4 per 1,000 for dementia of Alzheimer type, 6.3 per 1,000 for multi-infarct dementia, and 2.1 per 1,000 for secondary dementia.

In four of the cases, a non-psychotic form of organic mental disorder (ICD category 310) had been diagnosed at the first interview. In retrospect, it seems probable that each of these conditions represented the early stage of a dementing condition which subsequently became florid. If these are excluded from the group of new cases identified at follow-up, on the grounds that the illness had already declared itself at the time of first interview, the estimated incidence rate falls slightly, from 17.8 to 16.3 per 1,000. However, to be logically consistent, analogous mild disorders developing during the follow-up interval should then be included in the count, in which case the estimated incidence rate would rise again. On balance, it seems preferable to exclude from the at-risk sample only those persons whose mental condition was already severe enough at the outset to warrant a diagnosis of dementia or related organic psychosis (ICD categories 290–294) and to include only new cases with a similar degree of severity when calculating incidence rates.

In Table 4.1, the age-specific rates for both sexes combined are shown in conjunction with corresponding rates from field studies in a number of other west European countries, carried out during the past thirty years. The age-related trends can be seen to be similar in all these studies.

The disparities between their earlier and later survey findings, apparent in Table 4.1, led the research group in 'Lundby' to suggest that the incidence of late-life dementia may be declining (Hagnell *et al.* 1981). The data from other studies do not provide any evidence of a general decline in incidence over recent decades. They cannot, however, exclude the possibility, especially as ten-year age groups are rather too broad to correct any confounding effect due to a general ageing trend in elderly populations, and hence to ensure that the findings of the different studies are safely comparable with one another.

In Table 4.2, the male and female incidence rates are presented by ten-year age group. Viewed in this form, the data suggest a higher risk for dementing disorders among women, accounted for by a relative excess of new cases in the age range above 75 years. Below this age, the incidence rate for men is actually double that for women. However, the numbers of new cases are too small for these differences to achieve statistical significance.

An age-related increase in the incidence rate is clearly apparent only among the women, there being no corresponding male trend. Here again, the broadness of the age groups and the possibility of random variation do not allow any firm conclusions to be drawn. In a further step, therefore, the

Table 4.2 Age-specific male and female incidence rates for dementia in the community sample (N = 314)

Age group (yr)	Men (N=110)			Women (N=204)		
	Person-years at risk	New cases	Incidence rate per 1,000 (± S.E.)	Person-years at risk	New cases	Incidence rate per 1,000 (± S.E.)
65–74	265.4	4	15.1 ± 7.5	520.0	4	7.7 ± 3.8
75–84	324.4	4	12.3 ± 6.1	588.9	14	23.8 ± 6.3
85 and over	50.5	1	19.8 ± 19.6	162.5	7	43.1 ± 15.9
65 and over	640.3	9	14.1 ± 4.7	1,271.4	25	19.7 ± 3.9

risk for a new dementing illness was examined for each sex, with the aid of the Cox regression model. Application of this technique provided no evidence that the age of onset differs between the sexes, or that the relative risks for men and women vary with the age group: in short, the trends indicated by Table 4.2 cannot be substantiated.

The distribution of new cases was also analysed in relation to marital status, social class, and type of household group (i.e., whether the proband was living alone or sharing with one or more other persons). The findings are summarized in Table 4.3.

Table 4.3 Incidence rates for dementia, according to selected sociodemographic variables (N = 314)

Sociodemographic variable	Person-years at risk	New cases	Incidence rate per 1,000	Mean age in years at first interview
Marital status:				
– married	817.8	9	11.0 ± 3.6	72.3
– widowed	927.8	19	20.5 ± 4.7	74.8
– single or divorced	166.3	6	36.1 ± 14.5	73.8
Social class (Kleining and Moore):				
I–III	582.0	9	15.5 ± 5.1	73.5
IV	582.7	8	13.7 ± 4.8	73.8
V	557.4	12	21.5 ± 6.1	73.8
VI	189.7	5	26.4 ± 11.6	74.4
Type of household:				
– living alone	860.8	20	23.2 ± 5.1	74.3
– sharing household	1,050.9	14	13.3 ± 3.5	73.0

The size of the observed differences between marital-status groups was unexpected. Table 4.3 suggests, in particular, that single and divorced elderly persons are at increased risk for a dementing illness. While this finding could also be due to random fluctuation, it is the more remarkable in that unmarried persons with a high risk for dementia are as a rule over-represented in field surveys, being selectively removed out of the community by admission to long-stay care. This issue will be addressed again in relation to the home residents' sample.

Widowed persons have an incidence rate nearly double that for the married. This significant difference could be accounted for in terms of intervening variables, marital status being independent neither of age nor of sex. The group of the widowed consisted predominantly of women and had a mean age 2.5 years higher than that of the married. When the effect of these variables was held constant in the multivariate analysis, the difference in incidence rates largely disappeared. None the less, the relative excess of new cases among the unmarried, even if without causal significance, is large enough for marital status to be considered as one possible indicator of risk when strategies of case-finding are under review.

Similar conclusions may be drawn from the distribution of new cases according to type of household group. Here the observed difference in frequency is obviously related to that between married and unmarried persons, discussed above. Although it too ceases to be significant once the effect of age is partialled out, the disparity is large enough to make living alone an indicator of risk in purely predictive terms.

In the original survey, each proband was allocated to a social class category according to the hierarchical classification of Kleining and Moore (1968). In Table 4.3, the resulting distribution has been combined to give four groups, which correspond to the middle class, lower middle class, upper (skilled) working class, and lower (unskilled) working class respectively. The differences in incidence rate are small enough to be due to chance; nevertheless, the trend towards a higher risk in the working-class groups is noteworthy, since it is consistent with the finding in the original survey of a raised prevalence of organic mental disorders in this section of the elderly population (Cooper and Sosna 1983; Cooper 1986).

Although no physical examination or laboratory investigations could be undertaken as part of the field study, each respondent was scored on simple rating scales for impairment of mobility, vision, and hearing. In Table 4.4, the incidence rates for dementia are set out according to these earlier findings, using in each instance a basic dichotomy into impaired and unimpaired.

Table 4.4 Incidence of dementia, according to the presence or absence of physical and sensory impairment (N = 314)

Form of impairment	Person-years at risk	New cases	Incidence rate per 1,000 (± S.E.)	Mean age in years at first interview
Mobility:				
– impaired	408.3	8	19.7 ± 6.9	76.5
– unimpaired	1,503.4	26	17.3 ± 3.4	72.9
Vision:				
– impaired	245.4	6	24.4 ± 9.8	77.4
– unimpaired	1,666.3	28	16.8 ± 3.1	73.1
Hearing:				
– impaired	168.4	4	23.8 ± 11.7	78.8
– unimpaired	1,743.3	30	17.2 ± 3.1	73.1

Table 4.4 reveals a consistent trend for physical or sensory impairment to be associated with an increased risk of dementia, but the observed differences are not statistically significant. One must also bear in mind that there are appreciable differences in mean age between the groups, varying

between 3.5 and 5.7 years. Once these differences are controlled for, the associations with physical and sensory impairment almost disappear. One cannot, therefore, assume that the trends shown in Table 4.4 carry any aetiological importance.

Table 4.5 Incidence rates for dementia, according to psychiatric status at the initial interview (N = 314)

Psychiatric status	Person-years at risk	New cases	Incidence rate per 1,000 (± S.E.)	Mean age in years at first interview
No significant abnormality (N = 253)	1,575.7	25	15.9 ± 3.2	73.4
Functional mental illness (N = 43)	260.8	5	19.2 ± 8.5	73.0
Non-psychotic organic mental impairment (ICD 310) (N = 18)	75.2	4	53.2 ± 25.9	77.5

The predictive relevance of the psychiatric status at first interview was also assessed. At that time, forty-three of the following cohort had been diagnosed as cases of 'functional' mental illness, and an additional eighteen as cases of minor organic mental impairment (ICD category 310, or 'mild dementia'). Table 4.5 reveals no definite increase in dementia risk among the functionally mentally ill, such as would be expected, either if late-life dementia frequently declared itself as a functional mental disturbance, or if the presence of such a disorder were itself a risk factor for the development of a dementing condition.

As could be anticipated, those persons originally diagnosed as cases of mild organic impairment carried the highest risk for a dementing illness. Yet in this group of eighteen persons, definite evidence of dementia was confirmed at follow-up in only four instances. The main reason for this apparent anomaly was that the sub-group proved to have a low life expectancy, most of its members dying early in the follow-up period, before a florid dementia had had time to develop. Of the four still surviving at follow-up who could be interviewed, two were found to be clinically demented, one manifested an unchanged level of mild cognitive impairment, and the fourth had recovered from a reversible organic psycho-syndrome.

Incidence of dementia in the sample of elderly home residents

At the initial interview, thirty-eight home residents were diagnosed as cases of organic mental disorder (severe or moderately severe), and were therefore excluded from the subsequent analysis of new cases. Of the remaining 108 respondents, twenty-six had developed a clinically severe dementing condition during the follow-up interval: a number which, in 324.9 person-years at risk, represents an incidence rate of eighty per 1,000 annually. The six new male cases, occurring in 45.7 person-years, correspond to a rate of 131.3 per 1,000 annually, and the twenty new female cases, occurring in 279.2 person-years, to a rate of 71.6 per 1,000 annually. In view of the small number of male home residents, however, a comparison between the rates for the two sexes is hardly meaningful.

The disparity between the incidence rates for the community and home-residents' samples is very striking. Among the latter, the overall rate of eighty per 1,000 is over four times as high as the rate of 17.8 per 1,000 found among the elderly in private households. This unexpected finding calls for an explanation. Before a direct influence of the residential environment is invoked, the comparability of the two samples must be inspected with some care.

Most of the other characteristics which serve to differentiate the samples – notably the high proportions of women and of the physically impaired, as well as the overwhelming preponderance of unmarried persons, among the home residents – are too weakly associated with the risk for dementia to explain the major disparity in incidence rates. More directly relevant is the difference of 7.5 years between the mean ages of the two samples. An attempt to control for this factor by dividing the samples into ten-year age groups served to reduce the contrast between the incidence rates, but still left a threefold difference to be accounted for.

A question thus arises as to whether the high risk for dementia observed among the home residents is due, at least in part, to the effects of an institutional environment, or whether it can be explained entirely by a selective process. In the latter event, one would expect the home residents to have been characterized, already at the first interview, by a raised frequency of minor cognitive deficits, such as might indicate the early stages of a dementing illness, even though not yet necessarily interfering with everyday activities.

To test this possibility, we examined the respondents' scores on the simple, 14-item 'dementia scale' incorporated in the psychiatric interview. In Table 4.6, the findings for both samples are presented in the form of a dichotomy, a score of 0–3 points being taken to indicate normal cognitive functioning at the time of interview, and a score of 4 or more points to indicate some degree of cognitive impairment.

The cognitively unimpaired groups in the two samples do not differ significantly in their incidence rates, although there is a definite tendency for the home residents still to manifest a higher risk. The difference apparent in Table 4.6 can be ascribed to the fact that the mentally unimpaired home residents were on average some six years older than

Table 4.6 Comparison of the incidence rates for dementia in the community and home residents' samples, according to cognitive impairment scale scores at first interview (N=420)[1]

Age-group (yr.)	0 – 3 points on cognitive impairment scale		4 or more points on cognitive impairment scale	
	Community sample (N=283)	Home residents' sample (N=54)	Community sample (N=30)	Home residents' sample (N=53)
65 – 79	10.1 ± 2.8	13.0 ± 12.9	32.0 ± 22.3	0.0[2]
80 or over	27.4 ± 7.5	48.5 ± 19.3	74.8 ± 29.2	197.2 ± 41.6
65 or over	14.7 ± 2.9	34.8 ± 12.9	55.8 ± 19.2	147.7 ± 32.1

[1] no cognitive impairment scale score available for one member of each sample
[2] no new cases in this sub-group, which had only 30.6 person-years at risk

their counterparts living in private households (79.0 years as against 73.1 years).

The incidence rate of dementia among the cognitively impaired, whether living in institutions or in private households, is four times as high as among the unimpaired: a significant difference. Once again, the rate among home residents is higher, but this excess can be explained by their greater mean age (83.1 years, as against 78.3 years for the community residents) and, in addition, their greater severity of cognitive impairment. The mean score for this group at first interview was 10.0, compared with 5.8 for the corresponding community sub-sample.

The comparison set out in Table 4.6 cannot, however, resolve the question as to whether institutional admission and long-term care increase the risk of clinically manifest dementia in the elderly. It shows that the raised incidence among the home residents is related to abnormalities already detectable at the time of first interview; however, we do not know how many of these were present at the time of admission, or to what extent their greater severity had developed following admission. At present, the most plausible explanation of the findings is a selective tendency for old people in the early stages of a progressive dementing disorder to be admitted to long-term care, not because of the developing mental impairments alone, but because of some combination of chronic ill-health, disability, and lack of familial or social support. At the same time, it must be emphasized that the present study was not designed to study the effects of home admission or long-stay care, and that for this purpose a prospective controlled study would be required.

The unexpected association of incidence rate with marital status appears in a new light when the community and home residents' samples are compared; the observed trends are contrary in the two groups: in the community sample, single and divorced persons together display a markedly increased risk for dementia (an increase of 158 per cent), the widowed occupy an intermediate position, and the married are at least risk. In the home residents' sample, on the other hand, the risk is higher for married and widowed persons and low for the single and divorced. The order of difference is similar in each case, but the direction of the trend is different. This suggests that the apparent co-variation between marital status and the incidence of dementia is likely to prove an artefact, due to a selective tendency in admission to long-stay care. How this tendency operates is still far from clear, but it may be that single and divorced elderly persons are relatively more likely to enter home care for reasons unconnected to the development of mental infirmity.

The scope for prediction of dementing illness in the elderly

Up to now it has not proved possible by means of prospective studies to identify any variables, other than age, which are of predictive value with regard to the individual risk for dementia. Familial aggregation of cases, often cited in this context, has so far been demonstrated only in retro-spective studies, and appears to be of predictive importance only for dementia of pre-senile onset. In the present study, an attempt was made to find such variables, and to assess their relative importance, with the aid of the Cox regression model. In general, this procedure served to strengthen the tentative conclusions outlined above. Although weak associations were found between the incidence of dementia and social class, household type, and presence of physical impairments, these were too unspecific to be of any great practical value for assessment of risk in the individual case. Only three variables were identified which fulfilled this requirement: age, marital status and the presence of mild cognitive deficits at the first interview.

Table 4.7 Effect of selected variables on the incidence rate of dementia, estimates from the Cox regression model

Co-variate	Beta coefficient	Standard error	Significance level	Effect on incidence rate
(Community sample)				
Additional year of age	0.056	0.029	> 0.05	+ 6%
Cognitive scale score at first interview (dichotomized)	1.245	0.445	< 0.01	+ 247%
Marital status (single or divorced)	0.948	0.458	< 0.05	+ 158%
(Home residents' sample)				
Additional year of age	0.019	0.032	> 0.05	+ 2%
Cognitive scale score at first interview (dichotomized)	1.477	0.476	< 0.01	+ 338%
Marital status (single or divorced)	− 1.137	0.568	< 0.05	− 68%

The findings set out in Table 4.7 provide an overview of the strength of these associations, and the relative significance of the individual variables. Although in both samples age can be seen to have an influence on the incidence rate, this is actually quite modest once the other variables are held constant. The significance of marital status, as has been shown, is considerable, but varies according to the nature of the sample. Of greatest predictive power is the presence of mild cognitive deficits which, expressed in terms of a score of four or more on the clinical rating scale, increased the probability of a new dementing illness by 247 per cent in the community sample and 338 per cent in the home residents' sample. This means in effect that the predictive value of age becomes trivial once the effect of cognitive impairment has been controlled in the analysis. The presence of cognitive deficits is itself associated with age; nevertheless, even the oldest respondents are found to be at low risk for a dementing illness if they are cognitively unimpaired at the initial examination.

This conclusion is valid only for a certain period of time. Since cognitive decline is itself associated with age, one must assume that the oldest members of the sample have the strongest tendency for such a decline, and hence that their risk for a clinically manifest dementia will increase accordingly. In other words, the degree of individual risk cannot be established once and for all by a single test early in the senium, but would have to be reassessed from time to time. Examination of the cumulative incidence curves suggests that a realistic time interval for such a prognostic assessment would be of the order of two-and-a-half to three years, since over this interval the risk of dementia remains virtually independent of age, once the level of cognitive functioning is held constant. After this interval the risk for the different age groups within the senium begin to diverge, as the influence of age asserts itself.

Discussion

The epidemiological findings of this study are in broad agreement with the reports of other longitudinal investigations of the elderly population samples (cf. Table 4.1). An annual incidence rate of 17.8 per 1,000 for the cohort of elderly persons living in private households was computed. The morbid risk was related to age and tripled for each additional ten years of age over 65. The incidence rate is properly comparable only with other elderly samples having the same age composition. For greater accuracy, age-specific rates are required, but in this as in other, similar studies so far carried out, ten-year age groups are the smallest for which rates can be meaningfully computed. Since dementing illness is a relatively rare condition in all but the very highest age groups, the numbers of new cases identified, even over a period of six or eight years, will be small and the confidence intervals for the estimated incidence rates correspondingly wide. This problem becomes more acute in attempts to compute specific rates for SDAT, MID, or other sub-categories of dementia.

The general statistical difficulty was also apparent when trying to interpret associations with sociodemographic and other variables. The weak associations found between incidence rates, on the one hand, and social class, type of household group, and presence of physical impairment, on the other, pointed to a possible influence of the person's life conditions on the risk of emergence of a clinical dementia, but were not firm enough to be useful either in assessing individual risk or as pointers to a possible aetiology. A similar conclusion applies to the difference in incidence rates between community and home residents, which was very pronounced but probably largely accounted for by confounding variables. Here again, there is some degree of association still to be explained, which hints at an influence of environmental conditions but cannot demonstrate it satisfactorily. These trends towards association with exogenous variables are suggestive enough to warrant further investigation, preferably in the setting of multi-centred collaborative projects, or based on large population samples secured by other means.

The prediction of dementia in the elderly is still at a very early stage of development. Much greater accuracy will be attainable once account can be taken of relative exposure to aetiologically linked risk factors. It will also be necessary to try to differentiate between premorbid characteristics of the individual, such as intellectual and educational level, which may influence the risk for a dementing illness in late life (La Rue and Jarvik 1986), and cognitive deficits which represent the early prodromal signs of a dementing process. Even at the present stage of knowledge, however, there is scope for improved empirical prediction through the development of more discriminating and reliable test procedures. The fact that some measure of success was achieved in the present study, making use of a simple, unvalidated form of cognitive testing, suggests that there is a large potential for scientific advance in this field.

Acknowledgements

The original study of old people in Mannheim was carried out as a project within Special Research Programme 116 (Psychiatric Epidemiology), with the support of the German Research Association. The subsequent follow-up study was made possible by a grant from the Federal Ministry of Youth, Family Affairs and Health.

We are grateful to our co-workers in these research projects, and especially to Jutta Jaeger and Eva Nahme (both graduates in psychology), for their participation in the field work of the follow-up study.

References

Allgulander, C. and Fisher, L.B. (1986) 'Survival analysis (or time to an event analysis) and the Cox regression model: methods for longitudinal psychiatric research', *Acta Psychiatrica Scandinavica* 74: 529–35.
Bergmann, K. and Cooper, B. (1986) 'Epidemiological and public-health aspects of senile dementia', in A.B. Sorensen, F.E. Weinert, and L.R. Sherrod (eds)

Human Development and the Life Course: Multi-Disciplinary Perspectives, Hillsdale, NJ: Erlbaum, pp. 71–97.

Bergmann, K., Kay, D.W.K., Foster, E.M., *et al.* (1971) 'A follow-up study of randomly selected community residents to assess the effects of chronic brain syndrome and cerebrovascular disease', *Psychiatry II*, Proceedings of the 5th World Congress of Psychiatry, Amsterdam: Excerpta Medica, pp. 856–65.

Cooper, B. (1986) 'Mental illness, disability and social conditions among old people in Mannheim', in H. Häfner, G. Moschel, and N. Sartorius (eds) *Mental Health in the Elderly*, Berlin: Springer, pp. 35–45.

Cooper, B. (1988) 'Epidemiological research on dementia: problems of case-finding and diagnosis', *Zeitschrift für Gerontopsychologie und -psychiatrie* 3: 193–203.

Cooper, B. (1989) 'The epidemiological contribution to research on late-life dementia', in P. Williams, G. Wilkinson, and K. Rawnsley (eds) *The Scope of Epidemiological Psychiatry*, London: Routledge, pp. 264–86.

Cooper, B. and Schwarz, R. (1982) 'Psychiatric case-identification in an elderly urban population', *Social Psychiatry* 17: 43–52.

Cooper, B. and Sosna, U. (1983) 'Psychische Erkrankung in der Altenbevölkerung: eine epidemiologische Feldstudie in Mannheim', *Nervenarzt* 54: 239–49.

Cooper, B., Mahnkopf, B., and Bickel, H. (1984) 'Psychische Erkrankung und soziale Isolation bei älteren Heimbewohnern: eine Vergleichsstudie', *Z. Gerontol.* 17: 117–25.

Hagnell, O., Lanke, J., Rorsman, B., and Öjesjö, L. (1981) 'Does the incidence of age psychosis decrease? A prospective longitudinal study of a complete population investigated during the 25-year period 1947–1972: the Lundby study', *Neuropsychobiology* 7: 201–11.

Hughes, C.P., Berg, L., Danziger, W.L., *et al.* (1982) 'A new clinical scale for the staging of dementia', *British Journal of Psychiatry* 140: 566–72.

Kay, D.W.K., Beamish, P., and Roth, M. (1964) 'Old-age mental disorders in Newcastle-upon-Tyne, part 1: a study of prevalence', *British Journal of Psychiatry* 110: 146–58.

Kleining, G. and Moore, H. (1968) 'Soziale Selbsteinstufung. Ein Instrument zur Messung sozialer Schichten', *Kölner Zeitschrift für Soziologie und Sozial-psychologie* 20: 502–22.

La Rue, A. and Jarvik, L.F. (1986) 'Towards the prediction of dementias arising in the senium', in L. Erlenmeyer-Kimling and N.E. Miller (eds) *Life-span Research on the Prediction of Psychopathology*, Hillsdale, NJ: Erlbaum, pp. 261–74.

Last, J.M. (ed.) (1983) *A Dictionary of Epidemiology*, New York: Oxford University Press.

McKhann, G., Drachman, D., Folstein, M., *et al.* (1984) 'Clinical diagnosis of Alzheimer's disease: report of the NINCDS-ADRDA Work Group', *Neurology* 34: 939–44

Nielsen, J.A., Biorn-Henriksen, T., and Bork, B.R. (1982) 'Incidence and disease expectancy for senile and arteriosclerotic dementia in a geographically delimited Danish rural population', in J. Magnussen, J. Nielsen, and J. Buch (eds) *Epidemiology and Prevention of Mental Illness in Old Age*, Hellerup, Denmark: EGV, pp. 52–3.

Nilsson, L.V. (1984) 'Incidence of severe dementia in an urban sample followed up from 70 to 79 years of age', *Acta Psychiatrica Scandinavica* 70: 478–86.

Roth, M., Tym, E., Mountjoy, C.Q., *et al.* (1986) 'CAMDEX: a standardized instrument for the diagnosis of mental disorder in the elderly, with special reference to the early detection of dementia', *British Journal of Psychiatry* 149: 698–709.

Chapter five

Cognitive function and other indices of dementia in a rural elderly female population: preliminary findings

Carol Brayne

Summary

The study examined a representative population of women aged 70–79 in an English rural setting, using a modified version of the CAMDEX (Cambridge Disorders of the Elderly Examination: Roth *et al.* 1986). The aim of the study was to examine the relationship of dementia and cognitive impairment to normal ageing in a community sample. The distribution of characteristics associated with dementia was examined. The distributions of scores on cognitive and other scales used in the diagnosis of dementia were found to be unimodal, skewed, and smooth, as for most physiological variables. There was no clear disjunction between the demented and the normal on any of the scales. The effects of age, social class, education, IQ, and health on cognitive and non-cognitive scales are discussed.

Introduction

There have been many recent epidemiological studies of dementia and cognitive impairment in elderly populations. The prevalence of dementia and cognitive impairment has been found to vary according to the age groups examined and the methodology employed. Approaches to the identification of cases of dementia and cognitive impairment have differed, ranging from short scales testing cognitive function to full psychiatric interview. Scales such as the Mini-Mental State Examination (Folstein *et al.* 1975) have been employed in large studies, such as the Epidemiologic Catchment Area Study (Holzer *et al.* 1984). The rates produced are based on levels of cognitive impairment according to set cut-off points. An alternative approach has been to use a cognitive scale as a screening procedure for identification of a sub-sample to be interviewed more intensively. Morgan *et al.* (1987) in Nottingham, England, employed this strategy in a study of the elderly in the community.

Dementia is, by definition, a condition which affects global cognitive function, behaviour, and personality. Few scales or standardized schedules have been able to investigate all these aspects. The Geriatric Mental State

(Copeland *et al.* 1976) is a standardized psychiatric interview which identifies mental disorders in the elderly, and has been widely used in the community. It gives a range of possible psychiatric diagnoses, and dementia and confusional states are represented by a single organic dimension. A further approach is that by Mölsa *et al.* (1982) who investigated all the cases of dementia known to services in a defined geographical area. They were able to examine these cases in great detail and arrive at differential diagnoses, with *post mortem* validation in some cases. Their results suggested a higher level of severity than might have been expected from a truly representative community study, and may have been affected by referral bias. Thus, their rates for the different disorders cannot necessarily be applied to the general population.

With changes in the age structure of populations, the issue of dementia in the community is of increasing practical importance. There appears to have been a decrease in mortality rates from stroke over the last decades in many countries, although it is not certain whether this reflects a true decrease in incidence (Malmgren *et al.* 1987). Because of the difficulties of differential diagnosis of dementia in the community, it is not known if there has been a corresponding decrease in mortality from, or incidence of, multi-infarct dementia. Intensive study of cases of dementia identified in the community is needed, using validated techniques for differential diagnosis.

It is thought that senile dementia of Alzheimer type (SDAT) is the most frequently found type of dementia in the elderly in the community in Europe and the United States. The classic features of SDAT are senile plaques and neurofibrillary tangles (Tomlinson *et al.* 1970), and yet these are also found in normal aged brains (Tomlinson *et al.* 1968), albeit in smaller numbers. Miller *et al.* (1984), in an autopsy series, found a consistent rise in the numbers of plaques and tangles present in aged brains over the age of 71. The Blessed Dementia Scale has been found to correlate well with the numbers of plaques and tangles in the brain (Blessed *et al.* 1968). If there is a threshold effect such that no dementia is manifest until a certain number of plaque and tangles are present in the brain (Roth *et al.* 1966), the distribution of scores on the Blessed Dementia Scale and other scales which are correlated with neuropathological findings might be expected to be bimodally distributed in a community sample.

Despite increasingly detailed knowledge about the neurobiology of the dementia, there remains a need for detailed studies of truly representative populations of the elderly (Henderson 1986; Brody 1982).

Aims and method

The study examined a population of women aged 70–79 in an English rural setting. Its main aim was to examine the relationship of dementia and cognitive impairment to normal ageing in a community sample, using a detailed standardized psychiatric interview (CAMDEX), which incorporates known scales and can arrive at differential diagnoses based on stated criteria.

Location and sample

The study was conducted in the Fens, a rural area fifteen miles from the city of Cambridge, with a comparatively stable population and a low rate of migration of the elderly. The area included one small town and four villages, served by a single health centre with six general practitioners. There is little overlap with adjacent health centres. Residential accommodation for the elderly is available in the area.

All women registered as patients with the general practitioners on a census day (1 October 1985), aged between 70 and 79, were included in the sampling frame, whether living in private households or not. Only those who have been in institutions such as geriatric hospitals outside the area for long periods are taken off the practice register. A search of local long-stay care facilities revealed only two women not on the register.

The sample was divided into two age groups: one aged 70–74 and one aged 75–79. A random sample consisting of 203 of the 270 women in the age-group 70–74 years was drawn, and all 207 women aged 75–79 years were included in the study.

The interview procedure

The interview was based mainly on the CAMDEX and was carried out by the author. CAMDEX was developed by Roth *et al.* (1986) for use in the detection of dementia in the elderly, including minimal and mild degrees. It is made up of the following:

(a) a structured psychiatric interview with the subject;
(b) a short neuropsychological battery (CAMCOG), which includes subscales covering most aspects of cognitive function, and incorporates the items of the Mini-Mental State Examination (Folstein *et al.* 1975);
(c) a standard recording of observed mental abnormalities;
(d) a structured interview with an informant;
(e) a brief physical examination, including blood-pressure reading;
(f) information on current medication;
(g) laboratory investigations where relevant.

Within these sections there are several standardized scales: the Dementia Scale of Blessed *et al.* (1968), which is not based on cognitive items; an information-memory scale using the ten best items from Roth and Hopkins's (1953) test, which is equivalent to the Abbreviated Mental

Test Score of Hodkinson (1972), and the Ischaemia Score of Hachinski *et al.* (1975). In addition to CAMCOG, scales based on information other than cognitive function have been constructed from CAMDEX: an organicity scale and a further ischaemia scale, neither based on cognitive testing but on other aspects of the diagnosis of dementia, and hence referred to as 'non-cognitive' scales.

At present, a diagnosis is arrived at by a clinician using criteria laid down in CAMDEX which are similar to those in the psychiatric glossary to the International Classification of Diseases, 9th Revision – ICD–9 (WHO 1978). Using the clinician's diagnosis, the cognitive battery (CAMCOG), and the accompanying non-cognitive scales, it is possible to arrive at operational diagnoses laid down in CAMDEX.

In addition to CAMDEX, the information-memory sub-scale of the Clifton Assessment Scale (Pattie and Gilleard 1979) was administered in order to compare the prevalence estimates for cognitive impairment with those found in comparable studies in Melton Mowbray (Clarke *et al.* 1984) and Nottingham (Morgan *et al.* 1987). Verbal IQ was also estimated, using the National Adult Reading Test (Nelson and O'Connell 1978). This was intended to provide an estimate of the premorbid IQ in demented persons, using the stability of reading ability for irregular words. The technique has been validated on hospital population samples (O'Carroll and Gilleard 1986; Hart *et al.* 1986).

Reaction times, both choice and simple, were measured and blood was taken for the estimation of haemoglobin, urea and electrolytes, glucose, thyroid function, thyroid microsomal and thyroglobulin antibodies, antinuclear factor, and creatine kinase isoenzymes. These were measured either to screen for somatic diseases or because they have been implicated in studies of the aetiology of SDAT or of the ageing process itself.

In a random 10 per cent sub-sample, the hospital version of the Geriatric Mental State (Copeland *et al.* 1976) was administered within ten days by a consultant psychiatrist trained in its use.

The interviews were conducted between October 1985 and October 1986, mostly in the first seven months of this period. The subjects were sent a letter by their own general practitioner, indicating when the interviewer would call on them at their place of residence. If the subject agreed to take part, the interview schedule was administered immediately and lasted from one-and-a-half to two hours.

Research findings

Response rate

The response rate was 89.0 per cent of the total sample (365/410). Ten subjects died before the author was able to approach them, leaving 200 in each age group. Ninety-one per cent of these were interviewed (365/400). There was a slightly higher refusal rate for the older age group than for the younger (20/200, or 10 per cent, and 15/200, or 7.5 per cent, respectively). Of those who refused to take part the author met all but four, briefly. Although formal measures of comparison were not possible, there was no evidence from these meetings that the refusers constituted a special group in terms of the mental state.

Permission was requested to speak to someone close to the subject, preferably someone younger than 70 (in order not to be in the age range of the study itself). Only 5 per cent of the sample either refused to allow the interviewer to approach an informant or did not have anyone close enough to them. This interview lasted from twenty to forty minutes. Most of the interviews (76 per cent) were conducted by telephone, and the rest face to face. Only one of the informants refused to take part.

Sociodemographic features

Most of the sample were married (44.8 per cent) or widowed (49.7 per cent). Most lived either with their husbands or alone in private households (41 per cent and 38 per cent respectively). Only 10.5 per cent lived with other family members and among these were some who were still supporting their unmarried children or bringing up their grand-children. Thirty-five respondents (9.4 per cent) lived in sheltered residential accommodation.

Social class was assessed according to the Register General's guidelines. The women were therefore characterized according to their husbands' occupations, or their own if they were divorced or single. A small number were unable to give their husbands' or their own former occupations (1.6 per cent).

There were relatively few women in the highest social class, I (2.7 per cent), or the lowest, V (7.4 per cent); most were in the intermediate classes, II, III, or IV (17.8 per cent, 46 per cent and 24.4 per cent respectively). This distribution reflects the large numbers of local people employed in agricultural work. There was no difference in the social class distributions for the two age groups, 70–74 and 75–79 years.

Most members of the sample had left school at the statutory leaving age of 13 or 14 years (75.9 per cent). Very few had left school younger (2.7 per cent), but a somewhat larger proportion had left later than 14 (21.4 per cent), though only a small number had gone on to any kind of further education (5.8 per cent). More of the younger than of the older age group left school after 14, but more of the older group had gone on to further education than of the younger group.

Prevalence of dementia and cognitive impairment

The prevalence of organic brain syndromes according to level of severity is given for the two age groups in Table 5.1, which shows the expected increase with age. All the moderately to severely demented subjects were in the age group above 75 years. The prevalence estimates for organic brain disorder in this sample, using the diagnostic criteria laid down in CAMDEX are as follows: senile dementia of Alzheimer type 3.8 per cent; multi-infarct dementia 2.5 per cent; mixed SDAT and MID 0.3 per cent; dementia secondary to other causes 1.4 per cent; acute confusional states 0.0 per cent. These figures are weighted to give proportions expected for the entire age range 70–79. The only type of dementia which appears to increase in prevalence between the two age groups is SDAT. The numbers of subjects in the other categories are extremely small.

Table 5.1 Prevalence and severity of organic brain syndromes by age group

Severity	70 – 74 years	75 – 79 years
	%	%
No dementia	95.7	88.3
Minimal/mild	4.3	8.9
Moderate/severe	–	2.8
	100.0	100.0
No of persons	185	180

Table 5.2 shows the distributions of the cognitive function scores in the whole sample for the information-memory score (Roth and Hopkins 1953), the Mini-Mental State Examination (MMSE), and CAMCOG. These all show similarly shaped distributions, extended or compressed according to the range of scores. CAMCOG and MMSE scores were highly inter-correlated (Spearman's rho 0.8; $p < 0.001$).

Table 5.2 Frequency distributions of cognitive scale scores: cumulative percentages (N = 365)

(a) Information-memory scale		(b) Mini-Mental State		(c) CAMCOG Scale	
Score	cum.%	Score	cum.%	Score	cum.%
0	0.3	0	0.3	9	0.3
2	1.1	8	0.8	29	0.8
4	1.4	12	1.1	49	1.6
6	2.7	16	3.8	69	13.2
8	5.8	20	14.2	79	30.4
10	20.3	24	48.2	89	65.2
11	44.3	26	72.3	106	100.0
12	100.0	30	100.0		

Table 5.3 shows the distribution of scores for the Blessed Dementia Scale and the organicity scale of CAMDEX: their skew is the opposite to that of the cognitive scales, but the shapes of the distributions are otherwise similar. These scales contain many of the same items and are highly inter-correlated (Spearman's rho 0.7; $p<0.001$).

Table 5.3 Frequency distributions of non-cognitive scale scores: cumulative percentages (N = 365)

(a) Blessed Dementia Scale		(b) CAMDEX organicity scale	
Score	cum.%	Score	cum.%
0	50.6	0	34.6
2	87.9	2	71.7
4	95.0	4	84.6
6	97.6	6	92.0
8	98.5	8	96.3
10+	100.0	10+	100.0

The National Adult Reading Test score should estimate current IQ for the normal subjects and premorbid IQ for the demented subjects. In an unselected cross-section of the population a Gaussian distribution about a mean score of 100 would be expected; and is indeed found in this sample. There is a minimal correlation between age and estimated IQ (Spearman's rho 0.02; $p<0.05$).

The relationship between the severity of dementia and mean score of CAMCOG and MMSE is shown in Figures 5.1a and 5.1b. It can be seen that there is considerable overlap between the groups. There is, however, a clear and significant trend in the scales according to the clinical severity of dementia. A similar trend, with increasing scores, is seen for the Blessed Dementia Scale, shown in Figure 5.2.

In Figure 5.3, the frequency distributions for CAMCOG score for both demented and normal subjects are shown. The dementia cases lie on the skewed tail of the distribution of the normals. The organically impaired subjects on the right-hand side of the distribution are mainly those who are minimally or mildly affected.

In Figure 5.4, the frequency distributions for estimated IQ of those subjects diagnosed as normal can be compared with those diagnosed as demented. The distributions of the two groups are more similar than are those shown in Figure 5.3, although there is a small but significant downward shift in the median for the demented group.

The relationship between cognitive function, age, social class, and education is shown in Table 5.4. Age at interview shows a small but consistent association with the CAMCOG score, and education a more pronounced effect. The education effect is not explained by any age-related difference in age on leaving school.

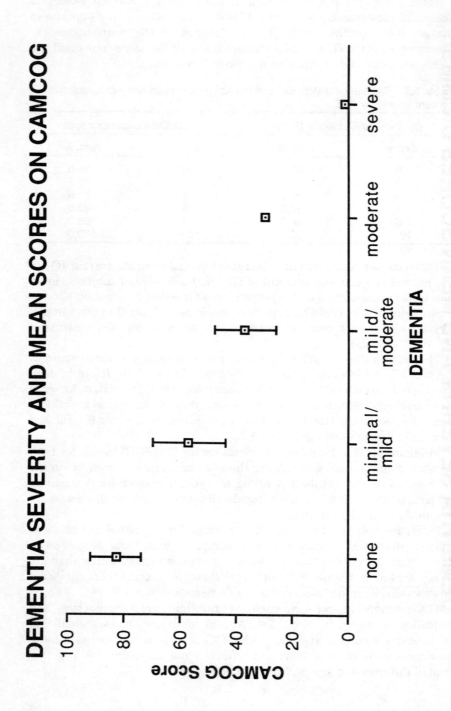

DEMENTIA SEVERITY AND MEAN SCORES ON CAMCOG

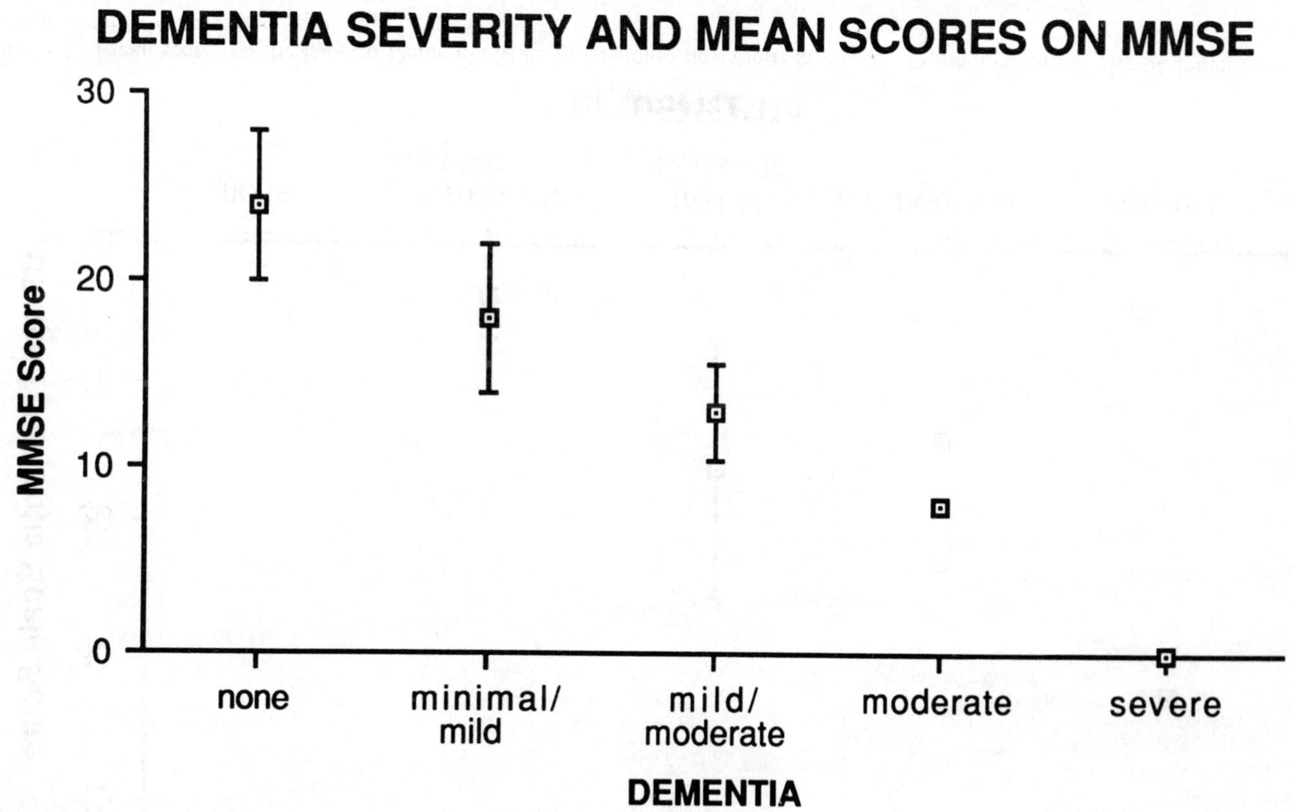

DEMENTIA SEVERITY AND MEAN SCORES ON MMSE

Figures 5.1a and 5.1b Mean scores on CAMCOG and MMSE (± standard deviation) in relation to the level of severity of dementia as diagnosed by CAMDEX

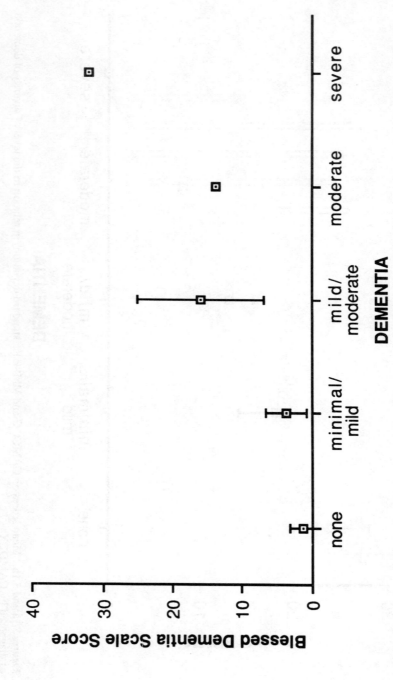

Figure 5.2 Mean scores on the Blessed Dementia Scale (± standard deviation) in relation to the level of severity of dementia as diagnosed by CAMDEX

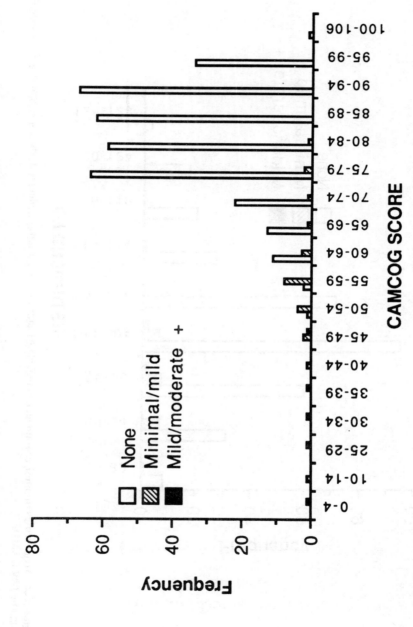

Figure 5.3 Frequency distribution of scores on CAMCOG in relation to the level of severity of dementia as diagnosed by CAMDEX

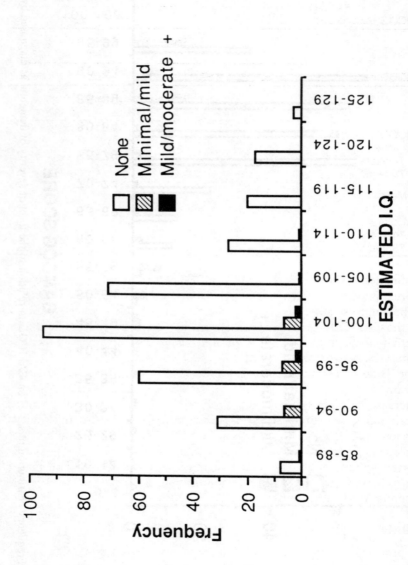

Figure 5.4 Frequency distribution of estimated verbal IQ (NART score) in relation to the level of severity of dementia as diagnosed by CAMDEX

Table 5.4 Cognitive scale scores according to selected sociodemographic variables (N = 365)

| | (a) Age group | | | |
	70 – 74 years		75 – 79	
CAMCOG mean score	86		80	

| | (b) Social class (R.G.) | | | | |
	I	II	III	IV	V
CAMCOG mean score	93	87	85	78	81

| | (c) School-leaving age | | |
	< 13 years	13 – 14 years	15 years+
CAMCOG mean score:			
70 – 74 years	79	85	90
75 – 79 years	70	79	86
Mini-Mental State mean score:			
70 – 74 years	23	24	26
75 – 79 years	21	23	25

Estimated IQ is correlated with CAMCOG score ($r = 0.53$; $p<0.001$). If a more homogeneous group is extracted of those who left school at 13 or 14 and belong to social class III, the estimated IQ is still strongly correlated with the CAMCOG score ($r = 0.50$; $p<0.001$). Neither reported limitation of activity through physical ill-health nor observed acute illness at the time of interview showed any relationship with cognitive scores.

The Blessed Dementia Scale and CAMDEX organicity scale scores show an inconsistent relationship to age, though with an overall tendency to increase with age. There is no manifest relationship to social class or educational level. Subjects with a current physical illness at the time of interview[1] had a higher mean organicity score than the remainder of the sample (3.8 compared wih 2.0, a highly significant difference). Those who reported limitation of activity due to physical ill-health also had higher mean scores on this scale (2.7 compared with 1.5) and on the Blessed Dementia Scale (1.3 compared with 2.5).

Discussion

The prevalence ratios found in this study using the CAMDEX clinical diagnosis are similar to those reported elsewhere for women of the age

---

[1] Current physical illness included a wide range of conditions, from acute exacerbation of chronic bronchitis and arthritis to pleural effusion, carcinoma, and myxoedema, which were not acute or severe enough to impair the ability to complete an interview.

groups under investigation. The rates of severe cognitive impairment are similar to those reported in recent studies in the United Kingdom (Clarke *et al.* 1984; Morgan *et al.* 1987), while the distributions of cognitive impairment are comparable to those reported by Kay *et al.* (1985) from Tasmania and by Folstein *et al.* (1985) from Baltimore. The distributions on the cognitive and non-cognitive scales, with the exception of estimated IQ, show a smooth, skewed, unimodal pattern. When more homogenous sub-groups are selected – for example, by age group and educational level – a similar type of distribution is found. The only difference between the curves is a shift in the median. The type of curve is similar to those found when the distributions of most physiological variables are measured in representative community samples.

Scores on the cognitive and non-cognitive scales are affected by different variables. Cognitive function tests, other than brief information and memory scales, are influenced by sociodemographic variables, particularly educational level. This has been commented on previously with respect to hospital patients and in more heterogeneous populations (Anthony *et al.* 1982; Folstein *et al.* 1985). Non-cognitive scores appear to be sensitive to different factors, such as perceptions of illness. When such scales are used alone to identify cases of dementia, it is important to be aware that those identified will constitute a biased group. The different scales will tend to identify different individuals, particularly at the less severe end of the spectrum. Even if a second-stage examination is used to confirm the diagnosis of dementia, the final case identification will still be biased by the initial screening method. Kay *et al.* (1985) showed that different individuals were identified as demented when different diagnostic systems were applied to the same population, despite similar overall prevalence estimates. They pointed out that the various systems might therefore tend to identify different risk factors.

It has been argued that researchers should correct for the effect on cognitive function scales of the major sociodemographic variables, such as educational level, by using regression or standardization techniques (Kittner *et al.* 1986). Jarvik (1986) argues that this would be premature, pointing out that these variables have not yet been excluded as risk factors. Indeed, Henderson (1986) includes them in his list of possible risk factors for Alzheimer-type dementia. The effect on the scale scores of these cultural factors is of importance in cross-cultural studies. Non-cognitive scales may be of greater use in these settings, if they prove to be less subject to the effects of educational differences.

In this study of elderly women, the scores for the National Adult Reading Test were found to be normally distributed about 100, which would be predicted for a cross-section of the population. The similar shape of the distributions of the mentally normal and demented subjects – with the medians only a few points apart – could be interpreted as evidence that the score for demented subjects is closer to premorbid levels than to the current level of functioning. The similarity of the medians of the distributions suggests that low premorbid IQ is not a risk factor for the development of dementia. It could be argued that the small shift downwards in the median score for the demented subjects represents a small influence of intellectual level on the likelihood of a dementing illness. On the other hand, the findings could also be due to sensitivity of the test to the dementing process, or to a tendency on the part of the interviewer to diagnose those with lower IQ as cases of dementia. Despite this uncertainty, NART may prove of use in the future in predicting an expected level of cognitive performance and therefore serve as a test sensitive to divergence of this estimated level from the observed current level. Since it can be calculated for each individual, it might sidestep the difficulties inherent in global correction procedures for variables such as social class and educational level. This possibility could, however, only apply in populations where a basic level of literacy can be assumed.

Longitudinal data will be necessary to show which of the subjects identified as cases of dementia by the various systems – cognitive scales, non-cognitive scales, and various diagnostic criteria – have the greatest predictive accuracy.

Finally, to return to the original aim of the study: Cooper and Schwarz (1982) commented that there was no evidence of discontinuity between the psychiatrically ill and healthy groups in a community sample of old people in Mannheim. The present study suggests that Cooper's view can be applied to dementia, no dichotomy between demented and non-demented groups being found with any of the scales employed. There is a gradual increase in the probability of being diagnosed as a case of dementia as the scores on the cognitive scales decrease and those on the non-cognitive scales increase. The pattern is the same for the Blessed Dementia Scale, which has been shown to correlate with the frequency of plaques and tangles found at *post mortem*. This suggests that in population studies of the elderly, more attention should be directed towards determinants of level and change of cognitive functioning, rather than simply to the presence or absence of dementia.

Acknowledgements

This study was conducted while the author was a Medical Research Council Training Fellow in Epidemiology, and was supported by the Mental Health Foundation. I am grateful to Professor J.R.M. Copeland and his colleagues for training Dr P. Calloway in the use of the Geriatric Mental State and for providing AGECAT computer diagnoses. Thanks are also due to Professor R.M. Acheson, Dr P. Calloway, Dr Felicia Huppert, Sir Martin Roth, Professor Anthony Mann, the general practitioners and staff of the health centre, and to all the old people who participated in the interviews.

References

Anthony, J.C., LeResche, L., Niaz, U., von Korff, M.R., and Folstein, M.F. (1982) 'Limits of the "Mini-Mental State" as a screening test for dementia and delirium among hospital patients', *Psychological Medicine* 12 (2): 397–408.

Blessed, G., Tomlinson, B.E. and Roth, M. (1968) 'The association between quantitative measures and degenerative changes in the cerebral gray matter of elderly patients', *British Journal of Psychiatry* 114: 797–811.

Brody, J.A. (1982) 'An epidemiologist views senile dementia–facts and fragments', *American Journal of Epidemiology* 115 (2): 155–62.

Clarke, M., Clarke, S., Odell, A., and Jagger, C. (1984) 'The elderly at home: health and social status', *Health Trends* 1 (16): 3–7.

Cooper, B. and Schwarz, R. (1982) 'Psychiatric case-identification in an elderly urban population', *Social Psychiatry* 17: 43–52.

Copeland, J.R.M., Kelleher, M.J., Kellet, J.M., Gourlay, A.J., Gurland, B.J., Fleiss, J.L., and Sharpe, L. (1976) 'A semi-structured clinical interview for the assessment of diagnosis and mental state in the elderly, the Geriatric Mental State Schedule, I: development and reliability', *Psychological Medicine* 6: 439–46.

Folstein, M.F., Folstein, S.E., and McHugh, P.R. (1975) 'Mini-Mental State: a practical method for grading the cognitive state of patients for the clinician', *Journal of Psychiatric Research* 12: 189–98.

Folstein, M.F., Anthony, J.C., Parhad, I., Duffy, B., and Gruenberg, E.M. (1985) 'The meaning of cognitive impairment in the elderly', *Journal of the American Geriatric Society* 33 (4): 228–35.

Hachinski, V.C., Illiff, L.D., Zilkha, E., du Boulay, G.H., McAllister, U.L., Marshall, J., Ross Russell, R.W., and Symon, L. (1975) 'Cerebral blood flow in dementia', *Archives of Neurology* 32: 632–7.

Hart, S., Smith, C.M., and Swash, M. (1986) 'Assessing intellectual deterioration', *British Journal of Clinical Psychology* 25 (2): 119–24.

Henderson, A.S. (1986) 'The epidemiology of Alzheimer's disease', *British Medical Bulletin* 42 (1): 3–10.

Hodkinson, H.M. (1972) 'Evaluation of a mental test score for assessment of mental impairment in the elderly', *Age and Ageing* 1: 233–8.

Holzer, C.E., Tischler, G.L., Leaf, P.J., and Myers, J.K. (1984) 'An epidemiologic assessment of cognitive function in a community population', *Research in Community Mental Health* 4: 3–32.

Jarvik, L.F. (1986) 'The association between educational attainment and mental status examinations: of etiological significance for senile dementias or not?', *Journal of Chronic Diseases* 39 (3): 171–4.

Kay, D.W.K., Henderson, A.S., Scott, R., Wilson, J., Rickwood, D., and Grayson, D.A. (1985) 'Dementia and depression among the elderly living in the Hobart community: the effect of the diagnostic criteria on the prevalence rates', *Psychological Medicine* 15: 771–88.

Kittner, S.J., White, L.R., Farmer, M.E., Wolz, M., Kaplan, E., Moes, E., Brody, J.A., and Feinleib, M. (1986) 'Methodological issues in screening for dementia: the problem of education adjustment', *Journal of Chronic Diseases* 39 (3): 163–70.

Malmgren, R., Warlow, C., Bamford, J., and Sandercock, P. (1987) 'Geographical and secular trends in stroke incidence', *Lancet* ii: 1196–200.

Miller, E.D., Hicks, S.P., D'Amato, C.J., and Landis, J.R. (1984) 'A descriptive study of neuritic plaques and neurofibrillary tangles in an autopsy population', *American Journal of Epidemiology* 3: 331–41.

Mölsa, P.K., Marttila, R.J., and Rinne, U.K. (1982) 'Epidemiology of dementia in a Finnish population', *Acta Neurologica Scandinavica* 65: 541–52.

Morgan, K., Dalloso, H.M., Arie, T., Byrne, E.J., Jones, R., and Waite, J. (1987) 'Mental health and psychological well-being among the old and the very old living at home', *British Journal of Psychiatry* 150: 801–7.

Nelson, H.E., and O'Connell, A. (1978) 'Dementia: the estimation of premorbid intelligence levels using the new adult reading test', *Cortex* 14: 234–44.

O'Carroll, R.E. and Gilleard, C.J. (1986) 'Estimation of premorbid intelligence in dementia', *British Journal of Clinical Psychology* 25: 157–8.

Pattie, A.H. and Gilleard, C.J. (1979) *Manual of the Clifton Assessment Procedures for the Elderly (CAPE)*, Sevenoaks, England: Hodder & Stoughton Educational.

Roth, M. and Hopkins, B. (1953) 'Psychological test performance in patients over 60:1. senile psychosis and the affective disorders of old age', *Journal of Mental Science* 99: 439–50.

Roth, M., Tomlinson, B.E., and Blessed, G. (1966) 'Correlation between scores for dementia and counts of "senile plaques" in cerebral grey matter of elderly subjects', *Nature* 209: 109–10.

Roth, M., Tym, E., Mountjoy, C.Q., Huppert, F.A., Hendrie, H., Verma, S., and Goddard, R. (1986) 'CAMDEX: a standardised instrument for the diagnosis of mental disorder in the elderly with special reference to the early detection of dementia', *British Journal of Psychiatry* 149: 698–709.

Tomlinson, B.E., Blessed, G., and Roth, M. (1968) 'Observations on the brains of non-demented old people', *Journal of Neurological Science* 7: 331–56.

Tomlinson, B.E., Blessed, G., and Roth, M. (1970) 'Observations on the brains of demented old people', *Journal of Neurological Science* 11: 205–42.

World Health Organization (1978) *International Classification of Diseases, 9th Revision (ICD–9)*, Geneva: WHO.

Chapter six

The Munich Alcoholism Test (MALT) as a diagnostic instrument in primary and secondary prevention of alcoholism

H. Dilling and A.M. Oschinsky

Introduction

The estimated number of alcohol-dependent persons in West Germany – 1.5 million, or 2–3 per cent of the population – shows that alcoholism is a major problem in our society (Dilling *et al*. 1987). Causing a high rate of hospital admissions (Vereinigung Schweizer Krankenhäuser 1987), it is now the most frequent of all psychiatric admission diagnoses; in Lübeck for example, the annual admission rate corresponds to 0.5 per cent of the population (Dilling *et al*. 1987)! Considering that alcoholics comprise 7–14 per cent of all admissions to general hospitals, according to our own investigations (Auerbach and Melchertsen 1981), while others put the rate as high as 20 per cent (Trojan 1980), and taking into account the hardships for the families of alcoholics, another three to five million persons, the demand for prevention is more than justified.

While other major public health problems, such as AIDS, cancer, cardiovascular diseases, and perhaps even drug dependency, are given much greater prominence in health politics, alcoholism is not so much in the focus of attention, possibly because here preventive measures would be too troublesome for all of us: physicians, patients, politicians, and the general public. As an example, one may mention the public acceptance of 400,000 to 500,000 persons injured in traffic accidents annually in our country, a high proportion of which are caused by alcohol-intoxicated persons (Emmerich 1984). Another neglected aspect of prevention is that of public attitudes to alcohol abuse in general, which in Germany is largely tolerated. The consumption of alcohol is in no way restricted, and the local press even praises social events in terms of flowing streams of beer. Unfortunately psychiatrists and health workers are a relatively small pressure group, and therefore cannot do much for primary prevention, for instance by regulation of alcohol prices (Häfner 1981), as this would be a political issue.

As the opportunity for primary prevention by general measures in the population is low at present, perhaps attention should be directed more to individual primary prevention by detecting heavy drinkers who are at risk for alcoholism, and to secondary prevention by early diagnosis of alcoholics not yet identified and by early treatment. The early detection of alcoholism is a more difficult problem than most physicians realize. In an Australian investigation (Reid *et al*. 1986), only one-fourth of the alcoholics identified were known to their general practitioners. Similar results are found when diagnosis of alcoholism in general hospitals is analysed (Athen and Schranner 1981).

The high rates of alcoholism in general practice and general hospitals demand that recognition and identification of alcoholism risk and alcohol dependency should not be delayed until psychiatric treatment becomes necessary. The ward physician as well as the general practitioner ought to be able to identify these patients and to introduce primary preventive measures or early treatment.

The so-called Alcoholism Tests, developed in the last two decades, can be of substantial help in recognizing alcoholism. They include the Michigan Alcoholism Screening Test MAST (Selzer 1971) in different versions, the CAGE (Mayfield *et al*. 1974), and since 1977 in the German-speaking countries the Munich Alcoholism Test, the MALT, which was developed by Feuerlein and his co-workers (Feuerlein *et al*. 1977, 1979). In the meantime the MALT has been translated into English (Feuerlein *et al*. 1980) and several other languages. A modification has been developed in New Zealand, the Canterbury Alcoholism Screening Test, the so-called CAST (Elvy and Wells 1984).

A number of studies have demonstrated the usefulness of MALT. For example, Bernitzki and Bernd (1983), using this method in a general out-patient setting, identified 30 per cent of the male and 7 per cent of the female patients as alcohol dependent. An investigation by Möller and others (1987) on a hospital surgical ward found that 14 per cent of the patients were alcoholic and an additional 12 per cent at risk.

The MALT consists of two parts: a physician assessment section consisting of seven questions and a self-assessment section of twenty-four questions to be completed by the patient (Appendix I). The physicians' rating consists of items on somatic complications due to alcohol, the level of alcohol consumption, and the question of *foetor alcoholicus*. The self-rating part covers drinking behaviour, various psychological and social impairments, and somatic complaints related to withdrawal states. In computing the total score, each item of the physician's assessment section is given four points (F-score), whereas each item of the self-rating part scores one point (S-score). The total score is an index of alcoholism or risk for alcoholism. A person with eleven or more points is diagnosed as alcoholic, a person with between six and ten points as at high risk, which means in considerable danger of becoming alcoholic.

According to Feuerlein *et al*. (1977) the MALT is sensitive enough to identify 90 per cent of alcoholics and a further 8 per cent rated as at risk, only 2 per cent remaining undetected. Feuerlein claims that the danger of being erroneously classified as alcoholic by this method is negligible.

Aims and method

As part of a larger epidemiological study, we wish to address the question of the potential value of the MALT in primary or secondary prevention. First, we report on its use as a screening instrument in the general hospital setting, and, second, we try to assess its prognostic significance by means of a six-year follow-up study. In this report the results of our investigation at two different times, 1979/80 and 1985/7, are given, the MALT being used on both occasions.

Validity of the MALT

In the period 1979–80, 371 patients admitted to three different departments of Lübeck University Hospital were examined: 124 in surgery, 123 in internal medicine, and 124 in psychiatry (Nieder 1985). The results of screening with MALT were analyzed with respect to specificity, sensitivity, and efficiency, in relation to the diagnostic assessment of the research psychiatrist.

The initial cross-sectional study (Time T1)

Between August 1979 and January 1980, 825 patients in the psychiatric and neurological departments of Lübeck University Hospital were examined and divided, according to the MALT scores, into three different groups: alcoholics, persons at high risk, and normals. In addition, the group of alcoholics was subdivided into those without and those with alcohol-related psychiatric and somatic diseases.

The six-year follow-up (Time T2)

Six to seven years later, between May 1985 and May 1987, the patients who at T1 had been alcoholic or at high risk (Figure 6.1) were re-examined. Of the fifty-eight persons at high risk, thirty-two were again scored on the MALT, while of 150 alcoholics seventy-two could be re-examined. Some of the former patients who responded at follow-up did not fulfil all requirements of the MALT, for example, for results of a liver function test. Hence the number of those who completed the MALT is somewhat lower than that of all responders. Both groups were re-analyzed according to the MALT scores at follow-up.

To test the predictive value of MALT, the alcoholics identified at T1

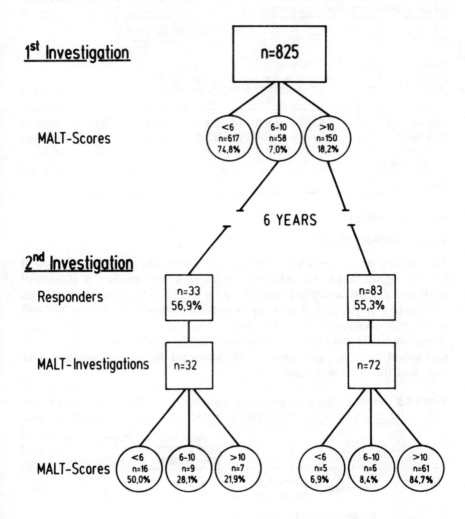

1ˢᵗ Investigation

Figure 6.1 Cross-section study and six year follow-up. MALT examination of alcoholics and persons at high risk in the departments of psychiatry and neurology of the Medizinische Universität zu Lübeck

were subdivided into two groups according to the MALT F-scores: one group without alcohol-related diseases (n=45) and a second group with alcohol-related diseases (n=105). At T2, more than half of these patients could be re-interviewed (Table 6.1), one-sixth had died, and one-third could not be contacted or refused the interview. We tried to compare the two groups with respect to their MALT scores and rates of abstinence.

Table 6.1 Follow-up investigation of 150 alcoholic in-patients without (I) and with (II) alcohol-related diseases diagnosed at T1

	Alcoholic in-patient groups					
	I *Without* *complications*		*II* *With* *complications*		*Total*	
Result of *follow-up*	n	%	n	%	n	%
Interviewed	25	55.5	58	55.2	83	55.3
Deceased	3	6.6	23	21.9	26	17.4
Refused	12	26.8	8	7.6	20	13.3
Not contacted	5	11.1	16	15.3	21	14.0
Total	45	100.0	105	100.0	150	100.0

Research findings

Validity of the MALT

The results of the preliminary study are given in Tables 6.2, 6.3 and 6.4. Taking the research psychiatrist's diagnosis as the standard of reference, we found a consistently high specificity for the MALT questionnaire, with a mean of 98.6 per cent. However, its sensitivity was lower (mean 74.2 per cent) and, moreover, varied widely as between the different hospital departments. It was highest in psychiatry and neurology, somewhat lower in internal medicine, and considerably lower on the surgical wards, where only half the cases were detected.

Table 6.2 Investigation in three clinical departments 1979/80: alcoholics and non-alcoholics according to ward physician and MALT versus research psychiatrist

			Research psychiatrist's diagnosis		
			Alcoholics	Non-alcoholics	Total
Ward physician's diagnosis	Psychiatry	Alcoholics Non-alcoholics	34 4	2 84	124
	Internal Medicine	Alcoholics Non-alcoholics	10 7	0 106	123
	Surgery	Alcoholics Non-alcoholics	1 8	0 115	124
MALT screening test	Psychiatry	Alcoholics Non-alcoholics	34 4	5 81	124
	Internal Medicine	Alcoholics Non-alcoholics	14 3	1 105	123
	Surgery	Alcoholics Non-alcoholics	4 5	1 114	124

Table 6.3 Investigation in three clinical departments 1979/80: alcoholics according to MALT, to the psychiatric researcher and to the ward physician (n =371).

	No. of cases of alcoholism detected		
	by MALT	by research psychiatrist	by ward physician
Surgery (n=124)	5 (4.0)	9 (7.3)	1 (0.8)
Internal Medicine (n=123)	15 (12.2)	17 (13.8)	10 (8.1)
Psychiatry (n=124)	39 (31.5)	38 (30.6)	36 (29.0)
Total (n=371)	59 (16.0)	64 (17.3)	47 (12.7)

The MALT questionnaire, as these findings emphasize, is clearly not independent of the diagnostic accuracy and attitudes of the treating physicians. The ward physicians in the psychiatric department detected nearly as many cases of alcoholism as were found either by MALT or by the research psychiatrist; the physicians in internal medicine detected relatively fewer of the cases and the staff on the surgical wards, where alcoholism is often not taken seriously or is dissimulated by patients, detected a much smaller proportion.

Table 6.4 Validity of MALT: case-finding in three clinical departments, 1979–80, compared with research psychiatrist's diagnosis

	Specificity (%)	Sensitivity (%)	Overall efficiency (%)
Surgery (n=124)	99.1	44.4	95.2
Internal Medicine (n=123)	99.1	82.4	96.7
Psychiatry (n=124)	94.2	89.5	92.7
Total (n=371)	98.6	74.2	95.5

Cross-sectional study at Time T1

The largest group, comprising three quarters of all patients in the psychiatric and neurological departments (74.8 per cent), consisted of persons with no detectable alcohol problem (Figure 6.1). This group was not followed up further. The second group, patients at high risk (score 6–10) constituted 7 per cent of patients in these departments. The third group, the alcoholics scoring 11 or more, represented 18.2 per cent of the patient sample.

For these three groups of patients we also tested the validity of the MALT by comparison with the diagnoses of the psychiatric ward physician (Riffert 1982). We found a high specificity of 95 per cent and a satisfactory sensitivity of 88 per cent, the overall efficiency of the instrument being 94 per cent. These results are closely similar to those obtained in the preliminary study, and confirm that the MALT score distributions correspond closely to clinical psychiatric diagnosis.

Follow-up study (Time T2)

Thirty-two of the fifty-eight persons at high risk could be re-examined using the MALT at T2 (Figure 6.1). Sixteen of these (50 per cent) scored below 6 points, 28.1 per cent scored as before between 6 and 10 points, and 21.9 per cent now scored more than 10 points, suggesting that they had become alcoholics.

Of 150 patients who scored above 10 points at T1, seventy-two could be included in the follow-up study. Of this group, 19.3 per cent had been abstinent since T1, 15.7 per cent more than one year and 13.2 per cent more than three months, while 51.8 per cent were not abstinent.

In order to examine for risk factors, we divided the group of alcoholics at T1 into those patients without and those with alcohol-related somatic or psychiatric diseases. At T1 these two groups showed considerable differences (Table 6.5): group I contained more female patients (1), younger patients (2) with a low MALT F-score (3), more patients with neurotic or psychogenic reactions and more persons who had attempted suicide. Group II contained more male patients (1) and older persons (2), fewer with neurotic disturbances (4) or a history of suicidal attempts (5), but more with high MALT F-scores (3). For (1), (2), etc., see Appendix II.

At the follow-up, twenty-five group I and fifty-eight group II patients could be re-examined, but the MALT could be repeated on only twenty-four and forty-eight patients respectively in these two groups.

The sex difference is still pronounced (6), with more females in group I. The mortality rate of group I was lower (7); the rate of

Table 6.5 Comparison of two groups of alcoholics without (I) and with (II) alcohol-related diseases according to MALT scores and rates of abstinence during follow-up

	I without complications		II with complications	
	T1 (1979/80)	T2 (1985/87)	T1 (1979/80)	T2 (1985/87)
n	45	25	105	58
male %	42.2	44.0	80.5	79.3
female %	57.8	56.0	20.0	20.7
age (x)	34.8	40.6	42.8	48.1
ICD–9 diagnosis 300 or 309 %	28.9		14.3	
suicidal attempt %	33.3		7.6	
MALT F (x)	4.7		10.8	
MALT S (x)	12.5		12.1	
Abstinence 1 year after T1 %		16.0		27.6
1 year before T2 %		28.0		37.9
6 years T1 – T2 %		16.0		22.4

persons who refused interview much higher in this group (8) (Table 6.1).

The abstinence rates were more favourable for group II than for group I. Only 16 per cent of group I and 22.4 per cent of group II remained abstinent over the follow-up period. During the last year prior to T2, only 28 per cent of group I and 37.9 per cent of group II remained abstinent. On the other hand, 84 per cent of group I and 72.4 per cent of group II showed a relapse in the first year after T1.

In the six-year follow-up, twenty-six of the 150 alcoholics examined at T1 died. Their mean age was six to seven years greater than that of the survivors (13), and 52 per cent had been divorced or separated compared to 19 per cent of the survivors (14). The MALT S-scores of the deceased patients averaged only 10.7 points, compared to 13.2 for those still alive at follow-up (15), which suggests a certain tendency to dissimulate on the part of those with a bad prognosis. On the other hand the MALT F-score was higher in the deceased group (16), as was the frequency of alcohol delirium (17), a diagnosis of polyneuritis (18), and a high gamma-glutamyl-transferase value (19): all features indicating an unfavourable prognosis.

Discussion

A special feature of our study concerns a characteristic of the population under investigation: the probands were not treated in the interval between first and follow-up examination; or, at least, they did not receive any special systematic treatment. This group can therefore be regarded as demonstrating the outcome of untreated chronic alcoholism with a low number of spontaneous remissions (Fahrenkrug 1987; Feuerlein 1987; Lemere 1953; Wieser 1966). The true outcome, however, may be even more adverse than this because of the exclusion of non-respondents at T2, who according to experience are mostly patients with an unfavourable course of illness (Jung *et al.* 1987).

In our study we are able to show that the MALT is a valuable screening instrument for use in the general hospital. This experience refers to the psychiatric, neurological, and internal medical departments. Although its sensitivity when used in the surgical department appeared much less satisfactory, even there more cases were detected by MALT than by the ward surgeons.

In a similar study, Möller *et al.* (1987) reported that the MALT also gives satisfactory results when used in surgical departments. This discrepancy may be at least partly due to the small number of alcoholics identified in the Lübeck department of surgery.

Our findings point to the presence in all the departments of a relatively high proportion of patients who are at risk for alcoholism as indicated by their scores. This group amounted to 9 per cent of the patients in internal medicine, 17 per cent of those in surgery and 15 per cent of those in psychiatry (Nieder 1985). This shows the extent of the problem which would be revealed by similar systematic enquiry in many general hospitals.

The follow-up of our patients from the psychiatric and neurological departments shows clearly that persons at high risk and alcoholics are most endangered. As a chronic disease alcoholism remits spontaneously in only a very small proportion of cases, and is characterized by a high rate of mortality (Feuerlein 1987; Lesch 1985; Oschinsky *et al.* 1986; Polich *et al.* 1980).

The identification of certain risk factors in our patient groups could facilitate prevention, and therefore deserves attention. Our findings concerning group I alcoholics suggest that these patients, mostly women, did not yet suffer from psychiatric or somatic complications, had been identified in hospital more or less by chance, but often had neurotic problems. This group, especially those persons described as 'rapid changers' (Vaglum and Vaglum 1987), at an early stage shows a type of drinking behaviour which is associated with an unfavourable prognosis. By using certain characteristic features, such as high S-score and low F-score, the MALT can thus help to identify a group of persons who ought to be singled out with special care because of a high risk of progressive alcoholism, but who on the other hand are only just beginning to develop dependency.

In considering the prospects for research in extramural settings, in general practice, and in field studies, one has to bear in mind that the group I alcoholics, a type highly represented in the general population, had a lower mean MALT S-score at T2, when examined in the community, than they had when examined in a clinical setting at T1. This suggests the possibility that many persons score lower than expected when they are tested outside the hospital environment. But even here the test produces enough positive evidence to indicate the need for more detailed examination. MALT-F on the other hand often cannot be applied in community studies for practical reasons.

Considering our findings under the aspect of prognosis we wish to emphasize the importance of certain variables which indicate the necessity of preventive measures, both in the high-risk group and in those who are already dependent. As a model for prophylactic measures, a long-term study in Malmö may be cited. For many years dependents and persons at risk received monthly consultations and their drinking behaviour was monitored by gamma-glutamyl-transferase (Kristenson and Trell 1982; Petersson *et al.* 1985). The results for the experimental group were much better than those for a control group. Even if the disease cannot be cured completely, the unfavourable course can be modified.

In conclusion, we are convinced that the use of MALT as a screening instrument offers a chance to non-specialists in particular for earlier and more effective diagnosis, and hence for preventive measures directed at abusers of alcohol, which can improve the prognosis of the disease. The study also indicates certain risk factors; for example, the prognosis for younger females with neurotic disturbances, often brought to attention by a suicidal attempt, must be regarded seriously. It seems to us of great importance to avoid the progression from high-risk drinking behaviour to alcohol dependency, and thus the emergence of a disease with serious consequences for the patients and their families.

Appendix I: The MALT Questionnaire

Items to be assessed by the physician (F-score)

1. Diseases of the liver (at least one symptom found on physical examination in addition to one positive laboratory test)

2. Polyneuropathy (only if no other cause, e.g., diabetes mellitus, is known)

3. Delirium tremens (on the present examination or previously)

4. Alcohol consumption of more than 150 ml (women 120 ml) of pure alcohol a day at least continued over several months

5. Alcohol consumption of more than 300 ml (women 240 ml) of pure alcohol at least once a month (alcoholic benders)

6. Foetor alcoholicus (at the time of medical examination)

7. Spouse, family members, or close friends have sought help because of alcohol-related problems of the patient (e.g. from a physician, social worker, or other appropriate facilities)

Items to be assessed by the patient himself as being 'true or 'not true' (S-score)

1. My hands have been trembling a lot recently.

2. In the morning I sometimes have the feeling of nausea.

3. I have sometimes tried to get rid of my trembling and nausea with alcohol.

4. At the moment I feel miserable because of my problems and difficulties.

5. It is not uncommon that I drink alcohol before lunch.

6. After the first glass or two of alcohol I feel a craving for more.

7. I think about alcohol a lot.

8. I have sometimes drunk alcohol even against my doctor's advice.

9. When I drink a lot of alcohol, I tend to eat little.

10. At work I have been criticized because of my drinking.

11. I prefer drinking alone.

12. Since I have started drinking I have been in worse shape.

13. I have often had a guilty conscience about drinking.

14. I have tried to limit my drinking to certain occasions or to certain times of the day.

15. I think I ought to drink less.

16. Without alcohol I would have fewer problems.

17. When I am upset I drink alcohol to calm down.

18. I think alcohol is destroying my life.

19. Sometimes I want to stop drinking, and sometimes I don't.

20. Other people can't understand why I drink.

21. I would get along better with my spouse if I didn't drink.

22. I have sometimes tried to get along without any alcohol at all.

23. I'd be content if I didn't drink.

24. People have often told me that they could smell alcohol on my breath.

Appendix II: Differences between alcoholics without (I) and with (II) alcohol-related diseases: results of statistical testing (cf. Table 6.5)

(1) sex I t1 / II t1	$p < 0.001$	$Chi^2 = 20.8944$	DF =	1
(2) age I t1 / II t1	$p < 0.001$	T = 3.6576	DF =	148
(3) MALT F I t1 / II t1	$p < 0.001$	T = 8.7665	DF =	148
(4) neurotics I t1 / II t1	$p < 0.025$	$Chi^2 = 5.7179$	DF =	1
(5) suicidal attempt I t1 / II t1	$p < 0.001$	$Chi^2 = 16.0439$	DF =	1
(6) sex I t2 / II t2	$p < 0.005$	$Chi^2 = 10.1251$	DF =	1
(7) deceased I t2 / II t2	$p < 0.025$	$Chi^2 = 5.1045$	DF =	1
(8) refused I t2 / II t2	$p < 0.005$	$Chi^2 = 8.8901$	DF =	1
(9) MALT-S II t1 / II t2	$p < 0.02$	T = 2.5452	DF =	68
(10) MALT-F II t1 / II t2	$p < 0.02$	T = 2.3912	DF =	68
(11) MALT-F I t2 / II t2	$p < 0.001$	T = 3.5260	DF =	81
(12) MALT-S I t2 / II t2	$p < 0.05$	T = 1.904	DF =	81

(13)–(19) deceased/living

(13) age	$p < 0.02$	T = 2.3731	DF =	148
(14) marital status	$p < 0.025$	$Chi^2 = 12.1401$	DF =	4
(15) Malt S	$p < 0.05$	T = 1.99862	DF =	146
(16) Malt F	$p < 0.05$	T = 2.0714	DF =	148
(17) withdrawal syndromes	$p < 0.001$	$Chi^2 = 4.5957$	DF =	1
(18) polyneuropathia	$p < 0.05$	$Chi^2 = 14.8972$	DF =	1
(19) gamma-GT	$p < 0.025$	$Chi^2 = 5.2791$	DF =	1

References

Athen, D. and Schranner, B. (1981) 'Zur Häufigkeit von Alkoholikern im Krankengut einer Medizinischen Klinik', in W. Keup (ed.) *Behandlung der Sucht und des Missbrauchs chemischer Stoffe*, Stuttgart: Thieme, pp. 43–7.

Auerbach, P. and Melchertsen, K. (1981) 'Zur Häufigkeit des Alkoholismus stationär behandelter Patienten aus Lübeck', *Schleswig-Holsteinisches Ärzteblatt* 34: 233–7.

Bernitzki, H.-G. and Berndt, H. (1983) 'Der nichterkannte Alkoholismus', *Zeitschrift für Ärztliche Fortbildung* 77: 729–33.

Dilling, H., Oschinsky, A.M., and Nieder, Ch. (1987) 'Trends in epidemiological and evaluative research on alcoholism in the Federal Republic of Germany', in B. Cooper (ed.) *Psychiatric Epidemiology*, London: Croom Helm, pp. 296–309.

Elvy, G.A. and Wells, J.E. (1984) 'The Canterbury alcoholism screening test (CAST): a detection instrument for use with hospitalized patients', *New Zealand Medical Journal* 97: 111–15.

Emmerich, E. (1984) 'Statistische Daten für die Jahre 1971–1982 über Kraftfahrzeugbestand, Verkehrsdisziplin, Strassenverkehrsunfälle, Fahrerlaubnis-Entziehungen, Fahrverbote und Mehrfachtäter im Strassenverkehr, unter Berücksichtigung von Trunkenheit am Steuer', *Blutalkohol* 21: 3–13.

Fahrenkrug, W.H. (1987) 'Amerikanische Langzeituntersuchungen zu Alkoholproblemen', in D. Kleiner (ed.) *Langzeitverläufe bei Suchtkrankheiten*, Heidelberg: Springer, p. 24–39.

Feuerlein, W. (1987) 'Langzeitverläufe des Alkoholismus (mit Literaturübersicht aus dem europäischen Raum)', in D. Kleiner (ed.) *Langzeitverläufe bei Suchtkrankheiten*, Heidelberg: Springer, pp. 40–54.

Feuerlein, W., Küfner, H., Ringer, Ch., and Antons, K. (1977) 'Der Münchner Alkoholismustest (MALT)', *Münchener Medizinische Wochenschrift* 119: 1275–82.

Feuerlein, W., Küfner, H., Ringer, Ch., and Antons, K. (1979) *Der Münchner Alkoholismustest (MALT) Testmanual*, Weinheim: Beltz.

Feuerlein, W., Ringer, Ch., Küfner, H., and Antons, K. (1980) 'Diagnosis of alcoholism: the Munich Alcoholism Test (MALT)', in M. Galanter (ed.) *Currents in Alcoholism VII*, New York: Grune & Stratton, pp. 133–47.

Häfner, H. (1981) 'Möglichkeiten wirksamer Prävention bei Alkoholismus und Drogenabhängigkeit', in H. Häfner and R. Welz, (eds) *Drogenabhängigkeit und Alkoholismus*, Köln: Rheinland-Verlag, pp. 11–23.

Hurt, R.D., Morse, R.M., and Swenson, W.M. (1980) 'Diagnosis of alcoholism with a self-administered alcoholism screening test', *Mayo Clinic Proceedings* 55: 365–70.

Jung, U., Köster, W., Schneider. R., Bühringer, G., and Mai, N. (1987) 'Katamnesen bei behandelten Alkoholabhängigen mit wiederholten Messzeitpunkten über 4 Jahre', in D. Kleiner (ed.) *Langzeitverläufe bei Suchtkrankheiten*, Heidelberg: Springer, pp. 89–114.

Kristenson, H. and Trell, E. (1982) 'Comparisons between a questionnaire (Mm-MAST), interviews and serum gamma-glutamyl-transferase (GGT) in a health survey of middle-aged males', *British Journal of Addiction* 77: 297–305.

Lemere, F. (1953) 'What happens to alcoholics?' *American Journal of Psychiatry* 109: 674–6.

Lesch, O. M. (1985) *Chronischer Alkoholismus, Typen und ihr Verlauf: Eine Langzeitstudie*, Stuttgart: Thieme.

Mayfield, D., McLead, G., and Hall, P. (1974) 'The CAGE questionnaire: validation of a new alcoholism screening instrument', *American Journal of Psychiatry* 131: 1121–3.

Möller, H.J., Angermund, A., and Mühlen, B. (1987) 'Prävalenzraten von Alkoholismus an einem chirurgischen Allgemeinkrankenhaus: Empirische Untersuchungen mit dem Münchener Alkoholismus-Test', *Suchtgefahren* 33: 199–202.

Nieder, Chr. (1985) 'Vergleichende Untersuchung über die Prävalenz und Diagnostik von Alkoholismus an drei Kliniken der Medizinischen Hochschule zu Lübeck', unpublished dissertation, Medical University of Lübeck.

Oschinsky, A.M., Schön, St., and Schnitzer, W. (1986) 'Mortality of a 6-year follow-up study of in-patient alcoholics', submitted for publication in the Proceedings of the 32nd International Institute on the Prevention and Treatment of Alcoholism, Budapest.

Petersson, B., Kristenson, H., Trell, E., and Hood, B. (1985) 'Screening and intervention for alcohol-related disease in middle-aged men: the Malmö Preventive Programme', in Ciba Foundation Symposium 110 (ed.) *The Value of Preventive Medicine*, London: Pitman, pp. 143–63.

Polich, J.M., Armor, D.J., and Braiker, H.D. (1980) 'Patterns of alcoholism over 4 years', *Journal of Studies on Alcohol* 41: 397–416.

Reid, A.L., Webb, G.R., Hennrikus, D., Fahey, P.P. and Sanson-Fisher, R.W. (1986) 'Detection of patients with high alcohol intake by general practitioners', *British Medical Journal (Clinical Research)* 293: 735–7.

Riffert, M. (1982) 'Methodische Probleme und Ergebnisse einer standardisierten psychiatrischen Untersuchung von Alkoholikern in den Kliniken für Psychiatrie und Neurologie der Medizinischen Hochschule Lübeck', unpublished dissertation, Medical University of Lübeck.

Selzer, M.L. (1971) 'The Michigan Alcoholism Screening Test', *American Journal of Psychiatry* 127: 1653–8.

Trojan, A. (1980) 'Epidemiologie des Alkoholkonsums und der Alkoholkrankheit in der Bundesrepublik Deutschland', *Suchtgefahren* 26: 1–17.

Vaglum, S. and Vaglum, P. (1987) 'Phases on the way to alcoholism in female psychiatric patients' *Acta Psychiatrica Scandinavica* 76: 183–92.

Vereinigung Schweizerischer Krankenhäuser (Association of Swiss Hospitals) (1987) *Diagnosendokumentation*, Aarau, Switzerland: Veska.

Wieser, S. (1966) 'Alkoholismus III: Katamnesen und Prognosen', *Fortschritte der Neurologie und Psychiatrie* 34: 566–88.

Chapter seven

Conceptual and methodological problems in estimation of the incidence of mental disorders from field survey data

William W. Eaton, Morton Kramer, James C. Anthony, Elsbeth M.L. Chee, and Sam Shapiro

Introduction

We address here two conceptual and two methodologic issues related to the estimation of incidence from field survey data. The conceptual issues are (1) the distinction of first from total incidence, and (2) the threshold at which disease is defined as present. The methodological issues are (1) the effect of systematic error in case detection on incidence, and (2) the effect of random error in case detection on incidence. Incidence data are presented for eight categories of mental disorder and examples are given from our work in psychiatric epidemiology.

Incidence data are crucial to the planning of effective intervention programmes. Risk factors can be credibly identified only in incidence studies, and these factors are critical to the identification of high-risk groups which can be targets of intervention programmes. The relationship of incidence to age is crucial also in guaranteeing that interventions take place before the population has entered into the period of the lifespan with high risk.

Many mental disorders do not come automatically to medical attention, in part because it can be difficult to differentiate symptoms of mental disorders from the non-specific distress and psychological upsets of every-day life. Also, there is considerable stigma and associated denial attached to many mental disorders, which act to keep them away from medical attention. As a result pyschiatric epidemiologists have long known that data based on treatment records provide incomplete and possibly biased information for estimating true prevalence or incidence data (Kramer 1969). In the case of prevalence, surveys of entire communities have been carried out which demonstrate that, except for the more severe mental disorders, most cases do not come to medical attention at all (Link and Dohrenwend 1980; Shapiro *et al.* 1984). In the case of incidence, the rates are so much lower than for prevalence that most community surveys do not examine a large enough sample to generate meaningful confidence intervals for rates, even if other conditions necessary for the estimation of incidence were met. Thus, in the field of pyschiatric epidemiology, incidence data from community studies are rare, despite the well-known advantage of incidence rates for studying risk factors.

One community study of the incidence of mental disorders exists that will be discussed briefly in this context: the study of the town of 'Lundby' in Sweden. A prevalence survey of the entire population of this town of about 2,500 persons was carried out by Essen-Moller in 1947, and a ten-year follow-up survey of the entire population was conducted in 1957 by Hagnell (1966). The 1947 survey allowed the population at risk to be identified, and the ten-year follow-up monitored about 25,000 person-years of risk, which is sufficient to estimate incidence rates for some mental disorders. Among those successfully followed up, the probability of developing a mental disorder within ten years following the initial survey – an approximation to the crude ten-year *cumulative* incidence – was estimated at 11.3 per cent for men and 20.4 per cent for women. Aside from Lundby and the ECA study, we know of only two other field studies with sample size sufficient to estimate incidence of specific mental disorders: Stirling County, Nova Scotia (Murphy 1980), and Traunstein in Bavaria.

Definition of prevalence and incidence

In order to avoid confu-ion, it is essential to distinguish *first incidence* from *total incidence*. The distinction itself is commonly assumed by epidemiologists but there does not appear to be consensus on the terminology. Most definitions of the incidence numerator include a concept such as 'new cases' (Lilienfeld and Lilienfeld 1980: 138), 'illness commencing' (Expert Committee 1959: 6), cases that 'come into being' (MacMahon *et al.* 1960: 54), or persons who 'develop a disease' (Mausner and Kramer 1985: 44), or 'have onset' (National Center for Health Statistics 1975: 129). Sartwell and Last (1980) imply total incidence when they state the necessity of allowing 'for an individual being counted more than once, if the condition is one for which this is possible (e.g., accidents, colds)'. Lilienfeld and Lilienfeld also occasionally equate 'incidence' with 'attack rate' (1980: 170). Kleinbaum *et al.* (1982) hint at the distinction between first and total incidence, but are not explicit on the issue. Morris (1975) defines incidence as equivalent to our 'first incidence', and 'attack rate' as equivalent to our 'total incidence'. Save for the latter text, in none of these definitions is it explicit whether or not an individual who is healthy now, but has had episodes of the disorder over the life course qualifies for a 'new' onset. First incidence corresponds to the most common use of the term 'incidence', but since the usage is by no means universal we prefer to keep the prefix.

The numerator of *first incidence* for a specified time period is composed of those individuals who have had an occurrence of the disorder for the first time in their lives and the denominator includes only persons who start the period with no prior history of the disorder. The numerator for *total incidence* includes all individuals who have had an occurrence of the disorder during the time period under investigation, whether or not it is the initial episode of their lives or a recurrent episode. The denominator for total incidence includes all population members except those cases of the disorder which are active at the beginning of the follow-up period. For the analyses presented below we have arbitrarily defined 'active' as having met criteria for the disorder during one's lifetime and having experienced some symptoms of the disorder during the year prior to baseline. This arbitrary definition corresponds to the structure of our interview (DIS) and to the expected length of our follow-up period.

The preference for first or total incidence in aetiologic studies depends on hypotheses and assumptions about the way causes and outcomes important to the disease ebb and flow. If the disease is recurrent and the causal factors vary in strength over time, then it might be important to study risk factors not only for first but for subsequent episodes (total incidence). For example, one might consider the effects of changing levels of stress on the occurrence of episodes of neurosis (Tyrer 1985) or of schizophrenia (Brown *et al.* 1972). For a disease with a presumed fixed progression from some starting point, such as dementia, the first occurrence might be the most important episode to focus on and first incidence is the appropriate rate. In the field of psychiatric epidemiology, there are a range of disorders with both types of causal structures operating, which has led us to focus on this distinction in types of incidence.

The two types of incidence are functionally related to different measures of prevalence. Kramer *et al.* (1981) have shown that *lifetime prevalence* (i.e., the proportion of persons in a defined population who have ever had an attack of a disorder) is a function of *first incidence* and mortality in affected and unaffected populations. *Point prevalence* (i.e., the proportion of persons in a defined population on a given day who manifest the disorder) is linked to *total incidence* by the queuing formula $P = f (I \times D)$ (Kramer 1957; Kleinbaum *et al.* 1982): that is, point prevalence is a function of the total number of cases occurring and their duration.

The *one-year prevalence* is a hybrid type of rate, conceptually mixing aspects of point and period prevalence, which has been found useful in the ECA Program (Eaton *et al.* 1985). It includes in the numerator all those surveyed individuals who have met the criteria for disorder in the past year, and as denominator all those interviewed. It is not a point prevalence rate because it covers a longer period of time, which can be defined as six months, two years, and so forth, as well as one year. But one-year prevalence is not a period prevalence rate because some individuals in the population who are ill at the beginning of the period are not successfully interviewed, because they either die or emigrate. As the time period covered in this rate becomes shorter, it approximates the point prevalence;

as the time period becomes longer, the rate approaches the period prevalence. If there is large mortality the one-year prevalence rate will diverge markedly from period prevalence.

Thresholds in identifying illness onset

Dating the onset of episodes is problematic for most mental disorders for many reasons. One is that the diagnostic criteria for the disorders themselves are not well agreed upon, and continual changes are being made in the definition of a case of disorder, such as the recent third revision of the *Diagnostic and Statistical Manual* (DSM-III) (American Psychiatric Association 1980). The DSM-III has the advantage that criteria for mental disorders are more or less explicitly defined, but it is nevertheless true that specific mental disorders are often very difficult to distinguish from non-morbid psychological states. Most disorders include symptoms that, taken by themselves, are part of everyone's normal experience; for example, feeling fearful, being short of breath or dizzy, and having sweaty palms are not uncommon experiences but they are also symptoms of panic disorder. It is the clustering of symptoms, often with the requirement that they be brought together in one period of time or 'spell', that generally forms the requirement for diagnosis. Although the clustering criteria are fairly explicit in DSM-III, it is not well established that they correspond to the characteristics generally associated with a disease, such as a predictable course, a response to treatment, an association with a biological aberration in the individual, or an associated disability. Thus, the lack of established validity of the criteria-based classification system exacerbates problems of dating the onset of disorder.

The absence of firm data on the validity of the classification system enjoins us to be very careful about conceptualizing the process of disease onset. One criterion of onset used in the epidemiology of some diseases is entry into treatment, but this is unacceptable in psychiatry since people with mental disorders so often do not seek treatment for them. Another criterion of onset sometimes used is detectability — that is, when the symptoms first appear — but this also is unacceptable because experiences analogous to the symptoms of most psychiatric disorders are so widespread. We prefer to conceptualize onset as a continuous line of development towards manifestation of a disease. At some point the development becomes irreversible, so that at some minimal level of symptomatology it is certain that the full characteristics of the disease, however defined, will become apparent. This use of irreversibility is consistent with some epidemiological uses (Kleinbaum *et al.* 1982). Prior to this point, the symptoms are thought of as 'subcriterial'. At the current state of knowledge in psychiatry, longitudinal studies in the general population, such as the ECA programme and others mentioned above, are needed to determine those levels of symptomatology at which irreversibility is achieved. To recapitulate: focus on population indicators for the force of morbidity leads us to consider explicitly the idea of a continuous line of development towards manifestation of disease with an as-yet-unknown point of irreversibility. At present we can only hypothesize where the disease begins, so that even the use of the word 'symptom' in the strict medical sense is problematic, since we cannot ascribe the complaint or behaviour to the disease with perfect accuracy.

There are at least two ways of thinking about the development towards disease. The first way is the increase in severity or intensity of symptoms. An individual could have all the symptoms required for diagnosis but none of them be sufficiently intense or severe: that is, the individual is not regarded as sick until the symptoms themselves are severe. The underlying logic of such an assumption may well be the relatively high frequency of occurrence of the symptoms in milder form, making it difficult to distinguish normal and subcriterial complaints from manifestations of disease. For many chronic diseases, it may be inappropriate to regard the symptom as ever having been 'absent', for example, personality traits giving rise to deviant behaviour, categorized as personality disorders on Axis II of the *Diagnostic and Statistical Manual* (APA 1980). This type of development we can refer to as 'symptom intensification', indicating that the symptoms are already present and have become more severe during a period of observation. This way of thinking leads the researcher to consider whether there is a crucial level of severity of a given symptom or symptoms in which the rate of development towards a full-blown disease state is accelerated.

A second way of thinking about progress towards disease is the occurrence of new symptoms where none existed. This involves the gradual acquisition of symptoms so that clusters are formed which increasingly approach the constellation required to meet specified definitions for diagnosis. 'Present' can be defined as occurrence either at a non-severe or at a severe level: thus, decisions made about the symptom intensification process complicate the idea of acquisition. This idea leads the researcher to consider the order in which symptoms occur over the natural history of disease, and, in particular, whether one symptom is more important than others in accelerating the process.

Figures 7.1 and 7.2 are adaptations of a diagram used by Lilienfeld and Lilienfeld (1980: Figure 6.3) to visualize the concept of incidence as a time-oriented rate. Here our adaptations give examples of the several distinct forms that onset can take when the disorder is defined by constellations of symptoms varying in intensity, as is the case with mental disorders. In both figures, the topmost subject ('A') is what we might consider the null hypothesis, and it corresponds to simple onset as portrayed in the original. Figure 7.1 shows how intensity, represented by

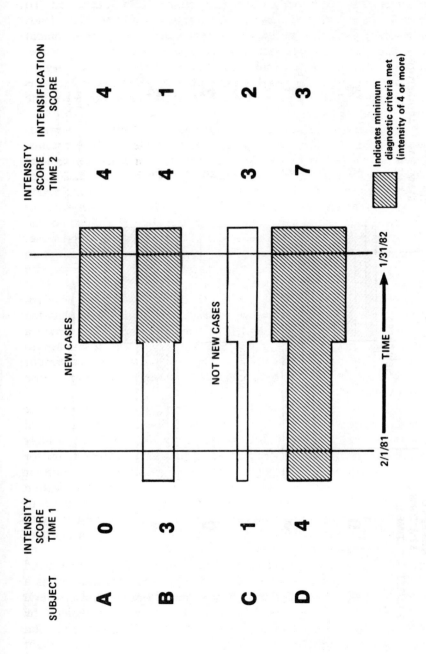

Figure 7.1 Incidence and symptom intensification

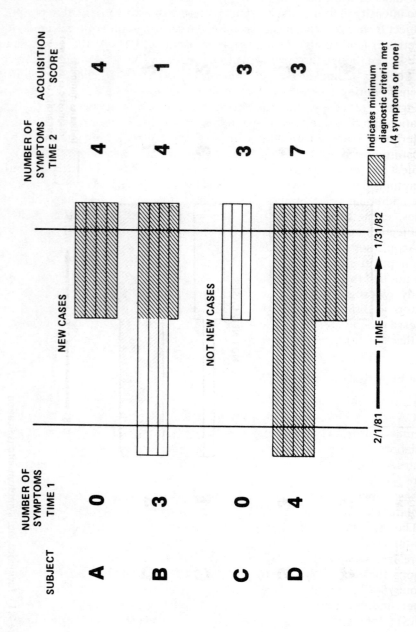

Figure 7.2 Incidence and symptom acquisition

the vertical width of the bars, might vary. The threshold of disease is set at four units of width, and in the null hypothesis subject A progresses from zero intensity to four units, becoming a case during the observation period. Subject B changes from nearly meeting the criteria (width of three units) to meeting it (four units) during the year. Both subjects A and B are new cases, even though the onset was more sudden in subject A than in subject B. Subjects C and D are *not* new cases, even though their symptoms intensify during the year more than do those of subject B.

Figure 7.2 adapts the same original diagram to conceptualize the relationship of acquisition of symptoms to incidence of disorder. Here the criterion of being a case is four or more symptoms, each represented by separate horizontal bars, and the null hypothesis is again represented by subject A, who displays the simultaneous onset of a cluster of four symptoms during the year. Subject B is also a new case, even though only one additional symptom has been acquired. Subjects C and D are *not* new cases, even though they have a larger acquisition of symptoms below (subject C) and above (subject D) the threshold.

Acquisition and intensification are indicators of the force of morbidity in the population, as are more traditional forms of incidence rate. But they are not tied to any one definition of caseness. Rather, these concepts allow study of progression of disease independently of case definition. Risk factors at different stages of the disease may be differentially related to disease progression only above or below the threshold set by the diagnosis. In this situation, we might reconsider the diagnostic threshold.

The ECA study as an example

One of the principle goals of the NIMH Epidemiologic Catchment Area (ECA) programme was to fill the gap in knowledge of incidence of specific mental disorders (Eaton *et al*. 1981). The ECA programme consists of five collaborative community surveys each in different locations in the United States, carried out by a university-based research team. Data are presented here for the site in Eastern Baltimore City (investigated by the team from Johns Hopkins University). In addition to a cross-sectional survey of each community sample, there was also a one-year follow-up interview.

The methods of the ECA surveys are more fully described elsewhere (Eaton and Kessler 1985). In brief, area probability samples of households were drawn and household members selected at random for interview from among those persons aged 18 years or older, achieving response rates of about 75–80 per cent. Persons agreeing to be interviewed participated in a ninety-minute interview which included the Diagnostic Interview Schedule (DIS) (Robins *et al*. 1985). This consists of pre-specified questions directly pertinent to DSM-III diagnostic criteria for a series of mental disorders. Diagnoses are made from the DIS symptom data by means of computer algorithms which simulate the application of DSM-III criteria (Boyd *et al.* 1985).

The case of panic disorders can serve as an example of the DIS method. The interviewer first asks: 'Have you ever had a spell or attack when all of a sudden you felt frightened, anxious or very uneasy in a situation when most people wouldn't be afraid?' If the answer to this question is affirmative, the interviewer asks whether any of a series of twelve autonomic symptoms were present in one of the worst such attacks, how frequently these occurred, the age at which the first attack occurred, how recently the most recent attack occurred, whether the attacks occurred only in the presence of phobic stimuli, and several questions to assess severity (whether the attack prompted seeking treatment or use of medicines; or whether the attacks interfered a lot with life or activities). If the attacks were accompanied by four or more autonomic symptoms, met operational criteria for severity and recurrence, and occurred in the absence of phobic stimuli, the disturbance was classified as DIS/DSM III panic disorder.

Table 7.1 presents estimates of prevalence and incidence for eight categories of mental disorder from the Eastern Baltimore Epidemiologic Catchment Area programme surveys. The columns of rates are arranged to allow comparisons between the various types of incidence and prevalence rates. The first column reproduces *lifetime prevalence* rates published elsewhere (Robins *et al.* 1984). For most disorders about half to two-thirds of the lifetime rate is made up of cases who met criteria during the prior year. This column closely approximates data published elsewhere using six months as the time period of recall (Myers *et al.* 1984).

Table 7.1 Prevalence and incidence rates for eight categories of DIS/DSM-III disorders per 1,000 population 18 years and over: Epidemiologic Catchment Area Program East Baltimore

DIS/DSM-III disorder category	Lifetime prevalence	One-year prevalence			Incidence	
		Full sample	Panel cohort		Total	First
			Wave 1	Wave 2		
Alcohol abuse/dependence	137	67	69	73	39	26
Drug abuse/dependence	56	28	26	19	14	13
Schizophrenia	16	11	11	8	6	5
Major depression	37	27	29	16	12	11
Phobia	233	160	161	74	45	39
Panic disorder	14	10	10	10	8	8
Obsessive-compulsive disorder	30	22	21	18	14	13
Any DIS disorder	380	267	267	197	116	95

After one year an attempt was made to interview the 3,481 original respondents again; 2,768 (79.5 per cent) were found and successfully interviewed: the so-called 'panel cohort' in Table 7.1. The follow-up interval, i.e., the interval between baseline and follow-up interviews, was not usually exactly 365 days; the total person-years of exposure for the 2,768 individuals in the panel cohort amounting to 2,812. Since this figure is close to the size of the cohort, we have used cohort sizes, and not years of exposure, as denominators. Attrition bias can be considered by comparing the one-year prevalence ratios for the full sample to those for the panel cohort, where the point in time of the interview is Wave 1 in both instances. If the 713 individuals not interviewed at Wave 2 were very different, in terms of frequency of disorder, from those successfully interviewed, the ratios would also be quite different.

In fact the estimates are similar, suggesting that attrition has occurred proportionately in numerator and denominator. The largest difference, for major depression, is two per 1,000, or about 7 per cent (2/27) relative difference. This lack of attrition bias is consistent with earlier findings from this and other survey sites showing a lack of strong bias due to non-response at Wave 1 (Von Korff *et al.* 1985; Cottler *et al.* 1987). The possibility exists that the *onset* of disorder during the panel interval, as opposed to status at Wave 1, affects attrition, but these data do not address this point.

The comparison of the one-year prevalence ratios for the same panel cohort at Wave 1 and Wave 2 (columns 3 and 4 of Table 7.1) shows that most ratios decline over the one-year period. The decline could be an effect of the maturation process of the individuals, or the consequence of a secular trend which affected the East Baltimore population during the year; or else it could be an effect of being interviewed a second time. One year seemed to be too short a period for maturation of such strong influence to occur, and we know of no important historical trend in East Baltimore that could have had such a beneficial influence. Further evidence about a possible test effect will be presented and discussed below.

The two columns on the far right in Table 7.1 present incidence rates. Persons with multiple episodes during the year enter the numerator only once, and it is assumed that individuals with active disorders at Wave 1 do not remit and become eligible for new onsets between baseline and follow-up. One reason that the total incidence rates differ from the one-year (Wave 2) prevalence rates is the episodic course of some disorders. The numerator of the one-year prevalence ratio includes all lifetime cases with active symptomatology during the follow-up year. Of these cases, some had active symptoms at Wave 1; these are excluded from both numerator and denominator of the total incidence rate, which measures the frequency of onset in the population only among those at risk for an onset. For disorders characterized by few, lengthy episodes, the numerator will be dominated by the active cases, and the one-year prevalence will be larger than the total incidence. For disorders characterized by multiple episodes, the one-year prevalence and the total incidence will be similar. The one-year prevalence rate for most of the disorders consists of individuals who are having new episodes of disorder or recurrences of disorder after a period of remission; for example, in Table 7.1 the total incidence rate is never less than half of the one-year prevalence rate. The comparison of the two incidence columns allows us to assess what proportion of episodes of disorders are new in the lifetime of the individual. There are surprisingly high proportions of apparently new episodes (the lowest proportion being 26/39 or two-thirds).

The concepts of intensification and acquisition can be operationally defined with the ECA data for diagnostic or syndrome groups or for the group of all DIS disorders. For a given syndrome – say, anxiety state – we can count the number of symptoms present at the non-severe level at Wave 1 (DIS code 2) which change to the more severe level at Wave 2 (DIS code 5). This count is an index of intensification, and can be calculated for each respondent by each syndrome or diagnostic area. The population as a whole and each sub-group have an average value for symptom intensification, which is analogous to the rate of incidence for the whole population. Indices of symptom acquisition can be estimated in similar manner, by counting for each subject the number of symptoms which change from 'not present' (DIS code 1) to 'present and severe' (DIS code 5). Analogous to the indices of intensification, there are first and total incidence forms of the acquisition indices, and population averages can be computed.

Systematic error

There is an epidemiological literature on the effects of systematic error on prevalence rates and measures of association (e.g., Link and Dohrenwend 1980). Here we focus on effects of systematic error on incidence.

As noted above, the survey data display a decline in reporting of symptoms between Wave 1 and Wave 2, probably not attributable to attrition, maturation, or historical effects. Table 7.2 presents a cross-classification of data obtained at the two waves of the ECA programme which allow us to examine incidence rates and possible sources of this decline in more detail. The two categories considered are 'DIS/DSM-III panic disorder' and 'Any DIS/DSM-III disorder'. These categories were chosen to represent polar opposites as regards breadth of disorder and magnitude of incidence. There are four categories of disorder status at each point in time: (1) the individual reports no symptoms of the disorder over the life course to the present time, or any symptoms reported are mild; (2) the respondent reports one or more severe symptoms of the disorder at some point over his lifetime, but does not qualify for the diagnosis (subcriterial); (3) the individual reports symptoms sufficient to meet diagnostic criteria at some time, but *not* at the time of the interview

Table 7.2 Panel analysis of DIS/DSM-III diagnosis and symptoms: Epidemiologic Catchment Area Program East Baltimore

Wave 1	Wave 2					
	No symptoms	No diagnosis; one or more symptoms	Past diagnosis	Present diagnosis	Completed interviews	Not interviewed or incomplete
Any DIS disorder						
No diagnosis; no symptoms	21 20.0%	77 73.3%	2 1.9%	5 4.8%	105 100.0%	33
No diagnosis; one or more symptoms	106 6.7%	1264 79.3%	71 4.5%	152 9.5%	1593 100.0%	412
Past diagnosis	10 2.5%	197 49.1%	100 25.0%	94 23.4%	401 100.0%	97
Present diagnosis	11 1.6%	292 43.7%	78 11.7%	288 43.0%	669 100.0%	169
	148	1830	251	539	2768	711
DIS panic disorder						
No diagnosis; no symptoms	2367 96.9%	66 2.7%	3 0.1%	7 0.3%	2443 100.0%	592
No diagnosis; one or more symptoms	126 70.4%	36 20.1%	4 2.2%	13 7.3%	179 100.0%	40
Past diagnosis	6 60.0%	2 20.0%	2 20.0%	0 0.0%	10 100.0%	2
Present diagnosis	14 46.7%	11 36.7%	1 3.3%	4 13.3%	30 100.0%	5
	2513	115	10	24	2662	713

or during the year prior to it; and (4) a sufficient number and severity of symptoms are reported to meet DSM-III criteria at the time of the interview. The table is set in the manner typical of crossover tables, with the percentage entries adding to 100 per cent across the rows.

The table allows estimation of lifetime and point prevalence of disorder, incidence for those with and without prior symptoms, recurrence, and certain important methodologic anomalies. For 'Any DIS disorder', the point prevalence at Wave 1 is 669/2,768 or 24.4 per cent. For panic disorder, the point prevalence at Wave 1 is 30/2,662, or 1.1 per cent. The lifetime prevalence rates of the two disorders are 38.6 per cent and 1.5 per cent respectively. The analogous prevalences at Wave 2 are substantially lower. For example, the point prevalence of 'Any DIS disorder' at Wave 2 is 19.5 per cent, representing a drop in magnitude of about 20 per cent. These figures differ slightly from those presented in Table 7.1 because here, in order to simplify the exposition, no sample weights are used.

The incidence estimate is in the top right-hand corner of the table. For example, of the 105 persons with no symptom of any DIS disorder, five, or 4.8 per cent, had a disorder at Wave 2; of the 2,443 person at Wave 1 with no symptoms of panic disorder over their lifetime, seven (0.3 per cent) had the disorder at Wave 2. The incidence estimates are higher for those with some symptoms at Wave 1, illustrating the accelerated development of disorder for those with some symptoms. The incidence rates for those with some symptoms are about twice as high for 'Any DIS disorder' (9.5 per cent compared to 4.8 per cent) and more than twenty times as high for panic disorder (7.3 per cent compared to 0.3 per cent). Of those eligible for first onset of panic disorder according to the criteria of Table 7.1 (i.e. 2,443 + 179 or 2,622), twenty had a first episode, giving an unweighted first incidence rate of about eight per 1,000 – a rate very similar to the figure in Table 7.1, which used weighted data.

The estimate for recurrence is found in the fourth entry in the third row of Table 7.2: of the 401 persons with a past history of 'Any DIS disorder', 94 (23.4 per cent) met criteria for diagnosis at Wave 2; of the persons with a past history of panic disorder at Wave 1, none qualified for this diagnosis at Wave 2. Finally, the estimate for continuation of disorder from Wave 1 to Wave 2 is found in the lower right cell of the table: of the 669 respondents with 'Any DIS disorder' at Wave 1, 288 (43 per cent) met criteria for one or more diagnoses at Wave 2; of the thirty respondents with a Wave 1 diagnosis of panic disorder at the time of the interview, four (13 per cent) had the disorder at the time of the second interview.

Five of the six cells below the diagonals in Table 7.2 theoretically ought to have zero frequencies. The exception is the cell in which the respondent reports symptoms consistent with a current diagnosis at Wave 1 and a past diagnosis at Wave 2. The other five cells record inconsistencies in the reporting of symptoms, and they have disturbingly high frequencies. For example, of 401 individuals who at Wave 1 reported 'Any DIS diagnosis' at some point in their lifetimes, more than half (207) did *not* meet the same criteria for lifetime diagnosis based on their reports at Wave 2: of ten respondents with a lifetime diagnosis of panic disorder at Wave 1, six reported no history of symptoms at all, and two others only symptoms not meeting the criteria for diagnosis, at Wave 2. In a separate paper, Anthony *et al.* (1988) present more detailed data on the other disorders one by one. The data on such inconsistencies in reporting shown in Table 7.2 are typical: about 50 per cent of the Wave 1 lifetime cases did not meet criteria for lifetime diagnosis at Wave 2.

The inconsistencies between Wave 1 and Wave 2 symptom-reporting appear to have both random and non-random components. If the lifetime prevalence estimates based on Waves 1 and 2 were roughly equal, the inconsistencies might be ascribed to (albeit unfortunately large) random error; but, since in fact the data show a sizeable drop in the lifetime prevalence ratios, there is considerable bias in the error as well.

We favour two hypotheses for how the effect of testing might have led to a decline in the reporting of symptoms. The first hypothesis is that the respondents learn that a positive response to a symptom is invariably followed by the detailed DIS probe questions, and a negative response is followed by a new symptom question – in other words, they learn that the interview will be much shorter if they answer 'no' and apply this knowledge in the second wave to shorten the interview. A second and related hypothesis is that the respondent's understanding of the purpose of the interview gradually evolves from a focus on physical health and minor emotional disturbances to a focus more exclusively on severe and bizarre disturbances. (In fact this hypothesized evolution of belief parallels, to some degree, the order of sections in the DIS, which begins with questions on somatic symptoms and relatively innocuous anxiety and depressive disorders, before asking questions relevant to schizophrenia, antisocial personality disorder and cognitive impairment.) As this evolution takes place, the respondent may re-evaluate the occurrence of symptoms in his or her own life history, and increasingly decide they are not relevant to the purpose of the interview. For some respondents, this re-evaluation may amount to denial of the occurrence of symptoms which have in fact occurred. Thus, systematic error in this case leads to underestimation of incidence.

Random error

The frequency of the inconsistencies in reporting is so large as to demand investigation before too much work on the analysis of incidence is performed. The justification for the investigation is that the frequencies of the inconsistent reporting are larger, by a factor of two or more, than the numerators for the incidence rates. How can we be confident in our estimates for incidence in the presence of so much error?

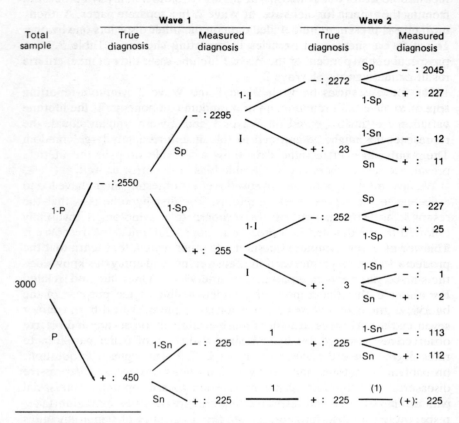

Figure 7.3 Relationship of measurement error to incidence in a hypothetical, two-wave field survey. Assumptions: True lifetime prevalence (P), Time 1 = 15%; True incidence (I) in one year = 1%, Sensitivity (Sn) = 50, and Specificity (Sp) = 90%

Figure 7.3 presents a simple model of the effects of error on the estimation of incidence. Others have shown how random measurement errors affect case ascertainment and prevalence estimates (Shrout and Fleiss 1981); Figure 7.3 shows that error which has little effect on prevalence can massively affect estimates of incidence when the incidence rates are low. Suppose a hypothetical sample of 3,000 persons has a lifetime prevalence ratio of 15 per cent for a given disorder, and an incidence rate of 1 per cent, and that case ascertainment at the first and second waves is imperfect, with a sensitivity of 50 per cent and a specificity of 90 per cent. There are twenty-six (i.e., 23 + 3) new cases of disorder and the screening process identifies eleven of them; but there are also 227 false positives identified as new cases, which result from lack of specificity of measurement at Wave 2; and an additional 112 false new cases which result from lack of sensitivity at Wave 1 and at Wave 2. The reported $T_1 - T_2$ incidence is 13.7 per cent (i.e., $11 + 227 + 112/2,550$); the incidence rate is grossly overestimated. If one were searching for causes of disorder in a prospective study many of the apparent new cases would be solely the result of measurement error (Schlesselman 1977; Yanagawa and Gladen 1984). Table 7.3 presents the percentage of observed new cases that are true new cases, i.e., the positive predictive values, as a function of variation in sensitivity, specificity, and incidence. In effect, Table 7.3 represents 108 measurement scenarios, each one analogous to Figure 7.3. The positive predictive values are generated as follows:

$$\frac{(1{-}P)\ (Sp)\ (I)\ (Sn)}{(1{-}P)\ (Sp)\ (1{-}1)\ (1{-}Sp) + (P)\ (1{-}Sn)\ (Sn) + (1{-}P)\ (Sp)\ (I)\ (Sn)}$$

This formula can be visualized from Figure 7.3: the numerator is the product of a single path ending in eleven cases; while the denominator is the sum of three separate paths, ending in 11, 227, and 112 respectively. For example, the conditions of Figure 7.3 show that 3 per cent (11 divided by 350) of the observed new cases would be true new cases. Only twenty-seven of the 108 measurement scenarios result in more than half of the observed new cases being true new cases, and all of these involve incidence rates above 5 per cent. For an incidence rate of 1 per cent, which is probably more realistic for psychiatric disorders, and, indeed, many other diseases as well, the highest positive predictive value is 30 per cent, even with an improbably high test sensitivity and specificity of 0.90 and 0.995, respectively. In contrast to positive predictive value as defined in studies of prevalence, here, even with a specificity of 100 per cent, there remains a sizeable upward bias in the rate.

It is important to realize that the discrepancies shown in Table 7.3 do not necessarily result from biased error. Random error of measurement has not been as clearly conceptualized in epidemiology as in psychometrics (see Schwartz 1986 for a review of this issue). If we adopt a definition of bias analogous to that used for continuous measures, we can define random or unbiased error as that in which mean observed value over many trials equals the true value. In respect of prevalence, error is random when the number of false positives equals the number of false negatives $[(P)\ (1{-}Sn) = (1{-}P)\ (1{-}Sp)]$. This situation is met for all the entries in Table 7.3, so long as the prevalence is allowed to vary.

Table 7.3 Percentage true new cases under varying assumptions about sensitivity, specificity, and incidence

	Sensitivity = 0.50					
	Specificity =					
	1.000	*0.995*	*0.990*	*0.950*	*0.900*	*0.800*
Incidence =						
0.000	—	00	00	00	00	00
0.005	05	05	04	02	02	01
0.010	10	09	08	05	03	02
0.050	36	34	32	21	15	09
0.100	53	51	48	35	26	18
0.200	69	67	66	54	44	32
	Sensitivity = 70					
	Specificity =					
	1.000	*0.995*	*0.990*	*0.950*	*0.900*	*0.800*
Incidence =						
0.000	—	00	00	00	00	00
0.005	09	09	07	04	02	01
0.010	16	14	13	07	05	03
0.050	48	45	43	29	20	13
0.100	65	63	60	45	35	24
0.200	79	77	75	64	54	40
	Sensitivity = 90					
	Specificity =					
	1.000	*0.995*	*0.990*	*0.950*	*0.900*	*0.800*
Incidence =						
0.000	—	00	00	00	00	00
0.005	22	18	15	06	04	02
0.010	36	30	26	12	07	04
0.050	74	68	64	41	28	18
0.100	85	81	78	59	46	31
0.200	92	90	88	76	65	50

The model used in Figure 7.3 and Table 7.3 is based on the assumption that error in measurement is unrelated to the size of the incidence rate, but this assumption may not be correct. For example, it seems plausible that false positives at Wave 1 might be subcriterial cases who are at much greater risk of developing the disorder before Wave 2 than the rest of the population. If for this group we assume an increase in the incidence rate by a factor of ten, there is very little effect on the bias in the rate itself – the true incidence is about doubled, but the observed incidence stays the same. (There will be no effect on the positive predictive value given in Table 7.3, because the affected cases are observed to be positive at Wave 1 and incorrectly judged not to be at risk for incidence.)

Several conclusions are possible from this analysis of random error:

1. error which has relatively innocuous effects on the estimation of prevalence can lead to gross overestimation of incidence;

2. even 'unbiased' error can have strong effects on the estimated incidence rate;

3. even with a specificity of 100 per cent there will be substantial upward biasing of the incidence rate; and

4. the presence of a raised incidence among false positives has little effect on bias.

None of these conclusions is unique to the DIS or the ECA programme. Measurement assumptions of models used to generate these conclusions are not inconsistent with known amounts of measurement error in the field of psychiatric epidemiology in general.

Conclusion

The purpose of the concept of incidence is to measure the frequency of onset of disease in populations. Incidence is central to much current research in epidemiology, but its value varies considerably, depending on the concepts of disease and disease onset and the quality of measures which are applied. In some situations, assiduously applying traditional concepts of incidence may lead researchers away from advances in the field of psychiatric epidemiology. In brief, three important problems with application of traditional concepts are: (1) the size of the force of error may be too large in relation to the force of morbidity; (2) the criteria for case definition may not be valid; (3) finally, for many psychiatric disorders, it is not yet clear that the approach which categorizes symptoms and diseases as 'present' or 'absent' is superior to approaches that specify psychopathology in relation to dimensions or continua.

References

American Psychiatric Association (1980) *Diagnostic and Statistical Manual, Third Revision (DSM–III)*, Washington, DC: APA.

Anthony, J.C. (1985) Presentation at the World Psychiatric Association, Community Psychiatry Section, Edinburgh (unpublished).

Boyd, J.H., Robin, L.N., Holzer, C.C., Von Korff, M., Jordan, K., and Escobar, J. (1985) 'Making diagnoses from DIS data', in W.W. Eaton and L.G. Kessler (eds) *Epidemiologic Field Methods in Psychiatry: The NIMH Epidemiologic Catchment Area Program*, New York: Academic Press.

Brown, G.W., Birley, J.L.T., and Wing, J.K. (1972) 'Influence of family life on the course of schizophrenic disorders: a replication', *British Journal of Psychiatry* 121: 241–58.

Cottler, L.B., Zipp, J.F., Robins, L.N., and Spitznagel, E.L. (1987) 'Difficult-to-recruit respondents and their effect on prevalence estimates in an epidemiological survey', *American Journal of Epidemiology* 125: 329–39.

Eaton, W.W. and Kessler, L.G. (eds) (1985) *Epidemiologic Field Methods in*

Psychiatry: The NIMH Epidemiologic Catchment Area Program, New York: Academic Press.

Eaton, W.W., Regier, D.A., Locke, B.Z., and Taube, C.A. (1981) 'The Epidemiologic Catchment Area Program of the National Institute of Mental Health', *Public Health Reports* 96: 319–25.

Eaton, W.W., Weissman, M.M., Anthony, J.C., *et al.* (1985) 'Problems in the definition and measurement of prevalence and incidence of psychiatric disorders', in W.W. Eaton and G.L. Kessler (eds) *Epidemiologic Field Methods in Psychiatry: The NIMH Epidemiologic Catchment Area Program*, New York: Academic Press.

Expert Committee on Health Statistics (1959) *Sixth Report*, Geneva: WHO.

Hagnell, O. (1966) *A Prospective Study of the Incidence of Mental Disorder*, Norstedts: Svenska Bokforlaget.

Kleinbaum, D.G., Kupper, L.L., and Morgenstern, H. (1982) *Epidemiologic Research: Principles and Quantitative Methods*, Belmont, Ca: Lifetime Learning Publications.

Kramer, M. (1957) 'Discussion of the concepts of prevalence and incidence as related to epidemiologic studies of mental disorders', *American Journal of Public Health* 47: 826–40.

Kramer, M. (1969) *Applications of Mental Health Statistics*, Geneva: WHO.

Kramer, M., Von Korff, M., and Kessler, L. (1980) 'The lifetime prevalence of mental disorders: estimation, uses and limitations', *Psychological Medicine* 10: 429–36.

Lilienfeld, A.M. and Lilienfeld, D.E. (1980) *Foundations of Epidemiology*, second edition, New York: Oxford University Press.

Link, B. and Dohrenwend, B.P. (1980) 'Formulation of hypotheses about the ratio of untreated to treated cases in the true prevalence studies of functional psychiatric disorders in adults in the United States', in *Epidemiological Estimates*, New York: Praeger.

MacMahon, B., Pugh, T.F., and Ipsen. J. (1980) *Epidemiologic Methods*, Boston, Mass: Little, Brown and Company.

Mausner, J.S. and Kramer, S. (1985) *Epidemiology: An Introductory Text*, Eastbourne, England: W.B. Saunders.

Miettinen, O. (1985) *Theoretical Epidemiology*, New York: Wiley.

Morris, J.N. (1975) *Uses of Epidemiology*, third edition, Edinburgh: Churchill Livingstone.

Murphy, J. (1980) 'Continuities in community-based psychiatric epidemiology', *Archives of General Psychiatry* 37: 1215–23.

Myers, J.K., Weissman, M.M., Tischler, G.L., *et al.* (1984) 'Six month prevalence of psychiatric disorders in three communities', *Archives of General Psychiatry* 41: 959–67.

National Center for Health Statistics (1975) *Health Interview Survey Procedures (1957–1974): Vital and Health Statistics*, Series 1, No. 11, Washington, DC: US Government Publishing Office.

Robins, L.N., Helzer, J.C., Orvaschel, H., *et al.* (1985) 'The Diagnostic Interview Schedule', in W.W. Eaton and L.G. Kessler (eds) *Epidemiologic Field Methods in Psychiatry: The NIMH Epidemiologic Catchment Area Program*, New York: Academic Press.

Robins, L.N., Helzer, J.E., Weissman, M.M., *et al.* (1984) 'Lifetime prevalence of specific psychiatric disorders in three sites', *Archives of General Psychiatry* 41: 949–58.

Sartwell, P.E., and Last, J.M. (1980) 'Epidemiology', in J.M. Last (ed.)

Maxcy-Rosenau Public Health and Preventive Medicine, eleventh edition, New York: Appleton-Century-Crofts, pp. 9–85.

Schlesselman, J.J. (1977) 'The effects of errors of diagnosis and frequency of examination on reported rates of disease', *Biometrics* 33: 635–42.

Schwartz, J.E. (1985) 'The neglected problem of measurement error in categorical data', *Sociological Methods and Research* 13: 435–66.

Shapiro, S., Skinner, E.A., Kessler, L.G., *et al.* (1984) 'Utilization of health and mental health services: three Epidemiologic Catchment Area sites', *Archives of General Psychiatry* 41: 971–8.

Shrout, P.E. and Fleiss, J.L. (1981) 'Reliability and case detection', in J.K. Wing, P. Bebbington, and L.N. Robins (eds) *What is a Case? The Problem of Definition in Psychiatric Community Surveys*, London: Grant McIntyre.

Tyrer, P. (1985) 'Neurosis divisible?', *Lancet* 1 (8430): 685–8.

Von Korff, M., Cottler, L., George, L.K., *et al.* (1985) 'Nonresponse and nonresponse bias in the ECA surveys', in W.W. Eaton and L.G. Kessler (eds) *Epidemiologic Field Methods in Psychiatry: The NIMH Epidemiologic Catchment Area Program*, New York: Academic Press.

Yanagawa, T. and Gladen, B. (1984) 'Estimating disease rates from a diagnostic test', *American Journal of Epidemiology* 119: 1015–23.

Part three

Identifying and assessing risk factors of mental disorders

Chapter eight

The aetiology of Alzheimer's disease: can epidemiology contribute?

A.S. Henderson

Introduction

For research on Alzheimer's disease (AD), the neurosciences and epidemiology are now in a position where mutual assistance towards progress is already taking place, a situation which has occurred before in psychiatry on only one occasion: the elucidation of pellagra (Goldberger 1914). The aims of this chapter are to review what is presently known about risk factors for AD and to consider what direction further epidemiological research should take. A stocktaking of the evidence now available may point towards testable hypotheses on aetiology. The information assembled here comes from three sources: surveys of general populations, descriptions of clinical series, and case-control studies. While the latter are the most efficient method for identifying risk factors, those conducted so far have been based on only moderately sized samples, with consequently limited power to identify risk factors with a high base rate in the controls. These are the studies by Bharucha *et al.* (1983), Heyman *et al.* (1984), French *et al.* (1985), Mortimer *et al.* (1985), Barclay *et al.* (1985), Amaducci *et al.* (1986), Shalat *et al.* (1986), and Chandra *et al.* (1986a, 1987). In this paper, AD occurring in the elderly will be referred to specifically as senile dementia of Alzheimer type (SDAT). Where no distinction is required, the generic term AD will be used.

Age

For the prevalence of undifferentiated dementia, there is agreement in all surveys that this increases with age. In a meta-analysis of twenty-two different studies, Jorm *et al.* (1987) found that the rate doubles every 4.5 years from 60–90 years of age for SDAT. An important question is whether the age-specific incidence rate also continues to climb, or if it decreases in late old age, as Gruenberg (1977) and Jarvik *et al.* (1980) suggested. There are two studies of the age-specific treated incidence of dementia: Helgason (1973) and Nielsen (1976), both reporting a steady rise with age. There are four sources of information on the age-specific incidence of specific dementias in general populations: Åkesson (1969); Mölsä *et al.* (1982); Hagnell *et al.* (1983); Rorsman *et al.* (1986). But these estimates are open to considerable lability, being based on very small denominators in the oldest age group. The conclusion must be that we do not yet know whether the incidence of AD does or does not decrease in the ninth and tenth decades of life.

At the level of neuropathology, Miller *et al.* (1984) reported changes with age in the density of both plaques and tangles in an autopsy series of 199 persons, finding that from age 71 years there was an abrupt, monotonic increase in the number of individuals with many of *both* lesions. On the basis of both the age-specific rates and the neuropathological findings, the conclusion must be that the process underlying Alzheimer-type dementia is increased in intensity with increasing age.

Sex

The meta-analysis by Jorm *et al.* (1987) found that the age-adjusted rates for women were significantly higher than for men. This female excess is confirmed by thirteen population surveys which report overall rates for AD by sex. The incidence data from Hagnell *et al.* (1983) and Rorsman *et al.* (1986) suggest a definitely higher rate in women. If this female excess in AD is accepted, the question for aetiology is what factors associated with being female could also promote the development of AD changes.

Ethnicity

Schoenberg *et al.* (1985) estimated the prevalence of AD (chronic progressive dementia) by clinical examination in the general population of Copiah County, Mississippi, finding higher prevalence rates for AD in Blacks. In their autopsy series, Miller *et al.* (1984) found no significant difference in the distribution of plaques and tangles in Blacks and in Whites. We shall return later to consider possible differences between Caucasian and Asian rates for AD.

Social class and education

Gurland (1981) has provided a lucid exposition of the evidence for a social-class gradient for dementia. He concluded that neither psychological tests nor clinical diagnosis can be accepted as culture-free indicators of a dementing process. The extent of their sociocultural biases is not known. Because of this, the new information, including the recent Epidemiologic Catchment Area (ECA) data, do not provide a conclusive answer. It is therefore an issue which deserves to be included in future surveys of dementia in general populations where the sample represents both those in the community and those in institutional care. A decisive study would be to investigate the mean density of plaques and of tangles across social classes, provided the autopsy material was on an unbiased sample.

Family history

It has consistently been found that first-degree relatives of AD cases have an increased incidence of dementia. This has been found for both presenile AD and SDAT, and has been taken to imply genetic transmission rather than some exposure shared by family members, although the latter is also conceivable. There is then the important question of what proportion of AD and of SDAT cases are sporadic, having no family history. At least half the cases seem to be sporadic (Heston et al. 1981). That is, a substantial number, possibly as many as half of all cases of AD and SDAT, may not have a primarily genetic basis. Some other pathogenic process, therefore, has to be invoked, although a genetic component is still possible.

Parental age

There are nine studies of parental age in dementia of Alzheimer type. All except one are of clinical samples. Only two of the nine studies have found positive results, with an upwards shift in maternal age which reached statistical significance. In the four studies where paternal age was examined, the findings were negative.

Fertility

In their Newcastle upon Tyne study, Kay et al. (1964) reported that their twenty-nine organic cases had had more children born than had normals or cases of functional psychiatric illness. Male organic cases had also had more children surviving. This is the only study which has reported such an increased fertility. Reduced fertility was found in the studies by Whalley et al. (1982), Coquoz (1984), and Gaillard (1984).

Down's syndrome in cases and in relatives

Heston et al. (1981) and Heyman et al. (1983, 1984) found an increased frequency of Down's syndrome in the families of Alzheimer-type cases of dementia, but there are five studies in which this association has not been found (Whalley et al. 1982; Nee et al. 1983; Barclay et al. 1985; Amaducci et al. 1986; Chandra et al. 1987).

Antecedents and co-morbidity

Information on antecedent diseases and co-morbidity may cast light on shared risk factors or aetiological processes. Larsson *et al.* (1963) asserted that 'There is no ground for concluding that previous somatic diseases are of any importance for the onset of senile dementia'. Kay *et al.* (1964) found that their organic cases had worse hearing and eyesight. Heyman *et al.* (1984) found a trend, not reaching statistical significance, towards a more frequent history of *herpes zoster*, blood transfusion, and previous psychiatric disorder in the cases. Analysis of the Framingham data by McWhorter and White (1987) revealed that in the cohort of 4,236 persons, the development of primary dementia was associated with a previous history of diabetes, inactivity, heart failure, or having less than one bowel movement a day. The relationship between AD and diabetes mellitus is unclear. While McWhorter and White found a positive association, Bucht *et al.* (1983) suggested the two conditions may not co-exist, having confirmed the observation by Adolfsson *et al.* (1980) that SDAT patients had higher insulin levels and appeared never to have diabetes.

Vascular dementia

Clinicians and neuropathologists are well aware that both AD and vascular dementia commonly co-exist, making for difficulty in clinical diagnosis. Tomlinson *et al.* (1970) estimated that about 18 per cent of their autopsy series of dementia were in this category. But it may be argued that if the two conditions are independent, their joint occurrence should be the product of their respective prevalence rates. This would be approximately 50 per cent $\times$ 17 per cent = 8.5 per cent using the Tomlinson estimates. Since the observed value is so much higher, it may be that the two dementias are not independent. One interpretation is that the clinical effects of mild AD and mild vascular dementia are additive, leading to an increased likelihood of recognizing their joint occurrence. An alternative hypothesis would be that the ischaemia of vascular dementia accelerates the pathogenesis of AD.

Thyroid disease

Heyman *et al.* (1983, 1984) reported an increased incidence of thyroid disease in the previous medical history of both their series. All of the AD cases who had had thyroid disease were female. This particular enquiry had been prompted by the finding of an association between Down's syndrome and thyroid disease in maternal relatives of people with the former (Fialkow *et al.* 1971). Six subsequent groups have included questions about thyroid disease, but had negative findings (Bharucha *et al.*

1983; French *et al.* 1985; Small *et al.* 1985; Barclay *et al.* 1985; Amaducci *et al.* 1986; Chandra *et al.* 1987).

Head injury

Three studies of AD have found an increased frequency of head injury in the previous history of cases compared to controls (Heyman *et al.* 1984; Mortimer *et al.* 1985; Shalat *et al.* 1986). In the study by Shalat *et al.* (1986), there was an increased frequency of head injury, but this did not reach statistical significance. Six other studies have not found the association (Soininen and Heinonen 1982; Bharucha *et al.* 1983; Sulkava *et al.* 1985; Barclay *et al.* 1985; Amaducci *et al.* 1986; Chandra *et al.* 1987). In the study by Soininen and Heinonen, a reverse association was found: six cases but thirteen controls had a history of head injury. Amaducci and his colleagues found more cases (n=13) than controls (n=5) with past head injury, but this difference did not reach statistical significance. Head injury has to be seen as a probable but unconfirmed risk factor in the light of the above evidence. In enquiring about previous head injury from relatives of a case of AD, there is a considerable risk of information bias.

Previous psychiatric disorder

A number of investigators have tested the hypothesis that the incidence of SDAT is higher in persons with a previous history of psychiatric disorder. Negative results have been reported by Larsson *et al.* (1963), Helgason (1973), and Soininen and Heinonen (1982). The latter study included information on previous use of major and minor tranquillizers. Heyman *et al.* (1984) noted a trend towards more previous psychiatric morbidity. French *et al.* (1985) found an odds ratio of 5.0 for depression compared to hospital controls. Barclay *et al.* (1985) also found an association with past depression.

Conditions associated with SDAT at death

Interest has been shown in those conditions which are present in persons dying of SDAT, in the expectation that these might provide a clue to the process of the dementia. The most comprehensive investigation has been by Chandra *et al.* (1986a, 1986b). They examined national data from death certificates in the USA in which AD and SDAT were mentioned. The increased prevalence of cataract and glaucoma are of interest since these are eye conditions associated with ageing, and the eye, like the brain, is ectodermal in origin.

135

Geographic distribution

Whalley and Holloway (1985) studied the spatial distribution of fifty-five cases of presenile AD in the city of Edinburgh, finding clustering in one postal sector. The evidence for urban-rural differences in dementia has been assembled by Jorm *et al.* (1987) in their meta-analysis of prevalence studies. They found three surveys of purely rural communities, each having significantly lower rates for dementia than in surveys of the urban elderly. These were the studies by Nielsen (1962), Jensen (1963), and Åkesson (1969). In the context of the ECA studies, Blazer *et al.* (1985) found a statistically higher rate for cognitive deficit on the Mini-Mental-State Examination in a rural compared to an urban population in North Carolina. But this difference was thought to be attributable to confounding by other variables, including age, race, and education, particularly the latter.

Regional variation

Gurland *et al.* (1983) and Copeland *et al.* (1987) reported the prevalence of dementia (not further differentiated) to be about twice as high in New York as in London. In the Mini-Finland Survey, Sulkava (1987) examined the prevalence of clinically diagnosed SDAT in persons aged 65 years and over in Finland. He reported higher rates in the north and the east of the country, both of which are more rural.

It is now widely recognized that a true difference may exist between Japan and western countries in the prevalence of SDAT and vascular dementia (WHO 1985). Jorm *et al.* (1987) found sixteen prevalence surveys which provided separate estimates for AD/SDAT and vascular dementia. The countries represented were Japan, the Soviet Union, Scandinavia, Britain, and the USA. They fitted a statistical model to these data, which showed that the Japanese and Russian rates were significantly higher for vascular dementia, the Finnish and US studies showed no significant difference, and the others showed an excess of AD/SDAT cases over vascular dementia. These regional differences could be due to diagnostic artefact. This could be excluded only by a specially mounted study which achieves standardized case-finding.

Exposures

A wide-ranging search has been made in several case-control studies into exposures such as farm animals, game, pets, viral infections, and travel in the South Pacific, all with negative findings. We now consider other exposures, summarized in Table 8.1.

Table 8.1 Proposed exposures in AD

Author	Exposure	Finding
Soininen and Heinonen (1982)	Smoking	−
French et al. (1985)	Smoking	−
Amaducci et al. (1986)	Smoking	−
Shalat et al. (1986)	Smoking	+
Chandra et al. (1987)	Smoking	−
Thygessen et al. (1970)	Malnutrition	+
Gibberd and Simmonds (1980)	Malnutrition	+
Abalan (1984)	Malnutrition	Hypothesis only
Murray et al. (1971)	Analgesics (phenacetin)	+
Heyman et al. (1984)	(phenacetin)	−
Amaducci et al. (1986)	(phenacetin)	−
Chandra et al. (1987)	(phenacetin)	−
Heyman et al. (1984)	Aluminium	−
Barclay et al. (1985)	Aluminium	−
French et al. (1985)	Aluminium	−
Amaducci et al. (1986)	Aluminium	−
Chandra et al. (1987)	Aluminium	−
Perl and Good (1987)	Aluminium	Hypothesis only
Axelson et al. (1976)	Organic solvents	+
Mikkelsen (1980)	Organic solvents	+
Nielsen et al. (1982)	Organic solvents	−
Heyman et al. (1984)	Organic solvents	−
Amaducci et al. (1986)	Organic solvents	−
French et al. (1985)	Organic solvents	−
Chandra et al. (1987)	Organic solvents	−
Deary et al. (1987)	Low calcium intake	Hypothesis only
Iivanainen (1975)	Vibratory tools[1]	+

[1] Proposed as a cause of cerebral atrophy, not specifically AD.

Smoking

Soininen and Heinonen (1982) found that smoking was more common in controls, but this did not reach statistical significance. In a comparison of ninety-two cases and 155 matched controls, Shalat *et al.* (1986) found an increased risk of AD among smokers, with an odds ratio of 2.3 and a statistically significant increase in risk with increased cigarette consumption. Three other studies have not found smoking to be a risk factor (French *et al.* 1985; Amaducci *et al.* 1986; Chandra *et al.* 1987).

Malnutrition

Cerebral atrophy with dementia has been reported in persons who have undergone extreme starvation, as in prisoner-of-war or concentration camps (e.g., Thygessen *et al.* 1970; Gibberd and Simmonds 1980). These observations have led Abalan (1984) to propose that an unrecognized state of malnutrition may be a cause of AD, though he did not make it clear how such malnutrition could take place in ordinary civilian life.

Analgesics

In an important paper, Murray *et al.* (1971) reported a high frequency of typical Alzheimer changes in patients who had ingested large amounts of phenacetin over many years. In an autopsy series, these changes were found to include plaques, tangles, and granulo-vacuolar degeneration, the distribution being characteristic of AD, with the hippocampus showing particular involvement. But in case-control studies following up this clue, no positive evidence has yet emerged. Neither Heyman *et al.* (1984), Amaducci *et al.* (1986), nor Chandra *et al.* (1987) found an increased frequency of analgesic use in their cases. On the other hand, no reports are yet available on the incidence of AD in cohorts of persons who have abused phenacetin.

Aluminium

The accumulation of aluminium in paired helical filaments has been well established since it was first reported by Crapper *et al.* (1973). It remains uncertain whether this is a primary or secondary phenomenon. Aluminium occurs as aluminosilicate in senile plaques (Candy *et al.* 1986). It has also been implicated in the dementia which follows renal dialysis (Dunea *et al.* 1978).

Heyman *et al.* (1984), Barclay *et al.* (1985), and French *et al.* (1985) found no increased frequency of peptic ulceration in their AD cases, a condition associated with the chronic ingestion of aluminium-containing antacids. Chandra *et al.* (1987) reported no difference for this exposure. Both Heyman *et al.* (1984) and Amaducci *et al.* (1986) enquired not only about stomach ulcer but also about habitual use of antacids, finding neither occurred more frequently in cases.

Concern about cooking pots as a source of aluminium was raised by Levick (1980). A crucial issue seems to be its bio-availability, little or no aluminium being absorbed from the gut (Mayor *et al.* 1977). Tennakone and Wickramanayake (1987) reported an experiment on leaching of aluminium from utensils, showing that this was enhanced nearly 1,000 times by the presence of trace quantities of fluoride. But this finding could not be replicated by Savory *et al.* (1987). Tap water may be another source of aluminium, particularly as many water supplies have large quantities of it added as a flocculant. The pH of water supplies, which will influence the solubility of aluminium, varies considerably. Acid rain in northern Europe has been considered as an aggravating factor (Pearce 1985; Samstag 1986).

Perl and Good (1987) have now proposed that AD involves a defect in the olfactory mucosa, leading to the influx of aluminium and possibly silicon into the brain. This suggestion is congruent with the finding by Serby *et al.* (1985) and others that there is olfactory dysfunction in AD.

Organic solvents

Some industrial solvents have neurotoxic properties (Browning 1965) and are therefore appropriate candidates as risk factors. Axelson *et al.* (1976) carried out a case-control study on 151 Swedish industrial workers registered with a pension fund and receiving a disability pension for some type of mental or neuropsychiatric disorder. Among the thirty-five persons exposed to organic solvents for thirty or more years, there were seven cases of presenile dementia. There were seventeen such cases in the 364 persons not exposed. This gives an odds ratio of 5.1. A major weakness in this study is the validity of the diagnosis of presenile dementia. This was apparently made by attending physicians, but no diagnostic criteria were specified.

Mikkelsen (1980) compared the incidence of neuropsychiatric morbidity, including presenile dementia, in a cohort of 2,601 male painters and 1,790 male bricklayers in Copenhagen, followed for five years. There was an increased incidence of presenile dementia recorded in the painters, but not of other neuropsychiatric disorders. The relative risk was 3.4. Both studies have the strength of being based on groups who may be at special risk, with a base-line exposure to a putative risk factor well above that likely to be encountered in a hospital-based case-control study. The positive finding for organic solvents in both studies has made it necessary to pursue this risk factor. Five subsequent studies have all had negative findings.

Calcium deficiency

Deary *et al.* (1987) have proposed that AD may be due to a low plasma calcium level, which in time causes disruption of intraneuronal microtubules. They reported a rank correlation of 0.488 between Mini-Mental State scores and serum calcium levels. A deficiency of calcium in soil and water has been implicated in the Guam Parkinson complex (Gajdusek 1985).

The contribution of epidemiology

In the array of possible risk factors reviewed here, the evidence from clinical epidemiology points to a number of hypotheses. The obvious relationship to age suggests that (1) in AD there is accumulation of some toxic substance; or (2) there is a time-dependent effect following the prior introduction of some toxic substance or infectious particle; or (3) there is an age-related decrease in a biological process necessary for normal neuronal function, and this may be accelerated by some environmental exposure or genetic vulnerability.

It is unlikely that an environmental exposure or genetic abnormality acts directly, but rather by accelerating some process which occurs in all ageing primate brains. For this it would be useful to know what structural and histochemical features there are in common for those brain areas selectively damaged in AD, and specifically, what is peculiar to the hippocampus.

There is then one further step which can be attempted in theory-building. The knowledge obtained so far about AD can be put to good use by our considering what some of the proposed risk factors have in common, as a single underlying process. One such process is proposed here, but it may be possible to identify several other candidates. Abnormal peroxidation with the formation of free oxygen radicals is known to increase with age, and with exposure to ischaemia, trauma, phenacetin, and organic solvents (Clark et al. 1985). Each of these occurs among the possible risk factors considered in this review. There are then a number of further observations, each consistent with the implication of free radicals in the pathogenesis of AD. The locus of the gene for superoxide dismutase is on the long arm of chromosome 21 near the Alzheimer locus (St George-Hyslop et al. 1987). Harman et al. (1976) earlier proposed a relationship between ageing of the brain and dietary fat. Harman (1985) suggested that lipid peroxidation may play a major role in the pathogenesis of AD, noting that lipofuscin is formed by the oxidative polymerization of lipids. He also noted that the brain is particularly vulnerable to free radicals. Next, lipofuscin has been found abundantly in cases of AD associated with phenacetin abuse (Murray et al. 1971). Harman (1985) also reported that free radical reactions are involved in the pathogenesis of amyloid. Clark et al. (1985) noted that insulin-dependent diabetes is associated with lipid peroxidation. Lastly, in their examination of the evidence from molecular biology, Beyreuther et al. (1988) conclude that 'theories and data which deal with lipid peroxidation, free radical attack and oxidative stress should be pursued'. Here is an example of a lead generated in the laboratory which could be pursued in epidemiology. Exposures should be sought which increase the likelihood of abnormal oxidative processes.

In short, there is both epidemiological and biological justification for testing the general hypothesis that risk factors for AD act by promoting the liberation of free oxygen radicals. Such a hypothesis is parsimonious in the light of the studies reviewed here; and it is useful as a guide to further work. It is known that free radicals can be trapped by substances such as Vitamin E (α-tocopherol) and selenium (Clark et al. 1985). If the hypothesis were upheld, therefore, it would lead to optimism for treatment and primary prevention. The latter, as Gruenberg has said in relation to pellagra, must be the ultimate service of epidemiology. It is nevertheless necessary to exercise caution about the free radical hypothesis, because abnormal peroxidation has already been widely invoked to explain a diversity of diseases besides AD. Alternative hypotheses are also needed, which must integrate the epidemiological findings. The latter are now substantial.

This paper is based on a larger review, published in *Acta Psychiatrica Scandinavica* (Henderson 1988).

References

Abalan, F. (1984) 'Alzheimer's disease and malnutrition: a new etiological hypothesis', *Medical Hypotheses* 15: 385–93.

Adolfsson, R., Bucht, G., Lithner, F., and Winblad, B. (1980) 'Hypoglycemia in Alzheimer's disease', *Acta Medica Scandinavica* 208: 387–8.

Åkesson, H.O. (1969) 'A population study of senile and arteriosclerotic psychoses', *Human Heredity* 19: 546–66.

Amaducci, L.A., Fratiglioni, L., Rocca, W.A., *et al.* (1986) 'Risk factors for clinically diagnosed Alzheimer's disease: a case control study of an Italian population', *Neurology* 36: 922–31.

Axelson, O., Hane, M., and Hogstedt, C. (1976) 'A case-reference study on neuropsychiatric disorders among workers exposed to solvents', *Scandinavian Journal of Work, Environment and Health* 2: 14–20.

Barclay, L.L., Kheyfets, S., Zemcov, A., Blass, J.P., and McDowell, F.H. (1985) 'Risk factors in Alzheimer's disease', in A. Fisher, I. Hanin, and D. Lachman (eds) *Alzheimer's and Parkinson's Diseases*, New York: Plenum, pp. 141–6.

Beyreuther, K., Beer, J., Hilbich, C., *et al.* (1988) 'Molecular pathology of amyloid deposition in Alzheimer's disease', in A.S. Henderson and J.H. Henderson (eds) *Etiology of Dementia of Alzheimer's Type*, Chichester: Wiley.

Bharucha, N.E., Schoenberg, B.S., and Kokmen, E. (1983) 'Dementia of Alzheimer's type (DAT): a case-control study of association with medical conditions and surgical procedures', *Neurology* 33: 85.

Blazer, D., George, L.K., Landerman, R., *et al.* (1985) 'Psychiatric disorders: a rural/urban comparison', *Archives of General Psychiatry* 42: 651–6.

Browning, E. (1965) *Toxicity and Metabolism of Industrial Solvents*, Amsterdam: Elsevier.

Bucht, G., Adolfsson, L.F., and Winblad, B. (1983) 'Changes in blood glucose and insulin secretion in patients with senile dementia of Alzheimer type', *Acta Medica Scandinavica* 213: 387–92.

Candy, J.M., Oakley, A.E., Klinowski, J., *et al.* (1986) 'Aluminosilicates and senile plaque formation in Alzheimer's disease', *Lancet* 15 February: 354–6.

Chandra, V., Bharucha, N.E. and Schoenberg, B.S. (1986a) 'Conditions associated with Alzheimer's disease at death: case-control study' *Neurology* 36: 209–11.

Chandra, V., Bharucha, N.E., and Schoenberg, B.S. (1986b) 'Patterns of mortality from types of dementia in the United States, 1971 and 1973–1978', *Neurology* 36: 204–8.

Chandra, V., Philipose, V., Bell, P.A., *et al.* (1987) 'Case-control study of late onset "probable Alzheimer's disease"', *Neurology* 37: 1295–300.

Clark, I.A., Cowden, W.B., and Hunt, N.H. (1985) 'Free radical-induced pathology', *Medical Research Reviews* 5: 297–332.

Copeland, J.R.M., Gurland, B.J., Dewey, M.E., *et al.* (1987) 'Is there more dementia, depression and neurosis in New York? A comparative community study of the elderly in New York and London, using the computer diagnosis, AGECAT', *British Journal of Psychiatry* 151: 466–73.

Coquoz, D. (1984) 'Epidemiology of senile dementia', in J. Wertheimer and M. Marois (eds) *Senile Dementia: Outlook for the Future*, New York: Alan R. Liss, pp. 427–41.

Crapper, D.R., Krishnan, S.S., and Dalton, A.J. (1973) 'Brain aluminium distribution in Alzheimer's disease and experimental neurofibrillary degeneration', *Science* 180: 511–13.

Deary, I.J., Hendrickson, A.E., and Burns, A. (1987) 'Serum calcium levels in Alzheimer's disease: a finding and an aetiological hypothesis', *Personality and Individual Differences* 8: 75–80.

Dunea, G., Mahurkar, S.D., Mamdani, B., and Smith, E.C. (1978) 'Role of aluminium in dialysis dementia', *Annals of Internal Medicine* 88: 502–4.

Fialkow, P.J., Thurline, H.C., Hecht, F., and Bryant, J. (1971) 'Familial predisposition to thyroid disease in Down's Syndrome: controlled immunoclinical studies', *American Journal of Human Genetics* 23: 67–86.

French, L.R., Schuman, L.M., Mortimer, J.A., *et al.* (1985) 'A case-control study of dementia of the Alzheimer type', *American Journal of Epidemiology* 121: 414–21.

Gaillard, M. (1984) 'Epidemiological elements in presenile Alzheimer's disease', in J. Wertheimer and M. Marois (eds) *Senile Dementia: Outlook for the Future*, New York: Alan R. Liss, pp. 411–25.

Gajdusek. D.C. (1985) 'Hypothesis: interference with axonal transport of neurofilament as a common pathogenetic mechanism in certain diseases of the central nervous system', *New England Journal of Medicine* 312: 714–19.

Gibberd, F.B. and Simmonds, J.P. (1980) 'Neurological disease in ex-Far-East prisoners of war', *Lancet* 19 July: 135–7.

Goldberger, J. (1914) 'The etiology of pellagra', *Public Health Report* 29: 1683.

Gruenberg, E.M. (1977) 'The failures of success', *Milbank Memorial Fund Quarterly* 55: 3–24.

Gurland, B.J. (1981) 'The borderlands of dementia: the influence of sociocultural characteristics on rates of dementia occurring in the senium', in N.E. Miller and G.D. Cohen (eds) *Clinical Aspects of Alzheimer's Disease and Senile Dementia: Aging 15*, New York: Raven Press, pp. 61–84.

Gurland, B., Copeland, J., Kuriansky, J., *et al.* (1983) *The Mind and Mood of Aging*, London: Croom Helm.

Hagnell, O., Lanke, J., Rorsman, B., *et al.* (1983) 'Current trends in the incidence of senile and multi-infarct dementia', *Archives of Psychiatry and Neurological Sciences* 233: 423–38.

Harman, D. (1985) 'Role of free radicals in aging and disease', in H.A. Johnson (ed.) *Relations Between Normal Aging and Disease,* New York: Raven Press, pp. 45–84.

Harman, D., Hendricks, S., Eddy, D.E. and Siebold, J. (1976) 'Free radical theory of aging: effect of dietary fat on central nervous system function', *Journal of the American Geriatric Society* 24: 301–7.

Helgason, T. (1973) 'Epidemiology of mental disorder in Iceland: a geriatric follow-up (preliminary report)', *Excerpta Medica International Congress Series* no. 274: 350–7.

Henderson, A.S. (1988) 'The risk factors for Alzheimer's disease: a review and a hypothesis', *Acta Psychiatrica Scandinavica* 78: 257–75.
Heston, L.L. Mastri, A.R., Anderson, V.E., and White, J. (1981) 'Dementia of the Alzheimer type: clinical genetics, natural history and associated conditions', *Archives of General Psychiatry* 30: 1085–90.
Heyman, A., Wilkinson, W.E., Hurwitz, B.J., *et al.* (1983) 'Alzheimer's disease: genetic aspects and associated clinical disorders', *Annals of Neurology* 14: 507–15.
Heyman, A., Wilkinson, W.E., Stafford, J.A., *et al.* (1984) 'Alzheimer's disease: a study of epidemiological aspects', *Annals of Neurology* 15: 335–41.
Iivanainen, M. (1975) 'Statistical correlations of diffuse cerebral atrophy, with special reference to diagnostic and aetiological clues', *Acta Neurologica Scandinavica* 51: 365–79.
Jarvik, L.F., Ruth, V., and Matsuyama, S.S. (1980) 'Organic brain syndrome and aging: a six-year follow-up of surviving twins', *Archives of General Psychiatry* 37: 280–6.
Jensen, K. (1963) 'Psychiatric problems in four Danish old age homes', *Acta Psychiatrica Scandinavica* Supplement 169: 411–19.
Jorm, A.F., Korten, A.E., and Henderson, A.S. (1987) 'The prevalence of dementia: a quantitative integration of the literature', *Acta Psychiatrica Scandinavica* 76: 465–79.
Kay, D.W.K., Beamish, P., and Roth, M. (1964) 'Old age mental disorders in Newcastle upon Tyne, part II: a study of possible social and medical causes', *British Journal of Psychiatry* 110: 668–82.
Larsson, T., Sjogren, T. and Jacobson, G. (1963) 'Senile dementia: a clinical, sociomedical and genetic study', *Acta Psychiatrica Scandinavica* Supplement 167: 1–259.
Levick, S.E. (1980) 'Dementia from aluminium pots?', *New England Journal of Medicine* 303: 164.
McWhorter, W. and White, L. (1987) 'Risk factors for dementia in a national longitudinal study: preliminary findings', paper presented to a NIMH Workshop, Bethesda, June.
Mayor, G.H., Keiser, J.A., Makdani, D., and Ku, P.K. (1977) 'Aluminium absorption and distribution: effect of parathyroid hormone', *Science* 197: 1187–9.
Mikkelsen, S. (1980) 'A cohort study of disability pension and death among painters with special regard to disabling presenile dementia as an occupational disease', *Scandinavian Journal of Social Medicine* 16: 34–43.
Miller, D.F., Hicks, S.P., D'Amato, C.J. and Landis, J.R. (1984) 'A descriptive study of neuritic plaques and neurofibrillary tangles in an autopsy population', *American Journal of Epidemiology* 120: 331–41.
Mölsa, P.K., Marttila, R.J. and Rinne, U.K. (1982) 'Epidemiology of dementia in a Finnish population', *Acta Neurologica Scandinavica* 65: 541–52.
Mortimer, J.A., French, L.R., Hutton, J.T., and Schuman, L.M. (1985) 'Head injury as a risk factor for Alzheimer's disease', *Neurology* 35: 264–7.
Murray, R.M., Greene, J.G., and Adams, J.H. (1971) 'Analgesic abuse and dementia', *Lancet* 31 July: 242–5.
Nee, L.E., Polinsky, R.J., Eldridge, R., *et al.* (1983) 'A family with histologically confirmed Alzheimer's disease', *Archives of Neurology* 40: 203–8.
Nielsen, J. (1962) 'Geronto-psychiatric period-prevalence investigation in a geographically delimited population', *Acta Psychiatrica Scandinavica* 38: 307–30.
Nielsen, J. (1976) 'The Samsø project from 1957 to 1974', *Acta Psychiatrica Scandinavica* 54: 198–222.

Nielsen, B., Gunner-Svensson, F., Friborg, S., and Olsen, J. (1982) 'Praevalens af svaer demens blandt aeldrei Odense kommune 1972', *Fagligt og Socialt* 144/146: 3455–7.

Pearce, F. (1985) 'Acid rain may cause senile dementia', *New Scientist* 25 April: 7.

Perl, D.P. and Good, P.F. (1987) 'Uptake of aluminium into central nervous system along nasal-olfactory pathways', *Lancet* 2 May: 1028.

Rorsman, B., Hagnell, O., and Lanke, J. (1986) 'Prevalence and incidence of senile and multi-infarct dementia in the Lundby Study: a comparison between the time periods 1947–1957 and 1957–1972', *Neuropsychobiology* 15: 122–9.

Samstag, T. (1986) 'Acid rain linked to senility disease', *The Times*, 4 November.

Savory, J., Nicholson, J.R., and Wills, M.R. (1987) 'Is aluminium leaching enhanced by fluoride?', *Nature* 327: 107–8.

Schoenberg, B.S., Anderson, D.A., and Haerer, A.F. (1985) 'Severe dementia: prevalence and clinical features in a biracial US population', *Archives of Neurology* 42: 740–3.

Serby, M., Corwin, J., Conrad, P., and Rotrosen, J. (1985) 'Olfactory dysfunction in Alzheimer's disease and Parkinson's disease', *American Journal of Psychiatry* 142: 781–2.

Shalat, S.L., Seltzer, B., Pidcock, C., and Baker, E.L. (1986) 'A case-control study of medical and familial history and Alzheimer's disease', *American Journal of Epidemiology* 124: 540.

Small, G.W., Matsuyama, S.S., Komanduri, R., *et al.* (1985) 'Thyroid disease in patients with dementia of the Alzheimer type', *Journal of the American Geriatric Society* 33: 538–9.

Soininen, H. and Heinonen, O.P. (1982) 'Clinical and etiological aspects of senile dementia', *European Neurology* 21: 401–10.

St George-Hyslop, P.H., Tanzi, R.E., Polinsky, R.J., *et al.* (1987) 'The genetic defect causing familial Alzheimer's disease maps on chromosome 21', *Science* 235: 885–90.

Sulkava, R. (1987) 'Epidemiology of Alzheimer's disease', paper presented to a NIMH Workshop, Bethesda, June.

Sulkava, R., Erkinjuntti, T., and Palo, J. (1985) 'Head injuries in Alzheimer's disease and vascular dementia', *Neurology*, 35: 1084.

Tennakone, K. and Wickramanayake, S. (1987) 'Aluminium leaching from cooking utensils', *Nature* 325: 202.

Thygessen, P., Hermann, K., and Willanger, R. (1970) 'Concentration camp survivors in Denmark', *Danish Medical Bulletin* 17: 65–108.

Tomlinson, B., Blessed, G., and Roth, M. (1970) 'Observations on the brains of demented old people', *Journal of Neurological Sciences* 11: 205–42.

Whalley, L.J. and Holloway, S. (1985) 'Non-random geographical distribution of Alzheimer's presenile dementia in Edinburgh, 1953–76', *Lancet* 9 March: 578.

Whalley, L.J., Carothers, A.D., Collyer, S., *et al.* (1982) 'A study of familial factors in Alzheimer's disease', *British Journal of Psychiatry* 140: 249–56.

World Health Organization (1985) *Dementia in Later Life: Research and Action*, Technical Report Series, 730, 7–77, Geneva: WHO.

Chapter nine

Family mobility as a risk for childhood psychopathology

Patricia Cohen, Jim Johnson, Elmer L. Struening, and Judith S. Brook

Introduction

Some of the earliest investigations in the field of psychiatric epidemiology included a major interest in the association between residential instability, migration, and mental illness (Malzberg 1940; Ødegaard 1932; Tietze *et al.* 1942). It has also long been known that there are mental health risks associated with refugee status, and the effects of separation of young children from their parents have been investigated consistently from the earliest studies of child psychiatric epidemiology. However, there has been relatively little investigation of the potential mental health risk to children associated with the more ordinary residential relocations of families. Yet residential mobility of individual family units is actually normative in some contemporary societies, as in the United States, where about half of all children in middle to late childhood have moved one or more times in a five-year period, and about 20 per cent in any given year. Although residential mobility rates are not increasing, this pattern is now an established part of American family life. As the problem of a shortage of low-income housing has become acute, both in the United States and in many European countries, it is increasingly important to understand the effects of residential instability on children, so that problems associated with this aspect of family homelessness can be estimated.

It seems likely that even when children are part of voluntary rather than forced family moves they may undergo some risk (Tooley 1970). Indeed, in middle-class America one frequently hears of families who remain in a location in order not to disrupt their children's school and social settings, on the assumption that these changes would involve some risk to the children. Moving companies publish recommendations to parents based on the assumption of risk for children (Jalongo 1985).

The literature on the effects of residential changes on children is fairly inconsistent. Several studies have identified a negative impact of frequent or recent moves on achievement levels (Feiner *et al.* 1981; Long 1975; Schaller 1975; Tetreau and Fuller 1942), whereas others have found no effect (Collins and Coulter 1974; Downie 1953) or even a positive effect (Goebel 1981) of residential change on academic achievement and measured intelligence. Similarly, although the majority of studies report associations between residential changes and indices of mental ill-health and negative self image (Gibbs 1985; Kroger 1980; Price 1965; Sagy and Antonovsky 1986; Schaller 1974; Shaw 1979; Shaw and Pangman 1975), as well as increased risk of accidents (Knudson-Cooper and Leuchtag 1982), there are also suggestions that such effects may be quite transitory (Sagy and Antonovsky 1986; Schaller 1974) or, in some circumstances, even positive (Tooley 1970; Van Dongen 1981). Some of these inconsistencies are doubtless due to the failure of the investigators to examine the issue of whether families who moved differed in relevant respects prior to the residential change, or whether the children's problems may have been present before the move.

Studies of effects of residential change on adults are similarly inconsistent (e.g., Ebata *et al.* 1983; Heller 1982; Schwab *et al.* 1978–9). Inferences drawn from investigations of residential change and instability in adults are inevitably constrained by the fact that mentally ill adults may move because they are mentally ill, rather than become mentally ill because they move. No previous studies have used a prospective longitudinal controlled design to investigate this problem. Furthermore, because children usually have little influence on decisions regarding family relocation, the potential problem of confounding the dependent variable with the risk factor is not present in these analyses.

There are a number of reasons why residential relocations may be a risk factor for childhood psychopathology. First, children, like adults, are likely to experience a loss of social network when the family moves (Donohue and Gullota 1983). It is this risk, as well as other adaptations required by a new setting (Northwood 1975), that accounts for the inclusion of moving as a potential stressful life event in all lists of such events (e.g., Coddington 1972).

Second, children are quite responsive to parental, and especially to maternal, depression and associated symptoms. For some of the same reasons as the children, and also because of the additional strains and stresses associated with moving and re-establishing the household, parents, particularly mothers, may be demoralized following a relocation. Therefore, either by direct modelling or as a consequence of a temporary decline in the quality of parenting, children may become symptomatic because a parent does.

A third reason for mental health problems is connected with the central role of school in the lives of children. Relocation, and especially frequent relocations, may cause difficulties at school, as curriculum and standards vary across settings. As is well known, scholastic problems are very often connected with a variety of mental health problems in children, including depression, separation anxiety, and conduct disorder (Berger *et al.* 1975; Rutter 1964).

Yet another potential reason for the association between relocation and disorder, and especially conduct disorder, lies in the weakening of social bonds and standards that is at least a temporary consequence of living in a district where one knows few people. A kind of 'mini-anomie' or loosening of the ties to society may often characterize the period following a relocation in an unfamiliar setting. If so, it is also plausible that children who experience frequent moves may develop less strong identification with the norms of the local community, and be at increased risk of conduct disorder, regardless of the timing of the most recent move. In these children, anomie may consolidate into more lasting attitudes of alienation from society.

In addition to these theoretical reasons why relocation itself may be a risk for children, there are also reasons why residential moves might be related to childhood psychopathology as an artefact of common causes. First, one time when children are more likely to move is when their parents divorce. Since divorce itself is a risk factor for childhood psychopathology (Guidubaldi *et al.* 1983; Hetherington *et al.* 1985; Wallerstein 1984), it follows that an apparent relationship between relocation and psychopathology may be attributed to that subset of children whose parents are separating.

Another possible artefact connecting childhood psychopathology and relocation is family poverty. If poor families are more likely to move often because of more tenuous connections to employment and housing, poverty could be the cause of a spurious relationship.

The present study was designed to explore these relationships, as well as the effects of potential moderating influences, in a large epidemiological sample of children. The analyses will examine effects of residential relocation on the frequency of psychopathology first in early and middle childhood, and then, using a longitudinal design, during late childhood and adolescence. The emphasis will be on the latter period, when it is easier to control for children's preceding problems.

Research method

The sample

Nine hundred and seventy-six mothers were successfully interviewed from a random sample of 1,141 families with one or more children between the ages of one and ten years living in two upstate New York counties, a response rate of 85.5 per cent (Kogan *et al.* 1977). In these interviews, completed in 1975, one randomly selected child was selected as the study child. Eight years later families were recontacted and asked to participate in further interviews with a parent and the selected child. Eighty-four per cent of the sample were traced, and 74 per cent successfully re-interviewed in their homes, wherever in the United States they were then living. Those lost to follow-up included proportionately more of the poor, urban dwellers, and families with children aged 1 to 4 at the time of the original interviews. Therefore a new random sample was drawn from poor, urban neighbourhoods in an attempt to improve the match of characteristics of the follow-up sample with those of the original geographical area. Fifty-four new families, each including a child between the ages of 9 and 12, the age of the youngest children in the follow-up sample, were interviewed.

Table 9.1 provides an overview of the demographic characteristics of the combined sample at the time of the 1983–4 interviews. With regard to parental education, occupation, family income, and marital status, the sample is broadly representative of families with children in the north-eastern section of the United States. Families ranged from the very poor to the wealthy, and lived in both urban and rural areas. However, only 4 per cent of the children were black and there was only one Hispanic child, limitations due to the characteristics of the sampled counties.

Table 9.1 Demographic characteristics of the follow-up sample (N = 778)

1983 Median family income	$23,000
% White	92
% Catholic	55
% Families intact	68
Maternal mean years of education	13
% mothers employed full time	41
% mothers employed part time	19
% mothers not employed	40

In the current analyses, only families in which both the child and a maternal caretaker could be interviewed were included. Children in paternal custody, or in the care of other relatives or non-relatives were excluded, as the effects of these special life circumstances would potentially have confounded the investigation of residential changes. The resulting sample was comprised of 711 children.

Methods of measurement

Residential mobility was measured by two questions answered by the mothers in each interview. The first concerned the number of years the family had lived at the current address. In this sample 7.3 per cent had moved in the previous year, nearly 10 per cent had lived in their current residence one to three years, 14 per cent three to five years, and 69 per cent more than five years. These rates of moving are lower than the national average, both because we were less likely to locate those who had moved, and especially frequent movers, and because the area sampled is somewhat more stable than other sections of the country or large metropolitan areas.

A second question asked how many times the family had moved in the previous eight years. On the average families had moved nearly exactly once. However, the distribution was quite skewed, with half the families not having moved at all, and over 5 per cent having moved four or more times. For the logistic regression analysis of diagnosis the measures were dichotomized according to whether or not the family had moved in the past year and whether the family had moved four or more times in the past five years. Logistic regressions were also carried out including additional categories of risk status, but without change in the findings reported here.

The measures of psychopathology in early childhood included conduct problems (including sub-scales of anger, aggression towards peers, temper-tantrums, and, for older children, pre-delinquent behaviours), anxiety, affective disturbance, and social isolation (with four questions regarding the child's contacts with peers), maternal psychiatric symptoms (as measured by the Hopkins Symptom Checklist (Derogatis *et al.* 1974)), and poor scholastic achievement as reported by both mother and child. Finally, the intervening variables and additional measures reflecting the quality of the parent-child interaction and parenting techniques were examined as potential moderators of stress associated with residential instability. These included communication with the mother, autonomy from the parents, power-assertive punishment by the mother, father involvement with the child, parental harmony, and the amount of time spent by the mother with the child.

Findings

Relationship of residential instability with other known risk factors

Early to middle childhood A history of frequent moves, though not recent moving, was found to be associated with divorce ($t = 5.39$, $657df$) and greater use of power-assertive punishment ($t = 2.40$, $657df$) in early and middle childhood once the effects of age and sex were partialled out. Neither relocation variable was significantly related to socio-economic status during that period. A history of frequent moves tended to be related to poor achievement ($t = 1.70$, 396 df. $p <.10$), although recent moving was not.

Late childhood and adolescence At the time of follow-up, frequent moves, though not recent moves, were related to socio-economic status, those of low status having moved more frequently (beta $= .11$, $t = 2.99$, $707df$.) Both recency and frequency of moving were related to divorce and remarriage. On average over the previous five years, divorced families had moved an additional half time more often than intact families, and had lived in their current residence about eight months less (ts = 3.70 and 7.47 respectively, 707 df); families with stepfathers had moved an additional one-quarter time and had lived in their current residence about six months less (ts = 1.29 and 4.04 respectively, 707 df).

Table 9.2 presents the relationships of residential change variables to some other possible risk factors. As can be seen, only one of these was significantly elevated in these logistic regression analyses. Social isolation was nearly 2.4 times as prevalent in children who had moved in the past year as for those without such a recent move (after controlling for age, sex, and socio-economic status). In ordinary regression analyses frequent moving was also found to be a weak predictor of maternal psychiatric symptoms (B = .08, p > .05). None of these relationships with other risks varied significantly as a function either of age or of sex.

Table 9.2 Prevalence ratios for other risk factors for children who have or have not moved home

	Total sample rate	Recent movers odds	Frequent movers odds
Friendless	0.06	1.72	0.46
Socially isolated	0.08	2.39[1]	0.76
Poor school achievement	0.18	1.36	1.12
Maternal high symptom score	0.17	0.98	1.51

[1]P < .05. All effects are comparisons with the residentially stable group, net of age, sex, and SES.

Relationship with psychopathology, controlling for age, sex, and socio-economic status

Early to middle childhood Frequent moving was related to immaturity assessed by maternal report when the children were ages one to ten (t = 2.49, 659 df). It was not, however, related to behavioural, anxiety, or affective disturbance (t = 1.15, 1.60, and 1.15 respectively, with 654 df). Furthermore, frequent moves during early childhood were not related to immaturity as assessed at follow-up; apparently, problems of immaturity reported for these children in the original interviews were only temporary, or at any rate did not last as long as eight years.

Recent moving was not related to any of the symptom measures as reported by mothers when the children were one to ten years old. Nor did any of the findings vary as a function of the age or sex of the child at the time of the original interviews.

Late childhood and adolescence Table 9.3 presents the relative risks for childhood psychopathology associated with frequent and recent changes in the family residence. As can be seen, only conduct disorder was significantly elevated, and both recent and frequent changes were found to be associated with the frequency of this type of disorder. However, when socio-economic status was held constant the association with frequent moving was found to disappear, and will therefore not be considered further here.

Table 9.3 Relative risk of psychopathology in late childhood and adolescence associated with recent and frequent moves

	Total sample rate	Recent movers odds	Frequent movers odds
Attention deficit	0.12	0.72	0.53
Oppositional	0.16	1.36	0.33
Overanxious	0.14	0.91	1.00
Separation anxiety	0.12	0.64	0.83
Conduct disorder	0.13	3.53[1]	2.45[1]

[1] $P < .05$, net of effects of age, sex, and SES.

Symptoms of depression measured in the follow-up interviews also tended to be related to frequent moving ($r = .08$, $p < .05$). This relationship also was entirely attributable to the relationship of low socio-economic status to frequent moving and depression, and we conclude therefore that it was not causal. Because major depression had been experienced by no more than 3 per cent of the sample, the number of cases was insufficient for logistic regression; therefore the relationship reported here is the correlation with the scaled measure of depressive symptoms.

Although we have argued that psychopathology in children is unlikely to be the cause of family relocation, severe conduct problems may constitute a possible exception. In order to check on this possibility we examined the relationship between conduct problems in early childhood and the recording of either frequent or recent family moves in the follow-up data. Although conduct problems were related to subsequent frequent moves, this relationship was also entirely accounted for by the relationship of both with low socio-economic status.

The relationship of recent moving with conduct disorder was found not only in the cross-sectional data, but even more strongly when early behavioural problems were taken into account, with the resulting provisional inference of a causal role of recent moving in conduct disorder. That is, a history of a recent change of residence is associated with a raised frequency of conduct disorders, and this finding appears to be due to an increase in conduct disorders among the children concerned following the move.

The above relationships did not vary as a function of the age or sex of the child. For the symptom measures in early childhood, increases in risk were similar for the different age and sex groups. During late childhood and adolescence the *relative risks* were similar for all ages and for boys as compared to girls. This is consistent with the observation that the *absolute* risk of conduct disorder went up more for boys than for girls, since the base rate for boys was about double that for girls.

Further analyses of the relationship of recency of moving to conduct disorder

Potential mediators   Table 9.4 presents the changes in relative risk associated with having moved in the previous year, controlling for potential confounding and mediating variables. In the first logistic regression equation, behaviour problems as measured in the earlier assessment were controlled, as well as age, sex, and socio-economic status. The risk of diagnosable conduct disorder in children who had moved in the previous year on these variables was over three times the risk of those whose families had not recently moved, but who were otherwise comparable.

Table 9.4 Changes in risk of conduct disorder associated with recent moving, controlling for potential confounding and mediating variables

Covariates	Relative risk	95% Confidence interval
Time 1 conduct disorder, age, sex, socio-economic status	3.14[1]	1.82 – 6.18
+ divorce, remarriage, poor school achievement	3.03[1]	1.38 – 6.68
+ maternal symptoms, social isolation	2.87[1]	1.27 – 6.47

[1] $p < .01$

Adding divorce and remarriage to the equation, as well as failure in school achievement, demonstrated that, although these characteristics were associated with residential instability, this relationship did not explain the distribution of conduct disorders. A third analysis, in which maternal demoralization and social isolation were added to the equation, again left the direct association between conduct disorder and a recent residential move only slightly reduced. Other known risks, originally hypothesized as potential mediators or moderators but not empirically related to recent moving, were also examined for their influence on the relative risk (analyses not shown here). Inclusion of these factors, which included duration of friendships, use of power-assertive punishment, presence of parental conflicts, and several aspects of parent-child relationships, left the estimation of relative risk essentially unchanged.

Potential moderators It was hypothesized that the children of families who had recently moved home would be at less risk for conduct disorder if they reported having many friends than if they were isolated. There were two reasons for this expectation, the first of which concerns the expected effect of low social support, while the second is of a more technical nature. Since we didn't know how far the family had moved, a high friendship index would serve to identify children whose families had relocated within the same community or school district, so that effects on the children should be minimal if present at all. However, contrary to expectation, the statistical findings suggested a very different explanation. Children who had lived many years at the same address, and yet had few friends, were at the greatest risk for conduct disorder. Those who had moved recently and had few friends were at less risk than this 'chronically' socially isolated group.

We also investigated potential interactions of several other variables with recent moving, to determine whether school failure, communication or involvement with parents, autonomy as compared to close supervision, or some other aspect of the family environment may moderate the risk of conduct disorder associated with having recently moved. None of these effects were statistically significant.

Thus we have no clear findings from among our measured variables to serve as a basis for recommending actions parents may take to mitigate the (temporary) risk of behaviour disorder symptoms following a residential move. Such potentially risk-moderating behaviours on the part of parents did not appear to be increased following a move, possibly because the parents were also experiencing increased stress and overwork at this time.

Summary and conclusions

One limitation on the current findings is posed by the fact that the portion of the sample lost to follow-up, all of whom had moved, may have included a higher proportion whose moves were traumatic for their children than did those actually examined in the present study. The families in this drop-out group were, on average, younger, more urban, and poorer than those on whom the data analysis is based. However, because the current findings are not conditional on either age or income, this bias may not be serious.

The analyses show that children in their early and middle childhood years living in families who moved frequently exhibited a variety of signs of immature behaviour, including attention-span problems and physical ineptitude. These problems appear to diminish over time and were no longer evident in late childhood or adolescence. In spite of the plausibility of the hypothesis, we found no evidence of an increased risk of psycho-pathology in older children in frequently moving families.

Children of ages 9 to 18 whose families had moved recently were about three times as likely to exhibit a diagnosable conduct disorder as those whose families had not, *ceteris paribus*. This risk was not an artefact of family dissolution or remarriage. It was associated with certain other risk factors, but its relationship to conduct disorder was not explained by them. Nor were any of the potential moderators of the impact of recent moving significant. Apparently this risk is not present in early childhood, probably because it involves behaviours that are uncommon at these ages.

The nature of the children's disturbance, and the apparent short period of vulnerability, leads us to hypothesize that relocation may lead to a temporary lessening of the constraints on behaviour usually associated with an extrafamilial environment that the child knows and in which the child and family are known. A number of authors have noted the importance of an attachment to the community and to its norms in prevention of behavioural problems (e.g., Wilson and Herrnstein 1985). In the period during which these attachments are being newly developed following a move, children may have a heightened risk for a variety of misbehaviours. Some of these may involve peers, either because the youth has not yet settled into a peer group or because deviant peers may be more accessible to young people who have recently arrived than are more socially normal peers. In these circumstances the recently moved child may exhibit symptoms of conduct disorder to a degree not predictable from other risks.

On the other hand, these findings suggest that we may have to think about residential change in a more differentiated fashion. On the whole children seemed to be resilient to such changes, even when they have occurred frequently. Of course it is likely that in many instances a family move will signal an improvement in living standards, and especially in the quality of housing. But even independently of possible improvements, residential changes give many children the opportunity for a fresh start. Particularly when children are having difficulties in school or with their peers, they may acquire a damaging reputation that is difficult to shake off without such a move. Perhaps, therefore, it is not surprising that potential increases in anxiety or problems in self-control associated with these changes should be offset by potential improvements in the same areas. In order to test this hypothesis, behavioural changes associated with moving will have to be investigated using a much shorter time frame than the eight-year interval used in the current study.

Acknowledgement

This study was supported by grants from the National Institute of Mental Health, the National Institute of Drug Abuse, and the William T. Grant Foundation, as well as by the New York State Office of Mental Health.

References

Berger, M., Yule, W., and Rutter, M. (1975) 'Attainment and adjustment in two geographic areas. II: The prevalence of specific reading retardation', *British Journal of Psychiatry* 126: 520–33.

Coddington, R.D. (1972) 'The significance of life events as etiologic factors in the diseases of children', *Journal of Psychosomatic Research* 16: 7–18.

Cohen, P. and Brook, J. (1987) 'Family factors related to the persistence of psychopathology in childhood and adolescence', *Psychiatry* 50: 332–45.

Cohen, P., O'Connor, P., Lewis, S.A., and Malachowski, B. (1987) 'A comparison of the agreement between DISC and K-SADS-P interviews of an epidemiological sample of children', *Journal of the American Academy of Child and Adolescent Psychiatry* 26: 662–7.

Cohen. P., Velez, C.N., Kohn, M., Schwab-Stone, M., and Johnson, J. (1987) 'Child psychiatric diagnosis by computer algorithm: theoretical issues and empirical tests', *Journal of the American Academy of Child and Adolescent Psychiatry* 26: 631–8.

Collins, J.M. and Coulter, F. (1974) 'Effects of geographic movement on the social and academic development of children of army personnel', *The Australian and New Zealand Journal of Sociology* 10: 222–3.

Costello, A., Edelbrock, C.S., Dulcan, M.K., Kalas, R., and Klaric, S.H. (1984) *Report on the NIMH Diagnostic Interview Schedule for Children (DISC)*, Department of Psychiatry, University of Pittsburgh.

Derogatis, L.R., Lipman, R.S., Rickels, K., Uhlenhuth, E.H., and Covi, L. (1974) 'The Hopkins Symptom Checklist (HSCL)', *Behavioral Science* 19: 1–15.

Donohue, K.C. and Gullota, T.P. (1983) 'The coping behaviors of adolescents following a move', *Adolescence* 18: 391–401.

Downie, N.M. (1953) 'A comparison between children who have moved from school to school with those who have been in continuous residence on various factors of adjustment', *Journal of Educational Psychology* 44: 50–3.

Ebata, K., Yoshimatsu, K., Miguchi, M., and Ozaki, A. (1983) 'Impact of migration on onset of mental disorders in relation to duration of residence', *American Journal of Social Psychiatry* 3: 25–32.

Feiner, R.D., Primavera, J., and Cauce, A.M. (1981) 'The impact of school transitions: a focus for preventive efforts', *American Journal of Community Psychology* 9: 449–59.

Gibbs, J.T. (1985) 'Psychosocial factors associated with depression in urban adolescent females: implications for assessment', *Journal of Youth and Adolescence* 14: 47–60.

Goebel, B.L. (1981) 'Mobile children: an American tragedy?', *Psychological Reports* 48: 15–18.

Guidubaldi, J., Cleminshaw, H.K., Perry, J.P., and Mcloughlin, C.S. (1983) 'The impact of parental divorce on children: report of the nationwide NASP study', *School Psychology Review* 12: 300–23.

Heller, T. (1982) 'The effects of involuntary residential relocation: a review', *American Journal of Community Psychology* 10: 471–92.

Hetherington, M.E., Cox. M., and Cox, R. (1985) 'Long-term effects of divorce and adjustment of children', *Journal of the American Academy of Child Psychiatry* 24: 518–30.

Jalongo, M.R. (1985) 'When young children move', *Young Children* September: 51–7.

Knudson-Cooper, M.S. and Leuchtag, A.K. (1982) 'The stress of a family move as a precipitating factor in children's burn accidents', *Journal of Human Stress* 8: 32–8.

Kogan, L.S., Smith, J., and Jenkins, S. (1977) 'Ecological validity of indicator data as predictors of survey findings', *Journal of Social Service Research* 1: 117–32.

Kroger, J.E. (1980) 'Residential mobility and self-concept in adolescence', *Adolescence* 15: 967–77.

Long, L.H. (1975) 'Does migration interfere with children's progress in school?', *Sociology of Education* 48: 369–81.

Malzberg, B. (1940) *Social and Biological Aspects of Mental Disease*, Utica, New York: State Hospital Press.

Northwood, L.K. (1975) 'The impact of urban removal from a child's point of view', *Journal of Sociology and Social Welfare* 3: 224–41.

Ødegaard, Ø. (1932) 'Emigration and insanity', *Acta Psychologica Neurologica*, Supplement No. 4.

Price, D.O. (1965) 'Next steps in studying mobility and mental health', in M.B. Kandtor (ed.) *Mobility and Mental Health*, Springfield Ill: Charles C. Thomas, pp. 238–47.

Rutter, M. (1964) 'Intelligence and childhood psychiatric disorder', *British Journal of Social and Clinical Psychology* 3: 120–9.

Sagy, S. and Antonovsky, H. (1986) 'Adolescents' reactions to the evacuation of the Sinai settlements: a longitudinal study', *Journal of Psychology* 120: 543–56.

Schaller, J. (1974) 'Experienced and expected problems reported by children after a family move', *Goteberg Psychological Reports* 4: 12.

Schaller, J. (1975) 'The relation between geographic mobility and school behavior', *Man-Environment Systems* 5: 185–7.

Schwab, J.J., Bell, R.A., Warheit, G.J., Schwab, R.B., and Traven, N.D. (1978–9). 'Some epidemiological aspects of psychosomatic medicine', *International Journal of Psychiatry in Medicine*, 9: 147–58.

Shaw, J.A. (1979) 'Adolescents in the mobile military community', *Adolescent Psychiatry* 7: 191–8.

Shaw, J.A. and Pangman, J. (1975) 'Geographic mobility and the military child', *Military Medicine* 140: 413–16.

Tetreau, E.D. and Fuller, V. (1942) 'Some factors associated with the school achievement of children in migrant families', *Elementary School Journal* 42: 423–31.

Tietze, C., Lemkau, P., and Cooper, M. (1942) 'Personality disorder and spatial mobility', *American Journal of Sociology* 43: 29–39.

Tooley, K. (1970) 'The role of geographic mobility in some adjustment problems of children and families', *Journal of the American Academy of Child Psychiatry* 9: 366–78.

Van Dongen, C.J. (1981) 'Relationships between attitudes toward family change of residence and children's post-move adjustment', *Issues in Mental Health Nursing* 3: 51–62.

Wallerstein, J.S. (1984) 'Children of divorce: preliminary report of a ten-year follow-up of young children', *American Journal of Orthopsychiatry* 54: 444–58.

Wilson, J.Q. and Herrnstein, R.J. (1985) *Crime and Human Nature*, New York: Simon & Shuster.

Chapter ten

The sociodemographic risk factors of depression in octogenarians

Hallgrímur Magnússon

Recently it has been pointed out that the influence of sociodemographic variables on the prevalence of depressive disorders may be age related. In a survey of almost 4,000 adults (Crowell 1986), the authors suggest that rural residence buffers young adults, rather than middle-aged and older adults, from major depression.

In this contribution the influence of some sociodemographic risk factors on the prevalence and incidence of depressive disorder in the very old population is studied.

Materials and methods

This is a birth cohort study. Its sample consists of all Icelanders born in the years 1895–7. This cohort was initially studied by Helgason (Helgason 1964) and since then three follow-up studies have been done. Two of these follow-up studies have been previously reported (Helgason 1971; Magnússon and Helgason 1981). In this chapter only the last two observation periods will be considered.

Table 10.1 shows the number of probands in the cohort surviving at the beginning and end of each of the last two observation periods, by sex. At the average age of 75 years the number of probands was 2,650 but at the average age of 87 years, by the end of the last observation period, the total number of probands alive was down to 1,049. It is noteworthy here that only one proband was not traced.

One of the most important issues in longitudinal studies is consistency in methodology, as the main purpose of such studies is to compare results at different points in time. Therefore, the information-gathering and the analysis of the data must be done in exactly the same manner in each follow-up period. The same method must be used throughout the study, even if the theoretical and technical background has changed while the study is going on. In the study presented here, great care has been taken to use exactly the same methods in collecting the data in each of the follow-up periods.

Table 10.1 Mortality and survival in the 1895–7 birth cohort during successive follow-up periods, according to sex

	Males	Females	Both sexes
Alive 1971 average age 75 years	1,207	1,443	2,650
Died 1971–1977	396	366	762
Not traced 1971–1977	0	1	1
Alive 1977 average age 81 years	811	1,076	1,887
Died 1977–1983	404	434	838
Not traced 1977–1983	0	0	0
Alive 1983 average age 87 years	407	642	1,049

Information on the mental health of each proband was collected from several sources. The main informant was the proband's family physician who was contacted by telephone, or visited, and with whom the mental and physical health of each proband was discussed along with the most important social and demographic variables. All records from nursing homes, residential homes, and hospitals were checked and every proband was looked up in the psychiatric register in Iceland. These sources of information were cross-checked, and, when they were inconsistent, further information was sought.

Several objections can be raised concerning the completeness of data collection and the validity of diagnosis. It has been shown (Williamson *et al.* 1964) that some important diseases of old age, including depression and dementia, are, in many cases, unknown to the family physician. In Iceland, however, a study of this question in a population aged 67 years and over (Haraldsson and Pengilsson 1979) found that seven out of fifty-seven patients with memory disturbance and three out of twenty-nine patients with depression were unknown to the family doctor. Nevertheless, it is probable that the prevalence and incidence of mental disorders estimated from the data collected in this manner are underestimates, since it is likely that some cases of the mental disorders were missed.

For this reason, it was decided, in the last phase of the study, to use a direct method of assessment of the surviving probands in addition to the original, indirect method. Therefore, interviews were carried out, using the community version of the Geriatric Mental State Schedule (GMS) (Copeland *et al.* 1976), when the probands were on average aged 87 years.

Of the 1,049 probands alive at the end of the follow-up period, 876 could be interviewed in this way.

The interviews were carried out by the author and five medical students, who had just finished their psychiatric training in the fifth year of medical school. The students were trained to use the GMS by videotaped interviews in addition to theoretical and practical instruction.

Table 10.2 Response rate in follow-up survey based on the Geriatric Mental State, according to sex

	Males		Females		Total	
	n	%	n	%	n	%
Participated in the interview	342	84.0	534	83.2	876	83.5
Refused interview	9	2.2	33	5.1	42	4.0
Not interviewed for other reasons	56	13.8	75	11.7	131	12.5
Total	407	100.0	642	100.0	1,049	100.0

The refusal rate was very low (4 per cent). It was not possible to interview an additional 131 probands, mostly because the location of their homes was very isolated and it was too expensive to visit them. Because of this, there is an over-representation of urban inhabitants among the probands who were interviewed.

The inter-rater reliability of the Icelandic translation of the GMS was studied and the inter-rater reliability between the raters was considered acceptable (kappa value 0.7). Computerized diagnosis based on the GMS interview scores was undertaken at the University of Liverpool, using the AGECAT algorithm developed by Copeland and Dewey (Dewey *et al.* 1986). The resulting diagnoses are hereafter referred to as AGECAT diagnoses. Diagnosis by the method regularly used in this study is hereafter referred to as the indirect method, since it is, in most cases, based on the medical records and interviews with the general practitioners, or other key informants, and only in a few cases with the probands themselves.

Research findings

Agreement between the diagnostic methods

Table 10.3 shows a comparison of the frequency of depression as diagnosed by the indirect method and by the AGECAT algorithm. The sensitivity and specificity of the indirect method, using AGECAT diagnosis as the criterion, are 69 per cent and 96 per cent respectively. Of the nineteen cases of depressive disorder identified by AGECAT and not by the indirect method, eleven (5.8 per cent) had been diagnosed as organic mental

Table 10.3 Comparison of depressive diagnoses made by the indirect method and the AGECAT algorithm

AGECAT diagnosis	Diagnosis by the indirect method		
	Depressive disorder	No depressive disorder	Total
Depressive disorder	43	19	62
No depressive disorder	29	709	738
	72	728	800

Indirect diagnosis: Sensitivity = 69%
Specificity = 96%

disorders, three as other mental disorders, and five had no psychiatric diagnosis. Of twenty-nine cases diagnosed as depressive disorder by the indirect method, but not identified by AGECAT there were seven with organic mental disorders, four with other mental disorders, and eighteen with no psychiatric diagnosis. The difficulty in differentiating between organic disorder and depression was thus the main source of disagreement.

Prevalence and incidence of depressive disorders

In Table 10.4 the prevalence of depressive disorder at the average age of 81 and 87 years is shown according to sex.

Table 10.4 Prevalence (%) of depression at the average age of 81 and 87 years, according to sex

	Diagnosis by the indirect method				AGECAT diagnosis	
	Age 80–83 years		Age 85–88 years		Age 85–88 years	
	n	%	n	%	n	%
Male	45	5.5	22	5.4	17	5.3
Female	104	9.7[1]	69	10.7	45	9.3
Both sexes	149	7.9	91	8.7	62	7.8

[1]Including two females in manic states.

Two women with bipolar affective disorder, who were manic at the time, have been included in the left-hand column of this table. No patient had manic symptoms at the end of the last follow-up period, i.e., at the average age of 87 years. The prevalence of depression, assessed by the indirect method, is shown as well as the computerized diagnosis of the AGECAT algorithm based on the GMS. Females show a higher prevalence of depression than males, as expected.

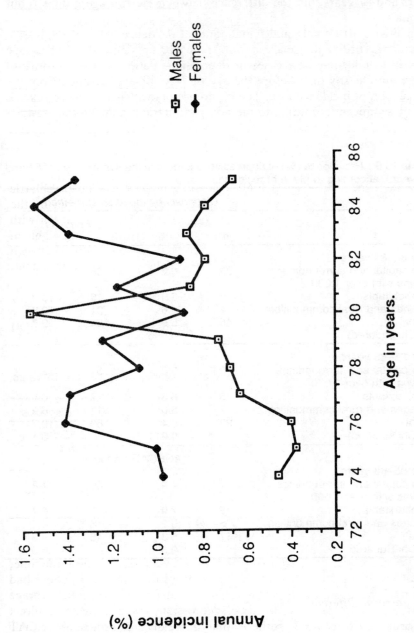

Figure 10.1 Incidence of depressive disorders according to sex

The difference between the sexes is significant at the 0.01 level at both 81 years and 87 years, but the difference between the two age groups is not significant.

In Figure 10.1, male and female annual incidence rates of depressive disorder according to age are shown. It must be emphasized that these age curves include only new cases of depression. Patients with a history of depression at any time before the age of 74 years are excluded from the calculation of incidence rate. The difference in incidence between sexes is highly significant according to the non-parametric Mann-Whitney test.

Table 10.5 Prevalence (%) of depressive disorders at the average age of 81 and 87 years, according to place of residence

| | \multicolumn{4}{c}{Diagnosis by the indirect method} | | | |
| | \multicolumn{2}{c}{Males} | | \multicolumn{2}{c}{Females} | |
	n	%	n	%
Age 80–83 years				
The capital and surroundings	23	6.2	55	9.0
Towns with over 1,000 inhabitants	8	5.9	18	10.2
Villages and rural communities	14	4.6	31	10.8
Total	45	5.5	104	9.7
P (Chi squared)		0.666		0.648
Age 85–88 years				
The capital and surroundings	10	5.3	51	12.7
Towns with over 1,000 inhabitants	5	6.3	7	6.5
Villages and rural communities	7	5.0	11	8.2
Total	22	5.4	69	10.7
P (Chi squared)		0.911		0.106
	\multicolumn{4}{c}{AGECAT diagnosis}			
Age 85–88 years				
The capital and surroundings	7	4.4	39	11.9
Towns with over 1,000 inhabitants	5	7.9	3	3.7
Villages and rural communities	5	5.2	3	4.2
Total	17	5.3	45	9.3
P (Chi Squared)		0.576		0.019

Urban-rural differences

In order to test the hypothesis that depressive disorders are equally prevalent in urban and rural areas, the country was divided into three parts:

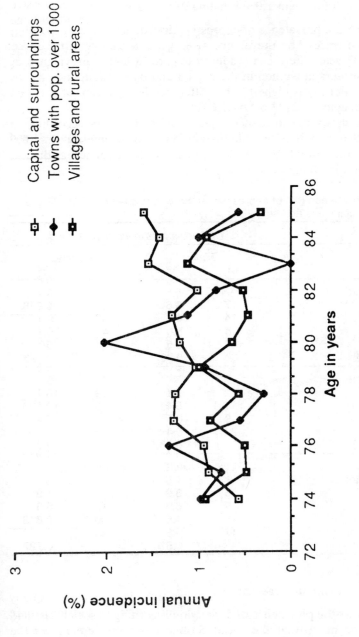

Figure 10.2 Incidence of depressive disorders according to place of residence

Capital and surroundings

Towns with pop. over 1000

Villages and rural areas

1. the capital and its surroundings, with more than 130,000 inhabitants or about 55 per cent of the total population of Iceland;
2. towns with over 1,000 inhabitants;
3. villages, with less than 1,000 inhabitants, and rural areas.

In Table 10.5 the prevalence of depressive disorders is shown according to place of residence. The prevalence at 81 years is similar in the three parts, but at 87 years there is a tendency towards a higher prevalence of depressive disorders in women in the capital and its surroundings, where the population density is highest. This difference is significant at the 0.02 level for the diagnosis based on AGECAT.

Figure 10.2 shows the incidence of depressive disorders according to place of residence. Using the Mann-Whitney non-parametric test, the incidence is significantly higher in the capital and its surroundings than in small towns and in villages and rural areas.

Table 10.6 Prevalence (%) of depression at the age of 80–83 and 85–88 years, according to social class and sex

| | Diagnosis by the indirect method | | | |
| | Males | | Females | |
	n	%	n	%
Age 80–83 years				
Social class 1	17	8.6	25	11.9
Social class 2	14	4.2	32	9.1
Social class 3	14	5.0	47	9.1
Total	45	5.5	104	9.7
P (Chi squared)		0.092		0.473
Age 85–88 years				
Social class 1	2	2.1	19	15.4
Social class 2	11	6.4	28	12.7
Social class 3	9	6.5	22	7.4
Total	22	5.4	69	10.7
P (Chi squared)		0.267		0.026
	AGECAT diagnosis			
Age 85–88 years				
Social class 1	3	3.9	11	11.5
Social class 2	9	6.9	14	8.9
Social class 3	5	4.5	20	8.8
Total	17	5.3	45	9.3
P (Chi squared)		0.576		0.727

Social class and living arrangement

Table 10.6 shows the prevalence of depression according to social class and sex. It must be noted that the social classes presented here reflect the

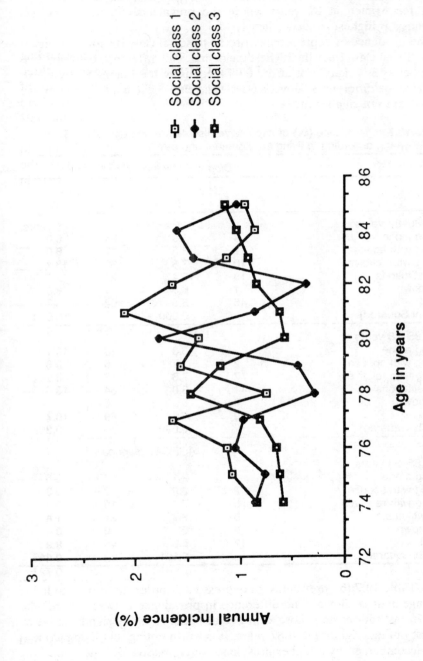

Figure 10.3 Incidence of depressive disorders according to social class

Social class 1
Social class 2
Social class 3

occupational and educational status at the age of 60 years. The difference in prevalence of depressive disorder between the social classes is significant only for women at 87 years where the prevalence based on indirect diagnosis is highest in social class 1.

The incidence of depression according to social class is shown in Figure 10.3. Social class 1 has the highest incidence. The difference between class 1 and class 3 is significant at the 0.05 level using the Mann-Whitney test, whereas the differences between class 2 and class 3 and between class 1 and class 2 are not significant.

Table 10.7 Prevalence (%) of depressive disorders at the age of 80–83 and 85–88 years, according to living arrangement and sex

	Diagnosis by the indirect method			
	Males		Females	
	n	%	n	%
Age 80–83 years				
Living alone	4	1.9	24	6.0
Living with spouse	12	3.5	17	8.9
Living with relatives	10	7.8	39	13.7
In institutions	18	15.4	23	12.3
Unknown	1	6.3	1	8.3
Total	45	5.5	104	9.7
P (Chi Squared)		0.000		0.004
Age 85–88 years				
Living alone	2	3.3	13	10.1
Living with spouse	2	1.7	5	9.8
Living with relatives	7	7.8	17	8.2
In institutions	11	8.0	34	13.3
Unknown	0	0	0	0
Total	2	5.4	69	10.7
P (Chi Squared)		0.090		0.352
	AGECAT diagnosis			
Age 85–88 years				
Living alone	1	2.1	7	6.5
Living with spouse	2	2.0	2	5.3
Living with relatives	5	7.7	15	9.9
In institutions	9	8.7	21	11.4
Unknown	0	0	0	0
Total	17	5.3	45	9.3
P (Chi squared)		0.101		0.445

In Table 10.7 the prevalence of depressive disorders according to living arrangement is shown. The difference in prevalence between those who live in institutions and those who live at home is highly significant at 81 years, but less significant at 87 years. It is worth noting that living alone is not accompanied by a higher prevalence of depressive disorders.

Discussion

In the present study, incidence rates are based on the indirect method of diagnosis and the same is true of the prevalence at 81 years. For the probands at 87 years, however, a new diagnostic method was also used and we therefore have two sets of diagnoses, each of which has been used to compute the frequency at this age. The prevalence by the indirect method is about 1 per cent higher than that based on the GMS and the sex difference in smaller towns and rural areas is reversed for the AGECAT diagnoses, as compared to the diagnoses by the indirect method. This is probably explained by the fact that the AGECAT diagnoses were made on a sample, which had a relative under-representation of inhabitants in small towns and rural areas. With this exception, the prevalence of depression derived by each method was similar.

One of the findings of this study is that the prevalence and the incidence rate do not change significantly with advancing age, at least not in the very old population. This finding is not consistent with those of other studies on the prevalence of depressive disorders in old age. Griffiths *et al.* (1987) report an increase in prevalence with age in a study of mobile old people in a rural community, while both Berkman *et al.* (1986) and Murrell *et al.* (1983) report a higher prevalence of depressive disorders for the age range over 75 years.

However, Kivelä *et al.* (1986), studying Finnish males from 65 to 84 years of age, found no significant difference in mean scores on the Zung self-rating depression scale between different age groups. In a study of old people in Gothenburg, Sweden, it was also found that the prevalence of affective psychosis and depressive neurosis was similar at the ages of 70, 75, and 79 years (Nilsson and Persson 1984).

The sociodemographic factors studied here seem to have a surprisingly small effect on the prevalence of depression among octogenarians. The urban/rural difference is only significant for women at the age of 85–87 years and only using the AGECAT diagnoses which are known to be based on a sample with over-representation of urban inhabitants. The type of living arrangement does not affect the prevalence, apart from the group in long-term institutional care, and this difference is significant only at the average age of 81 years. One can, therefore, speculate that depressive disorders in very old age may be less dependent on environmental factors than those found in younger age groups.

The incidence rate of depression between the ages of 74 and 85 years, unlike the prevalence, does vary both with social class and with area of residence. The incidence is higher in urban than in rural areas, but, as the prevalence is equal in both kinds of area, it appears that the excess is largely made up of cases which remit quite quickly. This finding is similar to those reported from a community survey in Florida where 'the urban residents did report a significantly higher number of depressive symptoms overall than did rural residents, though they did not report any more persistent depressive symptoms' (Neff 1983).

The frequency of new cases varies according to social status, class 1 having the highest incidence rate. On the other hand, the prevalence does not show any variation by social class except among women in the higher age group. Here again one may suspect that there is a higher frequency of depression in social class 1, but that the excess is among cases of good outcome, while chronic depression occurs with equal frequency in all classes. It is possible that the greater loss of occupational and financial status in social class 1 can lead to higher frequency of depression. With retirement the financial setback of people in social class 1 as well as the loss of status held by the professional and the managerial classes, by being forced to leave jobs to which they may have devoted their entire lives, can be a major life event of sufficient strength to precipitate a depression. Contributing to the financial setback are the modest pensions compared to earlier salaries which were, however, not sufficient to build up any capital reserve in order to maintain their standard of living.

There are many unanswered questions of this kind concerning depressive disorders in old age. In order to be able to apply preventive measures in this field, more research is needed into the risk factors of depression in the elderly.

References

Berkmann L.F., Berkmann, C.S., Kals, S., et al. (1986) 'Depressive symptoms in relation to physical health and functioning in the elderly', *American Journal of Epidemiology* 124: 372–88.

Copeland, J.R.M., Kelleher, M.J., Kellett, J.M., et al. (1976) 'A semi-structured clinical interview for the assessment of diagnosis and mental state in the elderly: the Geriatric Mental State Schedule', *Psychological Medicine* 6: 439–49.

Crowell, B.A., George, L.K., Blazer, D., and Landerman, R. (1986) 'Psychosocial risk factors and urban/rural difference in the prevalence of major depression', *British Journal of Psychiatry* 149: 307–14.

Dewey, M.E., Copeland, J.R.M., and Griffith-Jones, H.M. (1986) 'Computerized psychiatric diagnosis in the elderly: AGECAT', *Journal of Microcomputer Application* 9: 135–40.

Griffiths, R.A., Good, W.R., Watson, N.P., et al. (1987) 'Depression, dementia and disability in the elderly', *British Journal of Psychiatry* 150: 482–93.

Haraldsson, E., and Pengilsson, G. (1979) 'Könnun á högum aldradra i Kópavogi (A survey of the living condition and health of the elderly in the district Kópavogur)' *Læknabladid* (The Icelandic Medical Journal) Supplement 8: 32–4.

Helgason, T. (1964) 'Epidemiology of mental disorders in Iceland', *Acta Psychiatrica Scandinavica* Supplement 173.

Helgason, T. (1971) 'Epidemiology of mental disorders in Iceland: a geriatric follow-up', *Excerpta Medica*, International Congress Series No. 271, Amsterdam.

Kivelä S.L., Nissinen, A., Tuomilehto, J., et al. (1986) 'Prevalence of depressive and other symptoms in elderly Finnish men', *Acta Psychiatrica Scandinavica* 73: 93–100.

Magnússon, H., and Helgason, T. (1981) 'Epidemiology of mental disorders in the aged in Iceland', in G. Magnussen, J. Nilsen, and J. Buch (eds) *Epidemiology and Prevention of Mental Illness in Old Age*, Hellerup, Denmark: Nordisk samråd for eldreaktivitet (EGV), pp 29–33.

Murrell, S.A., Himmelfarb, S., and Wright, K. (1983) 'Prevalence of depression and its correlates in older adults', *American Journal of Epidemiology* 117: 173–85.

Neff, J. (1983) 'Urbanicity and depression reconsidered: the evidence regarding depressive symptomatology', *Journal of Nervous and Mental Disease* 171: 546–52.

Nilsson, L.V., and Persson, G. (1984) 'Prevalence of mental disorders in an urban sample examined at 70, 75 and 79 years of age', *Acta Psychiatrica Scandinavica* 69: 519–27.

Williamson, J., Stokoe, I.H., Gray, S., *et al.* (1964) 'Old people at home: their unreported needs', *Lancet* i: 1117–20.

Chapter eleven

Risk factors for AIDS-related bereavement in a cohort of homosexual men in New York City

John L. Martin and Laura Dean

Introduction

The AIDS epidemic has grown in the US from a few hundred cases in 1981 to over 80,000 in 1989. Specific groups have been designated as 'high risk', including homosexual and bisexual men, intravenous drug users (IVDUs) haemophiliacs, transfusion recipients, the sexual partners of these individuals, and children born to female members of these groups. Although transmission of HIV (Human Immunodeficiency Virus: the primary cause of AIDS) and AIDS illness can and do occur among individuals who cannot be categorized as belonging to one of these high-risk groups, the proportional distribution of AIDS cases within risk groups has remained remarkably stable over the first six years of this epidemic. Homosexual and bisexual males continue to be the most strongly affected sub-group, accounting for 70 per cent of the total number of US cases (CDC 1986). The case fatality rate is high: almost 50 per cent overall, and 80 per cent of these within 26 months. Although a number of drugs are under study as potential treatment candidates, their efficacy has not been fully demonstrated. There is no cure for AIDS.

The catastrophic experience of being sick with AIDS cannot be under-estimated. HIV-related neuropsychiatric impairment and dementia (Britton and Miller 1984; Hoffman 1984; Holland and Tross 1985; Faulstich 1986; Snider et al. 1983) represent particularly harsh disorders which will increase the demand for psychiatric services. Other physical, emotional, and social hardships wrought by this disease are tremendous and taxing. Thus, as the AIDS epidemic grows, the demand for psychological and mental health services will also grow. However, a substantial part of this demand may not come from those who are actually sick with AIDS but may come, instead, from the much larger group of individuals close to those who have developed AIDS, including those who have died. While not physically sick with AIDS, these friends and supporters are experiencing bereavement, each death being preceded by a protracted anticipatory bereavement period associated with the progression of what for most is a lethal illness. A recent comprehensive review of the clinical and epidemiological literature on bereavement by the Institute of Medicine (Osterweis *et al.* 1984) suggests that the experience of these losses, and the stresses associated with helping a loved one through the course of illness and death, may severely compromise an individual's health status. Extensive effects of bereavement on both mental health (Clayton 1974, 1979; Maddison and Viola 1968; Parkes and Brown 1972; Parkes and Weiss 1983; Parkes 1964; Paykel *et al.* 1969; Stein and Susser 1969; Thompson *et al.* 1984) and physical health (Bartrop *et al.* 1977; Chambers and Reiser 1953; Greene 1954, 1965; Schmale and Iker 1965; Stein *et al.* 1981; Thompson *et al.* 1984) have been documented.

The potential for widespread and growing psychiatric morbidity due to AIDS-related bereavement may best be appreciated by examining AIDS incidence rates over time. Since the Centers for Disease Control began surveillance and reporting of AIDS cases in the United States in 1981 (CDC 1981a), a distinctive feature of the epidemic has been the geometric increase in the number of case reports occurring within fixed periods of time. Although the doubling time for case numbers has increased from six months in 1983 to over thirteen months in 1986, the absolute number of cases is growing at a staggering rate. Almost as many new cases of AIDS occurred in the US in 1986 alone (roughly 15,000) as occurred in the prior five years, 1981 through 1985 (CDC 1986). It is now estimated that there will have been well over 270,000 cases of AIDS by the end of 1991, 74,000 of those occurring in 1991 alone (Institute of Medicine 1986: 8). Keeping in mind the fact that for most cases of AIDS there is a social network of persons who bear the anticipated and actual loss, the prevalence of bereavement-related distress and disorders may grow much faster than the actual rate of new AIDS cases. Thus, the potential demand for, and strain on, mental health services may also grow faster than one might predict from considering only the number of new AIDS cases.

Background and aims of the present study

In 1984 we initiated a community-based study designed to determine the behavioural and social risk factors for AIDS and document the impact of the AIDS epidemic on sexual behaviour, drug use, and mental health in the homosexual population. The theoretical framework for the study was derived from findings on the nature and effects of stressful life events (Dohrenwend and Dohrenwend 1974, 1978), the effects of social disorganization on mental health (Leighton 1955), and the key role of threat appraisal in determining the personal stressfulness of an event or experience (Lazarus 1966). We conceptualized the death of loved ones as one major type of stressor arising from the epidemic and fear for one's own life as a second major type of stressor arising from the epidemic. We

171

anticipated that these would be the two primary factors motivating behaviour change and influencing mental health and adaptation to the AIDS epidemic among homosexual men.

Although our long-term aim is to develop and test fully articulated, multifactorial models of the processes leading from the experience of bereavement stressors to psychological and behavioural changes, one preliminary question must first be addressed. Specifically, we need to determine who in the homosexual community is at highest risk for experiencing bereavement due to AIDS. Elucidating risk factors for any pathogenic substance, event, or behaviour is of interest in order (i) to define the population at risk, (ii) to specify possible causes of disease, and (iii) to locate points for intervention. Just as there is wide and systematic variation in risk of AIDS among homosexual men which is determined primarily by sexual behaviour factors, so there may be systematic variation in risk of bereavement due to AIDS. In light of the potential for morbidity and premature mortality associated with bereavement, it is of interest and value to attempt to locate and specify these risk factors.

It is important to note that AIDS-related bereavement is a growing public health problem not only among survivors in the homosexual community but also among the non-homosexual family members and friends of persons with AIDS. In addition, as the epidemiological trend in AIDS cases continues to shift towards socially and economically disadvantaged ethnic minorities and women, due to the transmission of HIV through drug abuse, problems associated with AIDS-related bereavement will also increase in these segments of the population. While we consider here only homosexual men, these results may be useful in planning for future social service and mental health needs in communities only now beginning to be affected by AIDS.

A further reason for exploring the question of risk factors is to know which variables must be controlled in analyses aimed at determining health consequences of bereavement. Should we find that AIDS-related bereavement is essentially an event randomly distributed in the community, future analyses of the relationships between bereavement and health outcomes will not have to consider determinants of bereavement itself in analytic models of this stress process. However, if AIDS-related bereavement is *not* randomly distributed in the community but rather is predictable from some set of personal or environmental factors, this information must be built into models designed to examine the mental health consequences of the stressful event.

This problem is an example of what Brown and Harris (1978: 73–4) and Dohrenwend and colleagues (in press) refer to as the question of 'independence' of events. To the extent that the occurrence of a life event is dependent on a characteristic of the individual, particularly that individual's psychological state, ascribing causal status to that event with respect to some health outcome becomes problematic due to circularity. That is to say, it could be that it was the individual's psychological or physical health status which brought about the occurrence of the event to begin with. In this study, since a key aim is to determine the impact of bereavement on mental and physical health, it is essential to determine whether or not factors related to health status are determinants of the bereavement itself.

The first clue about the potential non-random distribution of social losses grew out of preliminary work conducted in preparation for this study, in which it was found that AIDS-related deaths were concentrated in pockets of the community. Some men had lost entire groups of close friends while others had lost no one. Logically, it made sense that networks hit hard by AIDS would also be hit hard by bereavement among the survivors in the network. In addition, the fact that cases of AIDS tended to cluster within sexual-contact networks (CDC 1981b) was not only consistent with this naturalistic observation on the clustering of losses but also suggested that the behavioural risk factors for both AIDS and bereavement due to AIDS would be the same; namely, a history of high-risk sexual activity.

In this analysis we will evaluate the probability of being bereaved due to an AIDS-related loss as a function of sexual behaviour history. If bereavement and AIDS both share similar risk factors we should find that bereaved respondents are more likely to have engaged in sexual behaviour considered to be high risk – i.e., large number of partners and frequent anal intercourse (Kingsley et al. 1987; Martin 1986; Mayer et al. 1986; Polk et al. 1987; Stevens et al. 1986) compared to their non-bereaved counterparts. Should this hypothesis be confirmed, we would also expect to find that men who are bereaved will be more likely to have health problems associated with disturbed immunologic functioning as indicated by signs or symptoms of AIDS-related conditions (ARC) or HIV infection. We will test for this corollary also.

Method

Study participants

A total of 745 homosexual men make up the present sample. To be included in this sample a man had to reside in one of the five boroughs of New York City, be aged 20 to 65, have no diagnosis of AIDS, and identify himself as homosexual or bisexual. Since no sampling frame exists for enumerating homosexual and bisexual males in New York City we could neither draw a random sample of this section of the population nor evaluate the sample for representativeness once it was drawn. Recognizing this limitation, our goal was to generate a sample reflecting the diversity which exists in the male homosexual population, rather than a narrow sample of convenience (Martin and Vance 1984; Martin and Dean 1985).

An initial group of 291 men (39 per cent of the total sample) was recruited from the following channels: (1) gay organizations (n=131); (2) unsolicited volunteers (n=41); (3) pilot sample referrals (n=32); (4) the 1985 New York City Gay Pride Festival (n=72); (5) a public health clinic (n=15). The remaining 454 (61 per cent) respondents were recruited through personal referrals to the study by those 291 already interviewed. A summary of key demographic characteristics of this sample is shown in Table 11.1.

Table 11.1 Descriptive demographic characteristics of the sample (N=745)

Demographic variable	Sample value
Years of age[1]	35.7 (8.50)
Years of education[1]	16.3 (1.87)
Years in New York City[1]	7.97 (2.91)
% Black or Hispanic ethnic status	13
% Partnered with a lover[2]	37
% Manhattan resident	81

[1]Mean and (SD)
[2]A respondent qualified as having a lover if (1) he said he had a lover, (2) his lover viewed him as his lover (reciprocity), (3) friends viewed the two as a couple (public recognition), and (4) the relationship was extant for six months or more (duration).

Study design and data collection

This study is designed as a multi-wave panel study involving annual psychosocial assessments and semi-annual blood sampling on 44 per cent of the cohort for selected serologic and haematological characteristics. The present analysis is based only on the baseline data collected in the period June to October 1985, during which extensive historical information on social losses and sexual behaviour was collected. For many respondents this involved assessments of behaviour and losses occurring over the first four years of the epidemic. While we recognize the potential distortions, biases, and forgetting that can influence retrospective reports over such a long interval (Brown 1981; Jenkins et al. 1979) the deaths focused on are distinctive. The month and year of each occurrence are elicited and incidence rates compare closely (for the group as a whole) with surveillance statistics compiled by the CDC and the New York City Department of Health. For sexual behaviour measures, a test-retest reliability study was conducted which demonstrated an adequate degree of reliability for all measures of sexual behaviour of interest. Reliability coefficients are reported below.

All data were collected in face-to-face structured interviews, lasting two to four hours, usually in study participants' homes. Interviews were conducted by a total of ten trained interviewers: seven men and three women. No effects of interviewer bias have been detected to date on any variable used for any analysis. Written informed consent was obtained from all study subjects in accordance with procedures approved by the Columbia Presbyterian Medical Center Institutional Review Board.

Measures

HIV antibody status Six months after the interview took place 331 members (44 per cent) of the sample enrolled in a serological assessment in which they were evaluated for the presence of HIV antibody. Testing was conducted through the New York City Department of Health, Bureau of Laboratories, following the currently established and accepted protocols. Each blood sample was evaluated twice by the ELISA method (Abbott test kit) and all reactive specimens were further evaluated using the Western blot method of protein-based analysis. Individuals were designated as HIV antibody positive if they had two reactive ELISA assays and detectable antibody to two of the three major HIV proteins, p24, gp41 and gp120/160. As of mid-1986, the proportion of seropositive men in this study group was 36 per cent.

AIDS-related conditions (ARC) The measure of AIDS-related conditions (ARC) used here is a dichotomous indicator of the experience of at least one physical symptom associated with disturbed immunologic functioning. The conditions were ascertained through systematic inquiry about the occurrence of each of the following: oral or oesophageal candidiasis during the three years prior to the interview; a case of *herpes zoster* within three years prior to interview; unintentional weight loss of 10 pounds or more during the year prior to interview; unexplained diarrhoea persisting for two months or more during the previous year; unexplained fever persisting for two months or more; the presence of swollen lymph glands in two or more extra-inguinal sites for three months or more during the prior year. Any respondent who reported one or more of these problems received a score of one on the item, while all others received a score of zero. A subject is also given a score of one on this item if his physician has given him a diagnosis of ARC or a diagnosis of lymphadenopathy.

Sexual behaviour Four measures of sexual behaviour (Martin 1987) are used here, two of which refer to sexual activity occurring during the year before respondents first heard about AIDS ('pre-AIDS': predominantly 1980-1) and two identical measures which represent sexual activity in the year prior to the interview ('post-AIDS': 1984-5). *Total number of partners* is a count of the total number of partners with whom an individual had sexual contact in the 'pre-AIDS' and 'post-AIDS' time periods. The median number of partners for the pre-AIDS year was forty-one (inter-quartile range = 2,144), for the post-AIDS year the median was eleven (inter-quartile range = 1,27). The test-retest reliability for the pre-AIDS partner total is r=.503 (df=22, p < .01), and for the post-AIDS period, the test-retest reliability is r=.79 (df=22, p < .01). In this analysis, log transformations were applied to each of these measures in order to normalize the highly skewed distributions before employing parametric statistical techniques. *Frequency of receptive anal intercourse* is an index reflecting the number of sexual episodes in which an individual engaged in receptive anal intercourse within each of the two time periods. This particular sexual act is the one for which there is a consistently demonstrated relationship between its frequency of occurrence and the likelihood of current HIV antibody (Kingsley *et al.* 1987; Martin 1986; Mayer *et al.* 1986; Polk *et al.* 1987; Stevens *et al.* 1986). For this sample, the median pre-AIDS frequency of receptive anal intercourse was seventeen (IQ range = 1,71). For the post-AIDS year, the median frequency was four (IQ range = 0,19). The intra-class correlation coefficient (ICC) was used to assess test-retest agreement over time for the frequency of specific sexual acts. For receptive anal intercourse in the pre-AIDS year, ICC=.57 and for the post-AIDS year, ICC=.64. Both of these values indicate good reliability of these reports (Fleiss 1981: 225–6; Fleiss and Cohen 1973). As with partner totals, each measure of receptive anal intercourse was log-transformed in order to normalize the distributions for use in parametric statistical analysis.

The intercorrelations, means, standard deviations, and proportions of the risk-factor variables are summarized in Table 11.2.

Bereavement episodes We adapted Fischer's method for defining a social network (Fischer *et al.* 1977; Phillips and Fischer 1981) in order to inquire about the social network of persons with AIDS. Respondents were asked to name all men they knew who had died of AIDS since the beginning of the epidemic. (Interviewers recorded only first names or initials.) After all names were elicited, a set of ten questions was asked about each individual named, including the dates of diagnosis and death, the length of time the relationship had existed, the frequency of social and sexual contact (pre- and post-diagnosis), and the emotional closeness of the relationship specified in terms of (i) lover, (ii) close friend, (iii) friend, (iv) acquaintance, or (v) friend of a friend. Any individual who had lost a lover or close friend due to AIDS was designated as bereaved. Any individual who had lost no one or whose losses were limited to friends, acquaintances, or friends of friends was designated as not bereaved.

Since the start of the epidemic in 1981 up to mid-1985 when the baseline interview was conducted, 27 per cent (N=198) of this sample had experienced one episode of bereavement as defined above. Within this group of

Table 11.2 Intercorrelations[3] [off-diagonal elements] and means, (standard deviations) and percentages [diagonal elements] among six potential risk factors for bereavement (N=745)

	1	2	3	4	5	6
1. Number of sexual partners (pre–AIDS)[1]	3.31 (1.78)					
2. Frequency of receptive anal intercourse (pre–AIDS)[1]	0.48	2.77 (1.97)				
3. Number of sexual partners (post–AIDS)[1]	0.50	0.25	2.22 (1.31)			
4. Frequency of receptive anal intercourse (post-AIDS)[1]	0.12	0.38	0.17	1.71 (1.68)		
5. ARC symptom(s)[2]	0.08	0.19	0.05	0.12	21%	
6. Positive HIV antibody status[2]	0.23	0.38	0.14	0.27	0.23	34%

[1] Log transformation applied in all statistical analyses.
[2] Dichotomous variable.
[3] p < .05 for all correlations > | .07 |.

198 persons, 67 per cent (n=133) had experienced one such loss, 18 per cent (n=35) had experienced two losses, and 15 per cent (n=30) had experienced three or more losses, the maximum being six. In the analyses which follow, bereavement or no bereavement will be used as the dichotomous dependent variable.

Research findings

Demographic risk factors

As an initial step in the risk-factor analysis, bereaved respondents were compared with non-bereaved respondents on six demographic variables: age, ethnicity, education level, years of residence in New York City, residing in Manhattan as opposed to residency in one of the four other boroughs of New York City, and being in a primary relationship with a lover as opposed to being single. Using a simultaneous logistic regression model, controlling for all other demographic factors, only the number of years in New York City and Manhattan residency were found to be significantly predictive of being bereaved. Even these differences are not large, however. Bereaved respondents had lived in New York City approximately one year longer than the non-bereaved group, and 91 per cent of the bereaved lived in Manhattan compared to 78 per cent of the non-bereaved.

Although no linear relationship was found between probability of bereavement and age, a significant curvilinear effect was found. Both the observed and predicted probabilities of bereavement are shown in Figure 11.1.

It can be seen from Figure 11.1 that the 35–45 age group contains a disproportionately large number of bereaved subjects, compared with younger or older age groups.

Sexual-behaviour risk factors

Turning next to the question of sexual-behaviour risk factors, we again constructed and tested a logistic regression model predicting bereavement status from four sexual behaviour variables. Given the high inter-correlations between these predictors and the time sequence established by the pre-AIDS – post-AIDS measures, a hierarchical approach was used to test each term whereby the frequency of receptive anal intercourse and the number of partners during the pre-AIDS year were entered in that sequence, followed by frequency of receptive anal intercourse and number of partners during the post-AIDS year. The logistic regression results and descriptive statistics are shown in Table 11.3.

It can be seen from Table 11.3 that the two pre-AIDS variables are

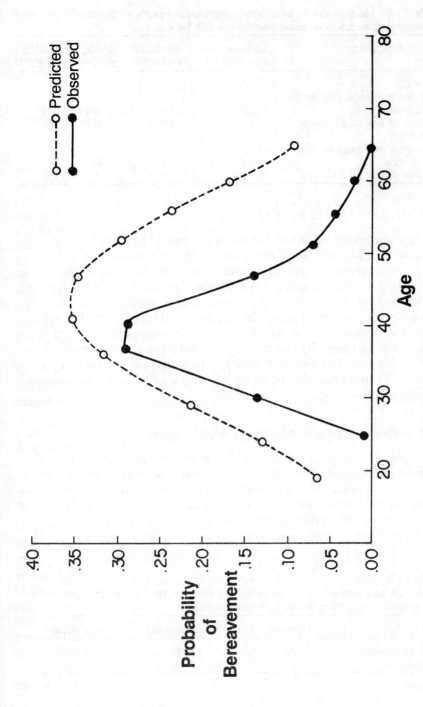

Figure 11.1 Relationship between age and bereavement

Table 11.3 Median values and logistic regression results of predicting bereavement status from sexual-behaviour risk factors

Sexual-behaviour factor	Bereaved (N=199)	Not bereaved (N=545)	Logistic regression coefficient (S.E.)
Pre-AIDS			
Frequency of receptive anal intercourse	30	14	0.16 (0.04)[1]
Number of sexual partners	51	19	0.37 (0.12)[1]
Post-AIDS			
Frequency of receptive anal intercourse	5	4	−0.01 (0.06)
Number of sexual partners	9	6	0.01 (0.14)

[1] p < .001

strongly predictive of current bereavement status. Bereaved respondents reported over two-and-a-half times the number of sexual partners and over twice the frequency of receptive anal intercourse episodes in the earlier time period, compared with the non-bereaved respondents. After controlling for both of these earlier risk factors, neither number of partners nor frequency of anal intercourse in the post-AIDS year predict current bereavement status. Although bereaved respondents as a group score higher on both post-AIDS variables, the differences are quite small. These findings indicate that men with a history of higher-risk sexual activity are significantly more likely to be bereaved compared to men with lower-risk sexual histories.

HIV antibody status and ARC status as risk factors

Since only 331 subjects enrolled in the serologic component of the study, we have information about HIV antibody status on only 44 per cent of the sample. In contrast, information about ARC status is available on the full sample of 745. Thus, evaluation of the relationship between each of these health factors and bereavement status was conducted using simple, one-degree-of-freedom chi-square tests. These results are shown in Table 11.4.

Table 11.4 Percentage of total sample (N=745) reporting one or more ARC symptoms and percentage of serology sub-sample (N=331) testing positive for HIV antibody, according to bereavement status

Risk factor	Bereaved	Not bereaved	Chi-square
ARC symptom(s)	29%	18%	11.03[1]
HIV positive	50%	29%	11.81[1]

[1] p < .001

It can be seen from Table 11.4 that there is a strong association between both HIV status and ARC status and the probability of having been bereaved. In the serology sub-sample (N=331), 50 per cent of those who are bereaved are HIV antibody positive, compared with only 29 per cent of those who are not bereaved. In the total sample (N=745), 29 per cent of those who are bereaved have experienced at least one clinically significant sign of ARC compared with 18 per cent of those who are not bereaved. These results indicate that men whose health status is complicated by either symptoms of ARC or infection with HIV are significantly more likely to be bereaved compared to men whose health status is not similarly compromised.

Discussion

Two main conclusions can be drawn from the foregoing results. First, the experience of bereavement is not a randomly distributed event among homosexual men, but can be predicted from a characteristic set of risk factors. One such risk factor which clearly predates the experiences of bereavement is a history of high-risk sexual activity early in the AIDS epidemic. The fact that a history of high numbers of partners and frequent receptive anal intercourse predicts not only AIDS morbidity (Polk *et al.* 1987) and HIV infection (Kingsley *et al.* 1987; Stevens *et al.* 1986) but also bereavement due to this illness illustrates the dual role of sexual behaviour as both an epidemiological and a psychosocial variable. It is because of this dual role that the second set of risk factors for bereavement emerged so clearly here: men who are HIV antibody positive or who have experienced one or more clinical symptoms associated with ARC are twice as likely to be bereaved as men who do not have evidence of compromised health or HIV infection.

The interdependence of high-risk sexual history, compromised health status and HIV antibodies as risk factors for bereavement is important to recognize in order to grasp the stressfulness of the AIDS epidemic for a particular sub-set of this population. In addition to the stress brought on by (a) knowing of one's high risk for AIDS due to prior behaviour patterns, (b) being anti-HIV positive, and (c) being clinically symptomatic, it is also highly likely that many of these men have lost one or more key persons since the epidemic began. Moreover, the disfiguring disease that killed these persons may also be in the process of killing their close survivors.

It is clear from these findings that AIDS-related bereavement is *not* a random event in this community and thus cannot be considered 'independent' of key personal characteristics of the affected individuals. Future studies aimed at determining the causal relationship between AIDS-related bereavement and either mental or physical health outcomes must take account of the fact that persons most likely to be bereaved are also more likely to develop AIDS in the future due to sexual behaviour histories resulting in elevated risk of HIV infection.

Acknowledgements

This research was supported by Grant MH39557 from the National Institute of Mental Health and by the New York City Department of Health. The authors would like to thank William Hall, Marc Garcia, Bruce Dohrenwend, Patrick Shrout, and Mary Clare Lennon for their thoughtful comments.

References

Bartrop, R.W., Lazarus, L., Luckhurst, E., *et al.* (1977) 'Depressed lymphocyte function after bereavement', *Lancet* 1: 834–6.

Britton, C. and Miller, J. (1984) 'Neurologic complications in immunodeficiency syndrome (AIDS)', *Neurologic Clinics* 2: 315–39.

Brown, G.W. (1981) 'Life events, pyschiatric disorder and physical illness', *Journal of Psychosomatic Research* 25: 461–73.

Brown, G.W. and Harris, T. (1978) *Social Origins of Depression: A Study of Psychiatric Disorder in Women*, New York: Free Press.

Centers for Disease Control (1981a) 'Kaposi's sarcoma and Pneumocystis pneumonia among homosexual men: New York City and California', *Morbidity and Mortality Weekly Report* 30: 305–8.

Centers for Disease Control (1981b) 'Pneumocystis pneumonia: Los Angeles', *Morbidity and Mortality Weekly Report* 30: 250–2.

Centers for Disease Control (1986) 'Update: AIDS – United States', *Morbidity and Mortality Weekly Report* 35: 17–21.

Chambers, W.N. and Reiser, M.F. (1953) 'Emotional stress in the precipitation of congestive heart failure', *Psychosomatic Medicine* 15: 38–60.

Clayton, P.J. (1974) 'Mortality and morbidity in the first year of widowhood', *Archives of General Psychiatry* 125: 747–50.

Clayton, P.J. (1979) 'The sequelae and non-sequelae of conjugal bereavement', *American Journal of Psychiatry* 136: 1530–43.

Dohrenwend, B.S. and Dohrenwend, B.P. (1974) 'Overview and prospects for research on stressful life events', in B.S. Dohrenwend and B.P. Dohrenwend (eds) *Stressful Life Events: Their Nature and Effects*, New York: Wiley, pp. 313–31.

Dohrenwend, B.S. and Dohrenwend, B.P. (1978) 'Some issues in research on stressful life events', *Journal of Nervous and Mental Disease* 166: 7–15.

Dohrenwend, B.P., Link, B.G., Kern, R., *et al.* (1987) 'Measuring life events: the problem of variability within event categories', in Cooper B. (ed.) *Psychiatric Epidemiology: Progress and Prospects*, London: Croom Helm.

Faulstich, M.E. (1986) 'Acquired immune deficiency syndrome: an overview of central nervous system complications and neuropsychiatric sequelae', *International Journal of Neuroscience* 30: 249–54.

Fischer, C.S., Jackson, R.M., Stueve, C.A., *et al.* (1977) *Networks and Places: Social Relations in the Urban Setting*, New York: Free Press.

Fleiss, J.L. (1981) *Statistical Methods for Rates and Proportions*, Second edition, New York: Wiley.

Fleiss, J.L. and Cohen, J. (1973) 'The equivalence of weighted kappa and the intraclass correlation coefficient as measures of reliability', *Educational Psychology Measurement* 33: 613–19.

Greene, W.A. (1954) 'Psychological factors and reticuloendothelial disease', *Psychosomatic Medicine* 16: 220–30.

Greene, W.A. (1965) 'Disease response to life stress', *Journal of the American Medical Women's Association* 20: 133–40.

Hoffman, R. (1984) 'Neuropsychiatric complications of AIDS', *Psychosomatics* 25: 393–400.

Holland, J. and Tross, S. (1985) 'The psychosocial and neuropsychiatric sequelae of the acquired immunodeficiency syndrome and related disorders', *Annals of Internal Medicine* 103: 760–4.

Institute of Medicine (1986) *Confronting AIDS: Directions for Public Health, Health Care, and Research*, Washington, DC: National Academy Press.

Jenkins, C.D., Hurst, M.W., and Rose, R.M. (1979) 'Life changes – do people really remember?', *Archives of General Psychiatry* 36: 379–84.

Kingsley, L.A., Kaslow, R., Rinaldo, C.R. Jr., *et al.* (1987). 'Risk factors for sero-conversion to human immunodeficiency virus among male homosexuals', *Lancet* 1: 345–9.

Lazarus, R.S. (1966) *Psychological Stress and the Coping Process*, New York: McGraw-Hill.

Leighton, A.H. (1955) 'Psychiatric disorder and the social environment: an outline for a frame of reference', *Psychiatry* 18: 367–83.

Maddison, D.C. and Viola, A. (1968) 'The health of widows in the year following bereavement', *Journal of Psychosomatic Research* 12: 297–306.

Martin, J.L. (1986) 'Demographic factors, sexual behavior patterns and HIV antibody status among New York City gay men', paper presented at the 94th annual convention of the American Psychological Association, Washington, DC.

Martin, J.L. (1987) 'The impact of AIDS on gay male sexual behavior patterns in New York City', *American Journal of Public Health* 77: 578–81.

Martin, J.L. and Dean, L. (1985) 'The impact of AIDS on New York City gay men: development of a community sample', paper presented at the 113th annual meeting of the American Public Health Association, Washington, DC.

Martin, J.L. and Vance, C.S. (1984) 'Behavioral and psychosocial factors in AIDS: methodological and substantive issues', *American Psychologist* 39: 1303–8.

Mayer, K., Ayotte, D., Groopman, J., *et al.* (1986) 'Association of human T lymphotropic virus type III antibodies with sexual and other behaviors in a cohort of homosexual men from Boston with and without generalized lymph-adenopathy', *American Journal of Medicine* 80: 357–63.

Osterweis, M., Solomon, F., and Green, M. (eds) (1984) *Bereavement: Reactions, Consequences and Care*, Washington, DC: National Academy Press.

Parkes, C.M. (1964) 'Recent bereavement as a cause of mental illness', *British Journal of Psychiatry* 110: 198–204.

Parkes, C.M. and Brown, R. (1972) 'Health after bereavement: a controlled study of young Boston widows and widowers', *Psychosomatic Medicine* 34: 449–61.

Parkes, C.M. and Weiss, R.S. (1983) *Recovery from Bereavement*, New York: Basic Books.

Paykel, E.S., Meyers, J.K., Dienelt, M.N., *et al.* (1969). 'Life events and depression: a controlled study', *Archives of General Psychiatry* 21: 753–60.

Phillips, S.L. and Fischer, C.S. (1981) 'Measuring social support networks in general populations', in B.S. Dohrenwend and B.P. Dohrenwend (eds) *Stressful Life Events and Their Contexts*, New York: Prodist, pp. 223–33.

Polk, B.F., Fox, R., Brookmeyer, R., *et al.* (1987) 'Predictors of the acquired immunodeficiency syndrome developing in a cohort of seropositive homosexual men', *New England Journal of Medicine* 316: 63–6.

Schmale, A. and Iker, H. (1965) 'The psychological setting of uterine cervical cancer', *Annals of the New York Academy of Sciences* 125: 794–801.

Snider, W., Simpson, D., Nielsen, S., *et al.* (1983) Neurological complications of acquired immune deficiency syndrome: analysis of 50 patients', *Annals of Neurology* 14: 403–18.

Stein, M., Schleifer, S.J., and Keller, S.E. (1981) 'Hypothalamic influences on immune responses', in R. Ader (ed.) *Psychoneuroimmunology*, New York: Academic Press.

Stein, Z. and Susser, M. (1969) 'Widowhood and mental illness', *British Journal of Preventive and Social Medicine* 23: 106–10.

Stevens, C.E., Taylor, P.E., Zang, E.A., *et al.* (1986) 'Human T-cell lymphotropic virus type III infection in a cohort of homosexual men in New York City', *Journal of the American Medical Association* 255: 2167–72.

Thompson, L., Breckenridge, J., Gallagher, D., *et al.* (1984) 'Effects of bereavement on self-perceptions of physical health in elderly widows and widowers', *Journal of Gerontology* 39: 309–14.

Chapter twelve

Seasonal variation in suicide in Italy

Christa Zimmermann-Tansella, Rocco Micciolo, Paul Williams, and Michele Tansella

The seasonal variation in suicide has been a topic of enquiry for many years. There is a general consensus among most published studies that deaths by suicide show a significant seasonal variation in incidence, the main peak occurring in the springtime.

Recently the possibility has been raised that there might be systematic differences in the seasonal variation depending on factors such as sex, geographical location, and sociocultural context.

As far as sex differences are concerned, analyses of suicide data from England and Wales for the years 1958 to 1974 (Meares *et al.* 1981) showed that women had a main peak in spring, but also a smaller subsidiary peak in November. Data from Finland on the suicide incidence during the years 1961–76 confirmed this secondary concentration of suicides in the autumn period for widowed and married women (Nayha 1982).

As far as geographical differences are concerned, it has been suggested that less seasonal variation occurs where there is less climatic variability throughout the year (Aschoff 1981). The importance of sociocultural factors is underlined by observations that the seasonal variation of suicide is higher in predominantly rural countries such as Finland and Greece compared to more industrialized countries such as Denmark or Sweden (e.g. Parker and Walter 1982) and that the spring peak in suicide is more characteristic of agricultural than of industrial occupations (Nayha 1982).

The possibility that the seasonal variation reported in previous studies is not directly linked to sex or to climate but may be mediated by the social environment, i.e., by the variation in social contacts over the different seasons of the year, should be considered. This hypothesis, if true, would have important implications for the prevention of suicide and would stimulate appropriate actions on high-risk groups.

To explore the sex differences in the seasonal variation in suicide and to evaluate the climatic factors in relation to urban-rural differences, we therefore investigated these issues using data on suicide in Italy for the years 1969 to 1981 (Micciolo *et al.* 1988, 1989).

Italy extends over ten degrees of latitude and there are significant climatic differences between the north/central and the southern parts. Season-related climatic differences are more marked in the upper part of the country (a long cold winter and a warm summer season) than in the south, where the winter is short and mild. Moreover both parts have some predominantly rural and some predominantly urbanized regions. These characteristics are ideal for analysing the effects of climatic and socio-cultural differences on the seasonal variation in suicide. With this aim, the monthly frequencies of suicide over the thirteen-year period were analysed for four sub-groups: north/central-urban, north/central-rural, southern-urban, and southern-rural.

Sex differences were explored by analysing the monthly frequencies for males and females separately over the same period.

Method

Monthly national data on suicide (defined according to the certified cause of death) were obtained from the Central Institute of Statistics (ISTAT) in Rome. The data were analysed in two ways. First, the frequency of suicide in each month was plotted for each sub-group separately and inspected. Second, harmonic analyses were conducted using the method described by Pocock (1974). This method was first applied to suicide data by Barraclough and White (1978) and has been used recently to study seasonal variation in affective disorders (Williams *et al.* 1987) and monthly variation in the pattern of extramural psychiatric care (Balestrieri *et al.* 1987). It describes the variation of the number of suicides among the months as a sum of sinusoidal curves (harmonics). Using this model it is possible to divide the total variance in a seasonal component (which consists of those harmonics which repeat themselves an exact number of times per year) and non-seasonal and random components. The contribution of individual harmonics (one cycle per year, two cycles per year, etc.) can also be estimated.

One basic assumption in applying harmonic analysis is that the number of suicides is constant over the years. Since this was not the case, the analysis was performed on the residuals obtained by subtracting the main effect of the years (estimated using an ANOVA approach) from the data.

Research findings

Sex differences

Figure 12. 1 shows the monthly suicide frequency for the thirteen years of the study. Rates for men were double those for women and there was an increasing rate from 1976 for each sex. Cyclical fluctuations in the number of suicides can also be seen.

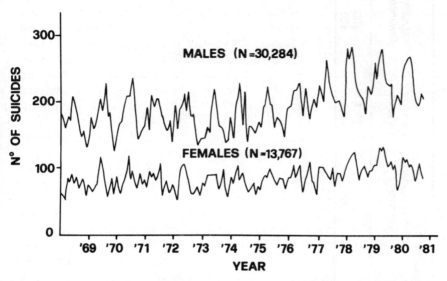

Figure 12.1   Monthly variation in the number of suicides for Italy, 1969–81

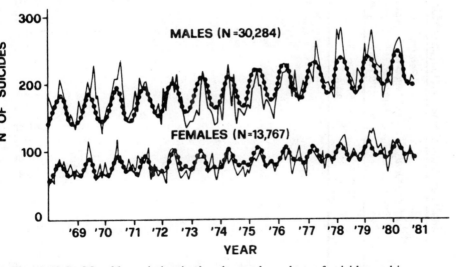

Figure 12.2   Monthly variation in the observed numbers of suicides and in expected numbers predicted by the first seasonal harmonic (males) and by the first and second seasonal harmonics (females). The trend over years was added to the expected numbers obtained from the harmonic analysis

Table 12.1 Harmonic analyses of male and female suicide incidence

		Percentage of variance explained by			
	All seasonal harmonics	First seasonal harmonic (one cycle/year)	Second seasonal harmonic (two-cycles/year)	Non-seasonal harmonics	Random variance	Total sample variance
Men	67.6	57.2	1.4	6.7	25.7	100
Women	50.6	30.6	13.3	8.6	40.8	100

Table 12.1 gives the results of the harmonic analyses. The seasonal harmonics accounted for 67.6 per cent of the variance in male suicides and it can be seen that the only important seasonal harmonic was the first (one cycle each year) accounting for 57.2 per cent of the total variance (84.7 per cent of the seasonal variance). The peak of this first harmonic occurred in May. We see also that the seasonal harmonics accounted for 50.6 per cent of the variance in female suicides. The first harmonic (one cycle each year) was the most important, accounting for 30.6 per cent of the total (60.5 per cent of the seasonal) variance, but the second harmonic (two cycles each year) was also substantial, accounting for 13.3 per cent of the total (26.3 per cent of the seasonal) variance in female suicides.

Figure 12.2 shows the expected values predicted by the first harmonic for males and those predicted by the first and the second harmonics for females. Examination of the expected values confirmed that the main peak was in May and that the subsidiary peak for women occurred in October–November. The differences between the maximum and the minimum number of expected suicides each month was fifty-four for males and twenty-five for females.

Geographical and urban-rural differences

This analysis used the data on the monthly frequency of suicides reported in each region of Italy for the years 1969–81. The regions were grouped according to the customary geopolitical division into north/central and south. North/central and southern regions were then divided into two groups, each depending on their location on the urban-rural continuum. This was done by ranking the regions according to the population density for 1974 (midpoint of the survey years).

Table 12.2 shows the annual suicide rates for the four different groupings. The rates are higher in the north/central than in the southern regions and the trend of increase is also greater in the upper part of the country. We see also that in both groups of regions suicide rates are higher in the less densely populated (rural) regions.

Figures 12.3 and 12.4 depict the monthly frequency of suicide in each of the four groups of regions. Cyclical fluctuations can be seen in each group and they appear consistent across the years. The trend of increase is also apparent and is greatest in the urban north and lowest in the rural south.

Harmonic analysis was used to cast light on the north/central-south difference in seasonality. As Table 12.3 demonstrates, the proportion of variance accounted for by seasonal harmonics was slightly greater for the north/central than for the southern region. In both cases only the first harmonic (one cycle each year) was important, and the amount of variance it explained did not differ between the two parts of the country. These early findings suggest, therefore, that climatic differences or differences in

Table 12.2 Annual suicide rates per 100,000 in Italy, 1969–81

	North/central regions		Southern regions	
	Urban	Rural	Urban	Rural
1969	6.18	6.93	3.50	4.56
1970	6.63	7.47	3.60	4.56
1971	7.03	7.15	3.62	5.27
1972	7.02	6.68	3.62	4.63
1973	6.68	6.82	3.39	5.27
1974	6.38	6.71	3.24	3.99
1975	6.50	6.26	3.77	4.63
1976	6.48	7.52	3.45	5.42
1977	7.43	7.52	3.70	5.44
1978	7.63	7.86	4.07	5.68
1979	8.38	8.78	4.12	5.91
1980	8.53	8.91	4.79	6.31
1981	8.04	8.44	4.47	6.17

climatic variability characteristic of the two parts of Italy exert no appreciable influence on the seasonal variation of suicide.

Table 12.3 also shows the results of the harmonic analyses conducted on the four sub-groups. Again in each case only the first harmonic was important. The seasonal variance was highest in the two urban groups and lowest in the rural regions, the seasonal variation in the rural south being the smallest. The peak of the first harmonic occurred always in May in urban regions, whereas in rural regions the peak occurred in June.

Table 12.3 Harmonic analyses on suicide incidence in different areas in Italy

	Percentage of variance explained by	
	All seasonal harmonics	First seasonal harmonic (one cycle/year)
North/central	69.1	50.5
South	55.9	48.0
Urban north/central	61.9	43.7
Urban south	52.6	41.9
Rural north/central	39.1	33.0
Rural south	18.9	18.8

Discussion

The reported findings demonstrate a marked seasonal variation in the incidence of suicide in Italy during the years 1969 to 1981. Moreover, they confirm observations from other countries (Meares *et al.* 1981; Nayha

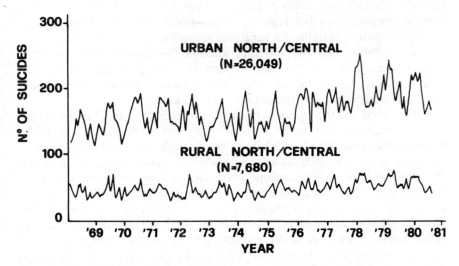

Figure 12.3 Monthly variation in observed numbers of suicides for urban and rural regions of north/central Italy

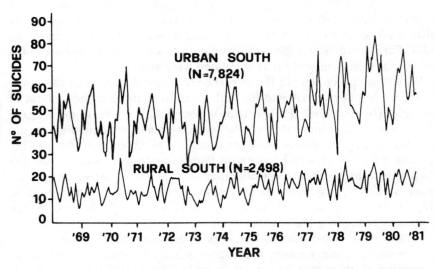

Figure 12.4 Monthly variation in observed numbers of suicides for urban and rural regions of southern Italy

1983) of important sex differences, with one cycle each year for men and two cycles each year for women.

No difference in seasonal variation was found between north/central and south Italy, thus excluding the hypothesis of a differential influence of climatic factors on seasonality. However, less seasonal variation occurred in rural compared to urban regions, a finding contrary to the observation of a higher seasonal variation in rural regions in Finland (Nayha 1982).

The possibility that the apparent seasonal fluctuation in suicide rates could be an artefact, due to seasonal fluctuation in recording and registration of suicides (as against accidents, natural causes of death, etc.), should be mentioned. However, this seems very unlikely.

The reasons for the seasonality of suicide incidence and for the sexual and sociocultural differences in seasonality are so far unknown. Links between the seasons and suicide have been sought for in the seasonality of depression. Several authors, analysing hospital admission data, found that the seasonality of suicide corresponds to the seasonal variation in affective psychosis (Eastwood and Stiasny 1978; Hare and Walters 1978). There is also evidence of seasonality in the occurrence of new episodes of affective disorders in the community (Williams *et al.* 1987), with some important sex differences. Males show a marked spring peak, and a lesser peak in late summer and autumn, in the occurrence of affective psychosis. The trends for women were similar, but seasonal variation was not significant and the amplitude of the spring peak was smaller than that for men despite the fact that women had a higher incidence rate for depression. No seasonal variation was observed in depressive neurosis for both sexes. In the present study a smaller seasonal variance in suicide incidence was observed for women as compared with men. Since the effects of seasonality are mainly attributed to climatic and natural environmental factors (Meares *et al.* 1981; Parker and Walter 1982) this would suggest a reduced responsiveness to natural factors in women as compared with men.

While the spring peak in the incidence of major depression and suicide incidence has been attributed for both sexes to changes in the amount of daylight (Nayha 1982; Parker and Walter 1982), there is no existing difference in circannual rhythms between men and women which could explain the autumn suicide peak for females. The hypothesis of a possibly greater influence of social factors on the incidence of female suicide has therefore to be taken into consideration. For example, the autumn peak, most marked among married and widowed women (Nayha 1982) could be due to sex-specific seasonal changes in social activity. Further studies are necessary to explore these possibilities.

As far as the urban-rural differences in the seasonality of suicide rates are concerned, the finding of a higher seasonal variation in urban as compared to rural regions was contrary to our expectations and needs comment. In Italy natural seasonal factors which should have their maximal impact in rural regions where people live in closer contact with their natural environment seem to be less potent than other season-related changes in urbanized areas in determining the annual rhythm in suicide incidence. This suggests the existence of environmental, non-natural rhythms coinciding with calendar-defined seasons which characterize urban life throughout Italy and which are less present in rural areas. Perhaps these patterns of seasonal change in urban regions (increased interaction in spring for example) are typical for Italy and may not be found in the same form in other countries with other types of urban, season-related social organization. This would explain the discrepancy with other reported findings. Further studies, comparing the monthly suicide variation in large cities with that in smaller towns within the same regions, are necessary to explore this issue.

Acknowledgements

This study was supported by the Consiglio Nazionale delle Ricerche (CNR, Roma), Progetto Finalizzato Medicina Preventiva e Riabilitativa. 1982–1987, Contract No. 86.01962.56.

References

Aschoff, J. (1981) 'Annual rhythms in man', in J. Aschoff (ed.) *Handbook of Behavioral Neurobiology: Biological Rhythms 4*, New York: Plenum, pp. 475–82.

Balestrieri, M., Williams, P., Micciolo, R., and Tansella, M. (1987), 'Monthly variation in the pattern of extramural psychiatric care', *Social Psychiatry* 22: 160–6.

Barraclough, B.M. and White, S.J. (1978) 'Monthly variation of suicide and undetermined death compared', *British Journal of Psychiatry* 132: 275–8.

Eastwood, M.R. and Stiasny, S. (1978) 'Psychiatric disorder, hospital admission and season', *Archives of General Psychiatry* 35: 769–71.

Hare, E.H. and Walter, S.D. (1978) 'Monthly variation of suicide and undetermined death compared', *Journal of Epidemiology and Community Health* 32: 47–52.

Meares, R., Mendelsohn, F.A.O., and Milgrom-Friedman, J. (1981) 'A sex difference in the seasonal variation of suicide rate: a single cycle for men, two cycles for women', *British Journal of Psychiatry* 138: 321–5.

Micciolo, R., Zimmermann-Tansella, C., Williams, P., and Tansella, M. (1988) 'Geographical variation in the seasonality of suicide', *Journal of Affective Disorders* 15: 163–8.

Micciolo, R., Zimmermann-Tansella, C., Williams, P., and Tansella, M. (1989) 'Seasonal variation in suicide: is there a sex difference?' *Psychological Medicine* (in press).

Nayha, S. (1982) 'Autumn incidence of suicides re-examined: data from Finland by sex, age and occupation', *British Journal of Psychiatry* 141: 512–7.

Nayha, S. (1983) 'The bi-seasonal incidence of some suicides: experience from Finland by marital status, 1961–1976', *Acta Psychiatrica Scandinavica* 67: 32–42.

Parker, G. and Walter, S. (1982) 'Seasonal variation in depressive disorders and suicidal deaths in New South Wales', *British Journal of Psychiatry* 140: 626–32.

Pocock, S.J. (1974) 'Harmonic analysis applied to seasonal variations in sickness absence', *Applied Statistics* 23(2): 103–20.

Williams, P., Balestrieri, M., and Tansella, M. (1987) 'Seasonal variation in affective disorders: a case register study', *Journal of Affective Disorders* 12: 145–52.

Chapter thirteen

Course and outcome of schizophrenia: a preliminary communication

Norman Sartorius

Introduction

The International Pilot Study of Schizophrenia (IPSS) demonstrated that transcultural comparative studies of mental disorders are feasible and that valid and reliable instruments for the assessment of these disorders in different cultures can be produced. It also showed that similar cases of schizophrenia exist in different cultures (WHO 1973, 1975). The most surprising finding of the IPSS, however, was that schizophrenic disorders in different cultures, although indistinguishable at the point of inclusion in the study, have a markedly different evolution and that the differences in their course and outcome are systematic, not random: favourable course and outcome of schizophrenia was significantly more frequent among patients in the developing countries than among patients in highly industrialized countries (WHO 1979).

This finding was of major significance: if it could be confirmed it would present a powerful argument in support of the thesis that sociocultural environment plays an important role in the development of schizophrenia and is to a large degree responsible for the impairment and disability which, according to reports from many countries over the years, often accompany or follow the schizophrenic syndrome.

Other hypotheses could also be offered to explain the difference. It could be, for example, that there are differences in the (biological or constitutional) ability of people to overcome an episode of schizophrenia. It could be that among people in the developing countries there were more who had a better capacity to recover from an attack of the disease. The higher prevalence of such people in developing countries could in turn be explained by high child mortality rates 'weeding out' most of the children with a lesser capacity to overcome stress or disease and increasing the proportion of those more able in the survivor-group.

A third hypothesis that could be built on an established difference in outcome in different cultures is that schizophrenia is not one but many diseases and that among them there are some with a more favourable course and outcome; the prevalence of these different diseases in the schizophrenia group may be different in different parts of the world.

But, interesting as these hypotheses may be, there was no point in launching studies to examine them until and unless the difference in the evolution of the illness in patients living in industrialized and other countries is firmly established. This consideration was at the basis of WHO's decision to initiate a second international and cross-cultural study which could establish beyond doubt whether there is a difference between the countries in the course of schizophrenia.

Design and method

The new study had to ensure that samples of patients with schizophrenia were not composed in a significantly different way in the various centres. It had to take the precautions usual in comparative cross-cultural studies, that is, (i) to use assessment instruments which were known to be applicable (and meaningful) in different cultures and (ii) to have investigators trained in the use of these instruments so that they could use them reliably. It also had to ensure that items likely to be helpful in the explanation of differences in course and outcome of schizophrenia were included in the examination and that their formulation was such that it could assure equivalence of responses across cultures.

The new study was therefore designed so as to include all new cases of schizophrenia contacting any helping agency in a geographically defined population. The instruments used for the assessment of the patients were those which had proved their value in the IPSS (complemented with additional questions or definitions where necessary) and a series of new instruments specifically developed and tested for this study. Among them the most notable were the schedules for the assessment of impairment and disability (Jablensky et al. 1980; WHO 1988). The investigators were trained in the use of all the instruments in joint training sessions and by circulation of taped interviews and written case histories. Reliability levels achieved in the assessment of the mental state and other characteristics of the patient were satisfactory at the beginning of the study and during its conduct.

The following field research centres participated in this project: Aarhus* (Denmark), Agra* and Chandigarh (India), Cali* (Colombia), Dublin (Ireland), Honolulu and Rochester (USA), Ibadan* (Nigeria), Moscow* (USSR), Nagasaki (Japan), Nottingham (UK), and Prague* (Czechoslovakia). The six centres indicated by an asterisk had taken part in the IPSS. The population size of each study area (total and in the 'risk' age group 15–54) is shown in Table 13.1.

Among the criteria for the selection of the centres to participate in the study were the existence of a well-trained team of investigators in the

Table 13.1 Catchment area populations

Centre	Total	Age group 15–54
Aarhus	574,000	314,000
Agra	2,806,346	1,426,755
Cali	1,347,466	784,009
Chandigarh/rural	103,865	61,642
Chandigarh/urban	348,609	205,786
Dublin	280,322	149,879
Honolulu	357,225	210,020
Ibadan	931,348	635,999
Moscow	392,097	231,866[1]
Nagasaki	447,444	267,149
Nottingham	380,023	202,214
Prague	1,114,809	578,379
Rochester	397,828	237,223

[1]Age 18–54

centre, the commitment of the centre staff to the investigation, and the support for the study of the institutions which housed the teams and of the governments concerned. These criteria had proved their value in previous studies, and in this study also all the centres invited to participate completed the work successfully. The design of the study is described in detail elsewhere (Sartorius *et al.* 1986; Jablensky *et al.* to be published).

Every resident of a given catchment area in the age range 15–54 who, at any time in the previous three months, had made a first contact with any 'helping agency' because of problems suggesting the presence of a psychotic illness was examined using a screening schedule which contained operationally defined criteria for inclusion in the study. Prior to the start of the case-finding process each project team had identified and contacted all services and agencies which were considered as likely sites of contact for potential study subjects. These ranged from local psychiatric facilities to non-specialist or alternative agencies which, in some of the areas, included traditional or religious healers.

Although complete uniformity in the composition of the case-finding networks and in the procedures leading to screening was impossible to achieve, the good co-operation that had been established between the project teams and the local 'helping agencies' resulted in a regular and uninterrupted inflow of cases in most of the centres. In order to insure against fluctuations in the case-finding rates because of extraneous, short-term disruptions, the case-finding process was extended over two or more years. The centres were also required to carry out additional small-scale studies to assess whether there was a significant 'leakage' of cases from the study.

With the exception of eighty-two cases who defaulted after screening, all patients who met the screening criteria were given a full clinical assessment by the area project team. This assessment included a mental state examination using the ninth edition of the Present State Examination (PSE) (Wing *et al.* 1974), and a detailed history interview (usually with a key informant) using the Psychiatric and Personal History Schedule (PPHS) constructed specifically for the study. A Diagnostic and Prognostic Schedule (DPS) which in addition to items about diagnosis also contained items concerning the estimated need for treatment and management measures, as well as a narrative summary of the case, was also filled in. Additional research instruments – for example, a Life Events Schedule, the Camberwell Family Interview, the Katz Adjustment Scales (KAS), and the WHO Disability Assessment Schedule (DAS) – were applied in centres participating in studies undertaken by sub-groups interested in special issues arising in the study. The results of these studies have been described elsewhere (Leff *et al.* 1987; Wig *et al.* 1987; Day *et al.* 1987; Katz *et al.* 1988; WHO 1988).

Copies of the research schedules or scoring sheets were mailed to the study headquarters in Geneva and checked for completeness, validity, and consistency. Each case was reviewed by headquarters investigators and consultants in order to ascertain that the inclusion criteria were met and that no exclusion criteria were present.

An important component of this central review of the material was the CATEGO reference classification of the cases which provided diagnostic assessment complementary to the clinical diagnosis.

Research findings

The total study population consisted of 1,379 subjects (745 men and 634 women). With the exception of one of the two catchment areas of the Chandigarh centre and the Agra area, the vast majority of the patients were urban residents. In Cali and Ibadan the samples included considerable proportions of inhabitants of the rapidly expanding peri-urban slum areas. With the exception of Ibadan, Cali, and the rural area of Chandigarh, where most patients came from very poor neighbourhoods, the socioeconomic status of the patients' neighbourhoods and households in the other centres was rated as 'average' in comparison with local standards in the majority of cases.

There was a marked predominance of single marital status among the male subjects in all centres except Agra, Chandigarh (rural), and Moscow; in contrast, relatively high proportions of the female subjects (with the exception of Cali, Dublin, and Nagasaki) were either married or divorced. While as many as 35 per cent of the patients in Aarhus were living alone, the proportion of single-person households was lower in the other centres, and virtually nil in Agra and Chandigarh.

The level of education varied markedly among the centres, the extremes being the high proportion of illiterate subjects (30–56 per cent) in Chandigarh (rural), Agra, and Ibadan, and the high percentages (10–23 per cent) of university graduates in Moscow, Chandigarh (urban), Prague, and Honolulu.

The great majority (86 per cent of the 1,218) cases in whom the beginning of the psychotic illness could be reliably dated had been identified by the case-finding network and assessed within twelve months of the onset of the disorder. The proportions of patients with a length of previous illness of less than six months and of six months and over did not differ between developed and developing countries.

The most common symptoms in all centres were those which could be seen as diagnostically non-specific indicators of a disturbed mental state, such as restlessness, poor concentration, subjective feeling of nervous tension, and social withdrawal. There was much similarity between symptom profiles of the patients in the developed and developing countries. There were, however, three points where the profiles differed: (i) there was a higher frequency of affective symptoms (mainly depressive) among patients in the developed countries; (ii) there was a higher frequency of delusional mood and 'thought insertion' in patients in the developed countries; and (iii) there was a higher frequency of 'voices speaking to subject' and of visual hallucinations in patients in the developing countries.

The incidence of schizophrenia was calculated for the eight catchment areas in which satisfactory coverage was achieved of the various 'helping agencies' which were thought likely to serve as first-contact points for most psychotic patients. It should be borne in mind that incidence in the present context refers to the rate of occurrence of first lifetime contacts with any service or agency by subjects (i) who presented evidence of having experienced psychotic symptoms during the previous twelve months and/or exhibited such symptoms on clinical examination close to the point of first contact, and (ii) who met specified diagnostic criteria for schizophrenia and related disorders. The population data for the denominator of the incidence rates were obtained from the census which was closest to the period of case-finding in each centre (1980 in most centres).

One-year rates per 10,000 population at risk in all age groups between 15 and 54 were calculated for a 'broad' diagnostic definition of the condition (i.e., all included cases except thirty-four on which insufficient data were available) and for a 'restrictive' definition based only on the presence of an initial clinical picture satisfying the criteria for CATEGO class S+. Among patients with a 'broad diagnosis' of schizophrenia, the majority fall into CATEGO classes S, P, or O+. The incidence figures for CATEGO class S+ patients were found to be very similar among the centres, ranging from 7/100,000 in Aarhus to 14/100,000 in Nottingham. The difference among the centres is not statistically significant (Table 13.2).

199

Table 13.2 One-year incidence rates, CATEGO class S+ per 100,000 population at risk (ages 15–54)

Centre	Male	Female	Total
Aarhus	9	5	7
Chandigarh (urban)	13	9	11
Chandigarh (rural)	8	11	9
Dublin	9	8	9
Honolulu	8	7	8
Moscow	10	14	12
Nagasaki	11	9	10
Nottingham	16	12	14

Follow-up examinations of patients, using the full battery of research instruments (including follow-up versions of the PPHS and the DAS), were carried out twice, at intervals of one year and two years following the date of initial screening and inclusion in the study. In addition to two cross-sections of symptomatology (assessed with the PSE) and one assessment of social disability (carried out with the DAS at two years), the longitudinal, month-by-month ratings and narrative notes on symptoms and behaviour provided the basis for an evaluation of the two-year (24 ± 6 months) pattern of course of the disorder.

Data sufficient for rating and categorizing the pattern of course were available on 1014 (i.e., 74 per cent) of the original 1,379 patients. Of those with completed follow-up, 600 subjects were assessed in centres in developed countries (76 per cent success at follow-up) and 414 in centres in developing countries (71 per cent success at follow-up). There were no significant differences in the demographic characteristics of the groups for whom follow-up data were available and the groups about which information was incomplete.

The findings of the analysis of the course of illness clearly confirmed those of the IPSS. Among patients in the developing countries there were significantly fewer who had a protracted course of illness. Nearly two-fifths of all patients in these countries had no further episodes of illness (nor any impairment) after the initial episode. Only one in ten patients with schizophrenia in the centres in developing countries showed an unrelenting course of illness over the two-year follow-up period. Of the patients who had further episodes of illness after they recovered from the initial episodes, half had good remissions in between (see Table 13.3).

Other characteristics of course and outcome supported the above finding: 38.3 per cent of the patients in the developing countries spent more than 75 per cent of the follow-up period in full remission; only 15.9 per cent had to be kept on antipsychotic medication over the two years and only 15.7 per cent had impaired social function (see table 13.4).

Table 13.3 Pattern of course, by centre

Pattern of course	Developed countries	Developing countries
	%	%
One episode, full remission	15.5	37.0
Several episodes, full remission	21.4	26.6
One episode, incomplete remission	17.2	11.6
Several episodes, incomplete remission	26.1	12.8
Continuous illness	19.8	12.1
No. of patients in this analysis	600	414

Table 13.4 Differences between patients in developed and developing countries on selected outcome variables

Variable	Developing country	Developed country
	%	%
Patients in full remission more than 3/4 of the follow-up time	38.3	22.3
Patients on anti-psychotic medication 76–100% of follow-up time	15.9	60.8
Patients never hospitalized	55.5	8.1
Patients with impaired social function, throughout	15.7	41.6

Total number of patients included in the study: 1,379
Number of patients included in this analysis: 1,014

Discussion

Detailed analyses of the course and outcome variables are now under way and their results will be published shortly. The preliminary examination of the data, however, already shows that the findings of this study confirm those of the IPSS: patients in developing countries experience a milder course of schizophrenia than do those in industrialized countries.

The full explanation of this finding may not be possible without further research; it is, however, important to note that the results of the present study can be of use for the planning of mental health services, particularly when they are considered jointly with other results of WHO studies (e.g., WHO 1984). A vast majority of patients in developing countries can be treated as out-patients and their disease does have a milder course under these circumstances. This does not mean that it is possible to organize an active and appropriate mental health service system without any in-patient facilities or rehabilitation programme. In a certain proportion of patients in the developing countries, schizophrenia does have a severe course and a poor outcome: though their numbers are smaller, appropriate facilities for their treatment and rehabilitation are of essential importance from the point of view of public health and for humanitarian reasons. Nevertheless, a different course of disease does mean that services for the mentally ill in developing countries have to be, to an extent, different in structure, function, and organization.

The possible explanations for the differences in course and outcome of schizophrenia sketched out at the beginning of this paper are not the only ones and future investigators will formulate others. The data from this study could be analysed to explore the probability of some of the hypotheses: it is, however, likely that further research into the course of schizophrenia will be necessary and that it requires longitudinal prospective studies of samples selected using epidemiological strategies.

Acknowledgements

The results presented here are a product of a joint effort of many individuals and institutions. Among them are A. Jablensky, Ailsa Korten, Gunilla Ernberg and other WHO staff, and the Heads of WHO Collaborating Centres, E. Strömgren (Aarhus), K.C. Dube (Agra), C. Leon (Cali), N.N. Wig and V. Varma (Chandigarh), D. Walsh (Dublin), A. Marsella and M. Kàtz (Honolulu), M. Olatawura (Ibadan), R.A. Nadzharov and N.N. Zharikov (Moscow), R. Takahashi and Y. Nakane (Nagasaki), J.E. Cooper (Nottingham), L. Hanzlicek and J. Gebhart (Prague), and L.C. Wynne and T. Gift (Rochester, N.Y.). This study was financed jointly by the field research centres, WHO and the National Institute of Mental Health, Washington, DC (mental health special grant MH 29969).

References

Day, R., Nielsen, J.A., Korten, A., et al. (1987) 'Stressful life events preceding the acute onset of schizophrenia: a cross-national study from the World Health Organization', Culture, Medicine and Psychiatry 11 (2), Dordrecht and Boston: D. Reidel Publishing Company.

Jablensky, A., Schwarz, R. and Tomov, T. (1980) 'WHO collaborative study on impairments and disabilities associated with schizophrenic disorders', in 'Epidemiological research as basis for the organization of extramural psychiatry', Acta Psychiatrica Scandinavica, Supplement 285, 62: 152–63.

Jablensky, A., Sartorius, N., Ernberg, G., et al. (in press) 'Schizophrenia: manifestations, incidence and course in different cultures: a report prepared on behalf of the collaborating investigators', Psychological Medicine.

Katz, M.M., Marsella, A., Dube, K.C., et al. (1988) 'On the expression of psychosis in different cultures: schizophrenia in an Indian and in a Nigerian community', Culture, Medicine and Psychiatry 12: 331–55.

Leff, J., Wig, N.N., Ghosh, A., *et al.* (1987) 'Expressed emotion and schizophrenia in North India, III: influence of relatives' expressed emotion on the course of schizophrenia in Chandigarh', *British Journal of Psychiatry* 151: 166–73.

Sartorius, N., Jablensky A., Korten, A., *et al.* (1986) 'Early manifestations and first-contact incidence of schizophrenia in different cultures: preliminary communication', *Psychological Medicine* 16: 909–28.

Wig, N.N., Menon, D.K., Bedi, H., *et al.* (1987) 'Expressed emotion and schizophrenia in North India, I: the cross-cultural transfer of ratings of relatives' expressed emotion', *British Journal of Psychiatry* 151: 156–60.

Wig, N.N., Menon, D.K., Bedi, H., *et al.* (1987) 'Expressed emotion and schizophrenia in North India, II: distribution of expressed emotion components among relatives of schizophrenic patients in Aarhus and Chandigarh', *British Journal of Psychiatry* 151: 160–5.

Wing, J.K., Cooper, J.E., and Sartorius, N. (1974) *The Measurement and Classification of Psychiatric Symptoms*, Cambridge: Cambridge University Press.

World Health Organization (1973) *The International Pilot Study of Schizophrenia vol. 1*, Geneva: WHO.

World Health Organization (1975) 'Schizophrenia: a multinational study: a summary of the intial evaluation phase of the International Pilot Study of Schizophrenia', *Public Health Paper* 63.

World Health Organization (1979) *Schizophrenia: An International Follow-up Study*, Chichester: Wiley.

World Health Organization (1984) 'Mental health care in developing countries: a critical appraisal of research findings', *Technical Report Series* 698, Geneva: WHO.

World Health Organization (1988) *WHO Psychiatric Disability Assessment Schedule (WHO/DAS)*, Geneva: WHO.

Part four

Finding ways to protect vulnerable groups and individuals

Chapter fourteen

Implications of a vulnerability model for the prevention of affective disorder

Tirril Harris

The translation of epidemiological findings into effective preventive strategies is rarely simple. In the case of affective disorder the task is doubly complicated. On the one hand, *psychiatric* unlike physical illness involves the individual's conscious interpretation of environmental factors. On the other hand, the multifactorial aetiology of depression, which has come to be generally acknowledged with the final common pathway model (Akiskal and McKinney 1973), introduces a variety of items which require intricate balancing in their combination. The aetiological model of depression which I shall discuss here – the vulnerability model outlined by George Brown and colleagues – focuses upon the intervening psychological process by which the grosser sociodemographic variables examined in epidemiological research become linked with depressive disorder. Moreover, by distinguishing provoking factors from vulnerability and symptom-formation factors, it allots weightings to the many variables proposed by multifactorial models. Aetiological models distinguishing provoking from vulnerability factors may perhaps be more familiar if described in terms of stress-diathesis or hazards versus resources (see Leighton in this volume). I shall argue that this distinction can deepen our understanding of the psychological process of depressive onset, thus throwing light on the topic of prevention of depression. The research I shall review will also have a more general bearing on the interpretation of epidemiological findings in prospective enquiries. Although an attempt will be made to set the theoretical model in the context of other research findings, limitations on space unfortunately may lend a certain parochialism to the discussion.

The initial vulnerability model

The early versions of the vulnerability model arose from findings in a random general population sample of 458 women in the inner London Borough of Camberwell in the early 1970s (Brown and Harris 1978a). The shortened version of the Present State Examination (or PSE, see Wing *et al.* 1974) was used to collect data on symptoms, and respondents with a number of such symptoms were subsequently given a clinical diagnostic interview by two collaborating psychiatrists. This allowed the distinction of cases (where symptoms were on a scale comparable to those among out-patient attenders) from borderline cases (where symptoms were present but less numerous and less severe). Although by the time of later surveys some of the better-known 'caseness' thresholds had been publicized (for example, the Index of Definition for use with the PSE), we continued to use the Bedford College threshold in order to ensure comparability with our own previous work. A discriminant function analysis performed on the PSE findings on 866 respondents rated according to the Bedford College system (Finlay-Jones *et al.* 1980) provided the basis for an algorithm which makes it possible for other PSE users to employ the same threshold (e.g., Bebbington *et al.* 1984). Their research suggests that this threshold for 'caseness' is comparable with, if perhaps a little higher than, others such as ID level-5 when using the CATEGO program with the PSE and the Research Diagnostic Criteria for major depression (Dean *et al.* 1983; Brown 1981; for further reference to CATEGO and ID level see Wing and Sturt 1978).

Using this threshold, chronic cases, whose episodes had begun more than twelve months before interview, were distinguished from onset cases, whose symptoms had begun only within that year. The former were then excluded from any analyses of possible aetiological factors. Variables considered included not only basic sociodemographic items such as social class, marital status, and so on, but also stressful experiences as measured by the Life Events and Difficulties Schedule or LEDS (for the most recent exposition see Brown and Harris 1989). This approach emphasizes the *qualitative* meaning of a life event rather than merely the amount of readjustment required by the experience. By rating such meanings con-textually, that is, in terms of the type of reaction to such a life event *expected* from the average person with the same biographical circum-stances, not in terms of the *actual* reaction of this particular respondent, the LEDS aims to reduce the degree of reporting bias attendant upon much stress research (Brown 1974). It emerged that events which were severe (that is, those which 10 to 14 days after their occurrence still threatened to have undesirable long-term consequences) were associated with onset of depression, as were major difficulties (ongoing problems of a certain contextual unpleasantness lasting at least two years and not involving physical health). The term 'provoking agent' was introduced to cover these two types of depressogenic stressor. Events where there was only a short-term threat or unpleasantness which had resolved within a few days were not associated with depressive onset.

The effects of these provoking agents seemed to be potentiated by four other sociodemographic factors, although the presence of these without a provoking agent did not increase the likelihood of depressive onset. This is the fundamental characteristic of a vulnerability factor. Table 14.1 illustrates this phenomenon for the most powerful of these factors, lack of an intimate, confiding relationship. It can be seen in the right-hand cell of the bottom row that lack of any confidant at all is not especially conducive to depression without the experience of a provoking agent. On the other hand, following the top row from left to right it is clear that women with a husband or boyfriend in whom they can confide (in the 'A' group) are less vulnerable than women with another confidant outside their household but seen at least once a week (the 'B' group) who in turn are less vulnerable than those with a confidant seen less frequently ('C' group) or no confidant at all ('D' group). Already the patterning of the epidemiological findings is hinting at the nature of the psychological process involved.

Table 14.1 Percentage of women in Camberwell who experienced onset of caseness in year, by whether they had a severe event or major difficulty and intimacy context (chronic cases excluded)

	Intimacy		
	'A' (high)	'B'	'C' OR 'D' (low)
	%	%	%
Severe event or major difficulty	10 (9/88)	26 (12/47)	41 (12/29)
No severe event or major difficulty	1 (2/193)	3 (1/39)	4 (1/23)

When the other three vulnerability factors are examined in addition we see further evidence of this kind of patterning (Table 14.2). The factors involved are, first, loss of mother in childhood before age 11 either by death or by a continuous separation of at least one year; second, the presence of three or more children under 15 at home, and, third, lack of employment (either full- or part-time) outside the home. Again, there is an effect which emerges only under certain conditions. Comparing the top row with the other two it is clear that only among those lacking a confiding relationship with husband or boyfriend does employment outside the home render women less vulnerable. If this can be correctly interpreted it may give clues to the intricacies of the psychic process by which employment and confiding somehow fend off the impact of provoking agents.

Our initial interpretation was presented in the schema below:

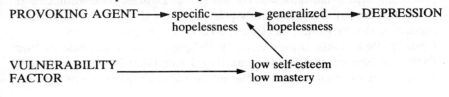

Table 14.2 Percentage of women developing depression among those with a provoking agent

	Employed	Not employed
	%	%
I 'A' intimacy	9 (4/43)	11 (5/45)
II No 'A' intimacy	15 (6/39)	30 (7/23)
III No 'A' intimacy; experience of either or both vulnerability factors 2 & 3 (early loss of mother, 3+ children under 15 at home)	63 (5/8)	100 (6/6)

Essentially this suggests, following Beck (1967), that cognitions concerning the future and its hopefulness are critical in terms of whether the vegetative symptoms of depression will overtake the subject. If she has only a low sense of self-worth she will be more likely to generalize any specific feelings of hopelessness about the provoking agent, and this generalization will be the critical step along the final pathway to depressive disorder. Three of the four vulnerability factors, it was argued, could contribute to a low level of ongoing self-esteem by involving roles where the subject had, or was prevented from having, an opportunity to enhance her self-esteem by successful performance: women with more than two young children would find it more difficult to leave the home to pursue such extra role identities, women with a job had exactly such an extra role area. A successful heterosexual partnership provided a similar opportunity, although there were alternative hypotheses which could explain how intimate confiding protected against depression – for example, a mechanistic process of ventilating dammed up feelings which might otherwise interfere with sleep or concentration. The fourth vulnerability factor, loss of mother in childhood, could also be linked with similar intrapsychic mediation involving the self-image, despite its distance in time from the onset period, if it was hypothesized that the sequelae of mother loss were likely to set in train a biography of role identities where performance could never be rewarded in the same way as if the original mother were still alive to praise any success.

Reflections on the initial model

Without replication, of course, this aetiological model was of little use for preventive work. A number of studies repeated the findings involving provoking agents and intimate confiding – in eight of nine studies (eight strict replications and one closely related), the patterning of data closely resembled that in Table 14.1 (Campbell *et al.* 1983; Brown and Prudo 1981; Costello 1982; Finlay-Jones 1988; Bebbington *et al.* 1984; Martin 1985; Parry and Shapiro 1986; Brown and Andrews 1985; Paykel *et al.* 1980). Thus, though the same success did not attend the replication of the other vulnerability factors, a basic version of the model seemed established as some kind of foundation from which to consider preventive implications – especially since there were good reasons to account for some of these failures (see Brown and Harris 1986a).

Initial reactions to this basic vulnerability model tended to involve recommendations to mitigate the vulnerability factors, on the grounds that little can be done to prevent life events such as the death of a key person, while other provoking agents of depression, such as redundancies at work or eviction from a house, are sociopolitically determined and can seldom be modified by clinicians. This line of approach was also supported by arguments that the model was wrongly formulated, the vulnerability factors being really risk factors of equal importance with provoking agents. These arguments were based on a particular type of multivariate analysis which pinpointed as the best fitting model one with two main effects but no interaction between the two types of factor (Tennant and Bebbington 1978). The statistical analysis at stake here involved *multiplicative* inter-action, but a comparable procedure using an additive approach would have revealed a significant interactive effect (Everitt and Smith 1979; Brown and Harris 1986b). Probably more important than statistical considerations, however, was the basic lack of refinement to the assumptions which underlie the move from epidemiological findings to policy recommenda-tions. It appeared logical to move from a finding – say, that lack of employment outside the home was a vulnerability (or, as was argued, a main risk) factor – to a preventive recommendation – say, that women should be encouraged to work outside the home.

Even in its initial version, however, the vulnerability model was more complicated than to permit such a simple, almost mechanistic move. First it should be emphasized that, even at the basic level of statistical association, lack of employment was emerging only as a second-order vulnerability factor (see earlier discussion of Table 14.2). Second, the speculative theoretical model invoked to explain the Camberwell findings (that is, the concepts – in small type – invoked to explain the associations – in capitals – in the model) was ambiguous about the time order of the relationship between the demographic factor and the low self-esteem considered crucial in explaining that factor's role. It was left open as to whether the low self-esteem predated the demographic factor, which would then be only an indicator of a pre-existing psychological vulnerability (model A below) or whether the factor actually itself lowered self-esteem (model B):

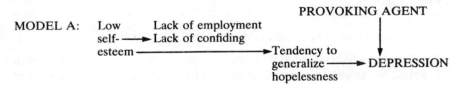

MODEL A:

PROVOKING AGENT

Low self-esteem → Lack of employment Lack of confiding

Low self-esteem → Tendency to generalize hopelessness → DEPRESSION

PROVOKING AGENT

MODEL B: Lack of employment Low ↓ Tendency to
            Lack of confiding ──▶ self- ──▶ generalize ──────▶ DEPRESSION
                                 esteem   hopelessness

Third, another complication involves the interrelationships of the factors over time. If vulnerability factors represent ongoing situations, is it not possible that they themselves may render it more or less likely that severe events will occur later? The vulnerability model as first presented was relatively static; thus, once a provoking agent occurred, vulnerability factors were found to act in synergy to potentiate its depressogenic impact. But, taking a more dynamic view, might it not be possible that over and above this process there is another, in which the occurrence of a provoking event or situation is made more likely later on by such a vulnerability factor, if a woman is not accustomed to it? Thus, cajoling mothers into full-time employment could have the effect of increasing their rate of ex-periencing provoking events: for example, by encroaching on the time they can devote to their teenage offspring these jobs might increase the numbers with events and difficulties involving children's truancy or delinquency. Similarly, a well-intentioned insistence on forced self-disclosure between spouses who have lived together without confiding might lead in the immediate period to an increased experience of severe revelation events, as earlier infidelities came to light rendering hitherto lukewarm marriages suddenly rejecting. All the good that might be achieved by a woman having an additional alternative role area as worker or confidante might be vitiated if the new role areas threatened her performance in the pre-existing role.

In sum then, without a closer grasp on the detailed historical develop-ment of the two types of factor it would be premature to derive conclusions about prevention from such a speculative causal model.

Later refinements of the model

Since the Camberwell survey it has been possible to explore this model of depressive disorder in more detail, on the one hand following up these particular questions and on the other gaining new insights into the psychological processes underlying the associations of the cruder socio-demographic variables. Two surveys in particular were able to throw light on the problems of biographical development and the time order of the various factors.

Vulnerability stemming from childhood: the conveyor belt

The first survey, carried out in 1978–9 in Walthamstow, London, was designed to explore the possible pathways by which the vulnerability factor 'loss of mother before age 11', identified by the Camberwell survey, could have an impact so many years later. It confirmed the earlier finding about prevalence of depression and also suggested that loss of mother between ages 11 and 17 could have an intermediate impact (Brown *et al.* 1986a). In examining the factors intervening between childhood loss and adult depression, the study pinpointed the quality of replacement care after the loss as the most important link in the causal chain (Harris *et al.* 1986). Another important link was the quality of any current relationship with a partner. This was expected in the light of the earlier research, but particularly interesting in terms of giving insight into the biographical development of vulnerability to depression was the finding that the women often appeared to have been trapped with these undependable partners as a result of the lack of adequate care shown them during childhood. Many had left home early to escape stepmothers and, having nowhere to go, had married before they had a chance to check on the suitability of their spouse. Even more often they had become premaritally pregnant, either as a result of inadequate instruction in sexual and contraceptive matters (yet another example of inadequate care) or, it seemed, because the sexual act had an aura of the physical affection which their upbringing had denied them (Harris *et al.* 1987). The couple forced to settle down to early child-rearing before they had had time to save enough resources seemed to be on a conveyor belt leading to the experience of the financial and interpersonal provoking agents so frequently producing depression:

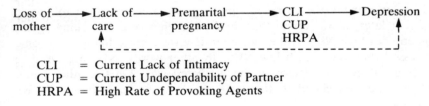

CLI   = Current Lack of Intimacy
CUP = Current Undependability of Partner
HRPA = High Rate of Provoking Agents

The second survey, carried out in Islington in the early 1980s, confirmed this set of links (Bifulco *et al.* 1987). It was further able to show that premarital pregnancy did not itself act as a current vulnerability factor. In other words the contribution of premarital pregnancy to depressive onset was only as a harbinger of later severe events and major difficulties, not also as a sign of some additional insensitivity to the impact of provoking agents. By contrast, lack of care contributed to depressive onset through both pathways (see dotted arrow above). Although the proportion with severe current life stress was much higher among those women with the two childhood and teenage experiences, those who had managed to avoid these provoking agents in the present period were rarely depressed despite their harsh biographies: they somehow seemed to have managed to get off the conveyor belt.

The focus on childhood lack of care in these two studies has parallels in other findings (Parker 1979, 1981, 1983; Adam *et al.* 1982; Kennard and Birtchnell 1982; Birtchnell and Kennard 1984) and is theoretically consistent with the model outlined, where self-esteem is given such a key role. It makes intuitive sense that nurturant attentiveness should convey to a child that the care-giver considers him worth caring for. Since the regard of others is the source of our own self-regard it is to be expected that deficient childhood care will result in a parallel deficiency in self-esteem which may persist into adulthood. It is to the examination of this that we now turn.

Testing the earlier speculations: self-esteem, positive versus negative

The great merit of the Islington study was that it was prospective and it was therefore possible to measure self-esteem before onset of depression, thus preserving any conclusions from the criticism that the findings were confounded by the impact of the episode itself. The measures of self-evaluation used were designed to cover as many as possible of the attributes and roles which go to make up the self-image and to allow for the fact that people may simultaneously feel highly positive about one aspect of themselves while feeling very negative about another. The two composite measures reported on here are basically summaries of all these aspects: positive evaluation of the self (PES) summarized all the comments made in the course of a three-hour interview which reflected definite self-approbation in the various areas, whereas negative evaluation of the self (NES) summarized the corresponding negative comments. At follow-up one year later, it was found that, in the presence of a provoking agent, women with high NES at the first interview were more likely to become depressed than those with low NES. In other words, NES appeared to act as a vulnerability factor in the predicted way. On the other hand, PES was not associated to the same extent with illness onset (Brown *et al.* 1986c).

Some overlap was found between NES and the presence of minor psychiatric symptoms at first interview, though less than expected. Of a total of 303 women at risk, sixty-five manifested *chronic* forms of these sub-clinical conditions, and thirty-three of these (51 per cent) had a high NES, compared with only forty-eight of the remaining 238 (20 per cent) who had no such symptomatology. The risk of onset of depression was also related to these sub-clinical conditions. By contrast, the history of a previous episode of affective disorder was found to be unrelated to the risk of a depressive episode. But when a more subtle approach was taken to the measurement of provoking agents it emerged that the vulnerability effect of chronic sub-clinical conditions, unlike the effect of NES, might be confounded by other factors, to which we now turn (see Brown *et al.* 1986b).

Further insights into provoking agents and their meaning

Already during the Camberwell study some provoking agents seemed more depressogenic than others, particularly if they involved loss (Finlay-Jones and Brown 1981). In the Islington survey, degree of loss was systematically rated on every severe event and was found to improve prediction of onset substantially: 27 per cent (24/88) of women with at least one loss event as compared with 12 per cent (5/42) of women with a non-loss severe event became depressed (Brown *et al.* 1987). The importance of loss for depressive onset has now been systematically established using another life event instrument (see Dohrenwend *et al.* 1986). The prospective nature of the Islington study allowed another refinement to the measure of events: knowledge of the subjects' commitments and role conflicts at first interview could be used to sharpen the ratings of threat in the follow-up period: severe events which 'matched' areas of earlier high commitment or high role conflict were more likely to produce depression, as were severe events which matched areas where the subject had already had a severe ongoing non-health difficulty lasting at least six months up to first interview. It was this last category of events – events matching an ongoing difficulty – which seemed to explain why women with chronic sub-clinical conditions were more likely to suffer depression. Those without matching events (but without NES) were no more likely to experience onset after a provoking agent than women without such a chronic minor condition (Brown *et al.* 1986b).

Perhaps even more striking than the importance of 'matching' was the overwhelming preponderance of events involving personal relationships: among the twenty-nine women with an onset of depression following a severe life event, 90 per cent of the events in question involved relationships (if pregnancies and births are counted) and only 10 per cent involved problems in other areas, such as work, finances, housing, or health; whereas among women experiencing severe life events who had no episode of depression, the corresponding proportions were 65 per cent and 35 per cent (Brown *et al.* 1987).

The significance of support within the setting of core relationships

This focus upon the importance of crises in relationships brings us back to the theme of the most important vulnerability factor in the Camberwell model, namely social support or intimacy. At the first Islington interview the women's social network and support system was rated on a whole range of measures by the SESS instrument (see Brown *et al.* 1986c). At the follow-up interview the crude Camberwell intimacy rating was applied retrospectively, and a new rating of crisis support also made in order to detail the actual mobilization of support to cope with the provoking agents which had occurred since the first interview. For crisis support to be rated as present not only did the woman have to have confided and received active emotional support, to at least a moderate degree, through a core relationship, but also there must have been no negative response (of the kind 'you have only yourself to blame' or 'anyone who worries about that sort of thing is a fool'). A core relationship involved either the partner or someone described by the subject as 'very close'.

Initial analysis of these data proved confusing: for single mothers the predictions of the model were confirmed, support recorded at the first interview being predictive of crisis support, and this in turn reducing vulnerability. For married women, highly negative measures predicted depression, but low positive ones did not; for example, among those with a provoking agent, 35 per cent (14/40) of those who reported negative interaction with the spouse – involving quarrels, threats of separation, or major tension – became depressed, compared with only 10 per cent (6/61) of those who had no such negative interaction. On the other hand, the presence of an intimate, confiding relationship (i.e., a positive measure) did not differentiate: compare the two row totals in Table 14.3. Furthermore, the two retrospective measures of support (an intimate, confiding relationship and the presence of crisis support during the follow-up period) fulfilled perfectly the requirements for vulnerability factors, as the column totals in Table 14.3 indicate. (See also Brown and Andrews 1985.)

Table 14.3 Confiding in husband at first interview, crisis support during the follow-up year and onset of depression among those with a provoking agent (97 married Islington women)

Confiding in husband at 1st interview	Crisis support from husband during follow-up		
	Yes % onset	No % onset	Total % onset
Yes	4 (1/28)	37 (7/19) 'let down'	17 (8/47)
No	25 (2/8)	24 (10/42)	24 (12/50)
Total	8(3/36)	28 (17/61)	21 (20/97)

Crisis support not known for 4

When both married and unmarried women were included in the analysis, the findings with regard to the retrospective measures were essentially similar, taking into account other core relationships as well as those with partners. Interestingly enough, however, a non-core relationship did not seem to reduce vulnerability: 58 per cent (7/12) with only such non-core support developed depression, compared to 33 per cent (14/42) of those receiving no support at all, and 10 per cent (9/92) of those receiving it from a core contact (p <.001, with four missing ratings). Crisis support from a member of a caring profession was also not associated with reduced vulnerability: 33 per cent (8/24) with and 18 per cent (22/122) without such support developed depression ($\chi^2 = 2.88$; $df = 1$; n.s.).

One possible explanation of these discrepancies is that retrospective reporting of intimacy and support cannot be trusted, being too subject to distortion as a result of depressed mood. But the successful prediction of depressive illness-onset by the prospective *negative* measures suggests that this is unlikely to be the main explanation. The confusion was clarified when two of the measures were examined simultaneously. Table 14.3 throws light upon a phenomenon of particular significance for depression; namely, being 'let down' by not receiving crisis support from someone from whom, because of a confiding relationship, there was reason to expect it. Table 14.3 presents data only for relationships with husbands and cohabitees, but a similarly high rate of depression was found among women who had been 'let down' in this way by other core relationships.

In terms of the theoretical model outlined above, it would make sense if the experience of being let down was even more likely to promote generalization of hopelessness (and thus depression) than the mere continuation of lack of support: it would act like another experience of loss. Particularly interesting here are the twelve cases of women who were let down by one core relationship, but found crisis support from another: 50 per cent (6/12) became depressed despite the support from a second person, compared with only 4 per cent (3/80) among the others who received crisis support.

Married women who neither confided in their husbands nor received crisis support from them did not have a high rate of depression if they received crisis support from another core contact: only 5 per cent (1/21) became depressed, compared with 43 per cent (9/21) with neither a confiding marriage nor support from another core contact (p < .01). In other words, if women have not recently been let down by their husbands, support from another person may prove to be protective: it is as if they became able to benefit from the support of another person once they had had time to adjust to expecting none from the marriage partner.

It is also important to consider here the suggestion of Henderson and his colleagues, that it is not the true availability of support which determines the risk of depression, but rather the 'plaintive style' of an individual. This infers a psychological predisposition, on the one hand, to complain of depression and, on the other hand, to perceive as unsupportive the behaviour of contacts whom less plaintive persons would consider adequately supportive (Henderson *et al.* 1981). While it is a plausible hypothesis that depressed women are more sensitive than others to being let down, a detailed examination of the descriptions of the experiences suggested that any but the most stoical women would have perceived these as unsupportive.

For example, one woman who had an ectopic pregnancy, thus losing her baby, was told by her husband that he might as well leave her now. Another husband refused to discuss their son's problems with his wife, despite repeated communications about him from the school, insisting that there was absolutely nothing wrong with the child. In the light of such findings, it seems unnecessary to invoke reporting bias to account for the different results obtained with the different measures.

The next step was to examine the relationship between self-esteem and social support. Whether a simple measure of crisis support from at least one core relationship was taken, or a more complex measure of being let down by any core contact, it was clear that the degree of support made a difference to those with a negative evaluation of self; whereas such a negative evaluation in itself made no difference to the risk of depression for those who had support during the follow-up period (Brown *et al.* 1986c). In short, the presence of support seemed to be more important in this respect than the self-esteem.

A caveat is required at this point, that the measures of support and self-esteem are not strictly comparable, since the former take account of changes after the first interview (i.e., being let down), while the latter on the other hand do not. It is possible to envisage various pathways by which changes in self-esteem during follow-up, uncharted by the measures in this study, could alter the picture of causal priority:

(i) No NES→Severe event→Let down→NES→Depression

(ii) No NES→Severe event→NES→stimulates others to let one down →Depression

(iii) No NES→Severe event→NES→Too diffident to ask for support →No crisis support→Depression

Since self-evaluation is a much 'softer' measure than crisis support it would be possible to collect information relevant to deciding between these models only if there were frequent interviews over the follow-up period, managing to catch the subject at a time when self-evaluation had become negative but before depressive onset with its possible attendant reporting bias. Until such evidence has been reviewed, therefore, it would be premature to rule that NES is of less importance than support.

Further exploration of other previously identified vulnerability factors: work and number of children at home

The Islington study also gave an opportunity to explore the earlier speculations that the relationship between the other vulnerability factors and self-esteem accounted for their role in predicting onset. This task turned out to be fruitless largely because there was little initial relationship between the factors and depression. The presence of three or more children under 15 at home seemed, if anything, to indicate resilience rather than vulnerability, and a detailed exploration of the women's child-rearing suggested that changes in contraceptive and child-minding practices in the decade between the Camberwell and Islington studies appeared to underlie this replication failure. It was argued that far from jeopardizing the vulnerability model, this kind of shift in levels of association between *demographic* indicators and disorder would be expected when broad social changes altered the psychological meaning of such indicators (Harris *et al.* 1989).

As emphasized earlier, lack of employment had originally emerged only as a second-order vulnerability factor and it was therefore not surprising that interpretation of the Islington data was not simple: full-time employment produced rates of onset no different from those of women without any work, but given small numbers it was not possible to conclude that part-time work offered any protection to those in poor marriages, once other important factors such as matching events were controlled (Brown *et al.* 1989). Interestingly, however, there was no relationship between employment and NES. In terms of the two models suggested on p. 211–12 model A can therefore be ruled out, whereby the link between low self-esteem and depression rendered spurious any link between lack of employment and depression. More thought may be needed, however, before all forms of Model B are dismissed. In a concluding discussion Brown and Bifulco focus on the fact that nearly all the Islington women had succeeded in obtaining the work status of their choice: that is, those without a job had chosen not to work. Thus, in other samples where lack of employment *had* seemed to act as a vulnerability factor, the absence of a job per se, with a daily routine to prevent depressive preoccupations, may have been less important than the fact that women had been unable to take up a chosen role. Speculatively, if a person's preferred self-image is as a working woman, not having a job may be important in promoting depression because it lowers self-evaluation, along the lines of model B2(i) below, whereas if she has chosen not to work there will be no effect either on NES or on depression, as in the Islington findings:

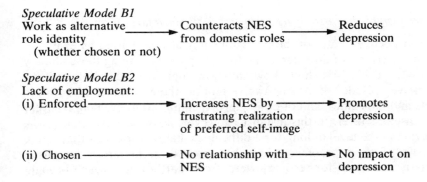

Speculative Model B1
Work as alternative ⟶ Counteracts NES ⟶ Reduces
role identity   from domestic roles   depression
   (whether chosen or not)

Speculative Model B2
Lack of employment:
(i) Enforced ⟶ Increases NES by ⟶ Promotes
                  frustrating realization   depression
                  of preferred self-image

(ii) Chosen ⟶ No relationship with ⟶ No impact on
                  NES   depression

Formulating the problem in this way is essentially similar to the interpretation given to the results concerning three or more children under 15 at home, where it was clear that in the 1980s most women had *chosen* their actual family size, unlike their counterparts in the 1960s. And upon reflection it was clear that the social changes behind the employment phenomenon to a large extent coincided with the changes behind the number of children phenomenon – the increasing availability of easy contraception, child-minding facilities and part-time jobs had extended the range of women's rights to choose their family size and employment status.

At this point it is worth drawing attention to another study of very similar prospective design to the Islington study in Edinburgh (Surtees *et al.* 1983, 1986; Ingham *et al.* 1986, 1987; Miller *et al.* 1987). Using the LEDS, this explored the relationship of the Camberwell vulnerability factors to self-esteem as measured by the Rosenberg scale (Rosenberg 1965). As in Islington, the negative items on the scale were separated from the positive ones and at first interview were found to relate to the vulnerability factors concerning quality of relationships (current intimacy and experience of at least one year's separation from mother in childhood), but not to current employment or number of children at home (Ingham *et al.* 1986).

Analysis of illness-onset by the time of follow-up interview, about one year later, suggested that this negative self-esteem scale was of definite predictive value for major depression, although the interpretation was complicated by the fact that provoking agents were not considered: in other words, the authors carried out an ordinary risk factor rather than a vulnerability factor analysis (Ingham *et al.* 1987). Another complication is that in Edinburgh, unlike in Islington, a previous episode of depression was of predictive importance. However, with the small numbers involved in the Edinburgh study it was difficult to disentangle the effects of previous depression from those of low self-esteem in the pre-onset period. Nevertheless, this problem apart, the degree to which the findings of the two studies correspond is impressive.

Further insights from studying recovery: a mirror image of onset

The prospective nature of the Islington study also permitted an examination of the course of disorder in the follow-up period among those already depressed. Table 14.4 shows how among women with quite longstanding depressive episodes of at least twelve months the experience of both life events and difficulties, and of crisis support, combined to promote recovery from caseness level. In this instance, however, it was the experience of a *reduction* in the level of long-term difficulties that was critical – that is, the opposite of their presence which had proved so important in onset. Similarly important for recovery were 'fresh start' events, which brought about change that heralded new hope, such as finding a job after months without one, being rehoused, or receiving a proposal of marriage from a new boyfriend, again the opposite of those loss events so crucial for onset. Once again crisis support appeared to compound the effect of the events and difficulties (Brown *et al.* 1988a). The process of recovery thus seemed the mirror image of the process of onset.

Table 14.4 Percentage of women in Islington with recovery or improvement from chronic depression in terms of experience of difficulty reduction or a fresh start event and social support (47 cases with episodes > 1 year)

		Fresh start or difficulty reduction	
		Yes	No
		%recovered	%recovered
Crisis support	Yes	83 (10/12)	43 (6/14)
	No	62 (8/13)	25 (2/8)

Implications of the revised vulnerability model

The 'sandcastle effect': prospective epidemiology and prevention

These findings have some general implications for the value of preventive work derived from prospective studies. The Islington survey highlighted the way in which first-interview material may need supplementing with further information about developments during the follow-up period if valid conclusions are to be drawn about state at second interview. Life events need little time to occur and can radically alter the whole context of a person's life, rendering it tumultuous although it was correctly documented as running smoothly at first interview. Similarly, relationships which have proved supportive hitherto may change under other circumstances, causing the person to be let down. Particularly noticeable is the fact that for both self-evaluation and quality of support negative measures appear to act as better predictors than positive ones, and this seems consistent with this recommendation to treat prospective studies with caution if they have not supplemented their data with retrospective probing at follow-up about changes since initial interview.

This picture of the different impact of changes upon positive and negative factors follows what we call the 'sandcastle effect': just as sandcastles can be knocked down in only a fraction of the time they take to build, so positive self-evaluation can be undermined in a few seconds, while negative self-evaluation may need months to be reversed or positive self-evaluation months to be built up. In a similar way, a simple negative remark can destroy trust in a relationship while building such trust again

221

can be a very slow process. If conclusions about preventive action are to be drawn, then it is vital that a critical approach should be taken to the prospective studies on which such conclusions are to be based, with an awareness that statistically significant associations with negative factors are likely to be more trustworthy than statistically non-significant associations with positive factors.

Preventive strategies for depression

Perhaps what stands out most in these data is the overriding importance in depression of attachment – the preponderance of relationship crises among the recent severe events, the close association between self-evaluation and the quality of relationships rather than between NES and aspects of employment or housework, the relative importance of crisis support as compared with self-evaluation, and the necessity for such support to come from a core tie and to be continuous, without 'let down'. It is not enough to get support from a non-core tie or from a care-giving professional, like a fire engine only rushed in during emergencies. There are various possible explanations for this, some giving greater emphasis to ongoing cognitive dispositions – for example, that people who are forced to call on professional services or neighbours, rather than on friends of their own, feel somehow inferior, or that it is because they are helpless personalities that not only are they prone to depression but also unable to find core contacts. Other explanations would emphasize the nature of the core relationship: many of the husbands of the depressed women were exceptionally undependable, while the friends of those who showed resilience in the face of a provoking agent were often tried and trusted over many years and made it clear that they did not mind being called upon for help at any time of day or night. The importance of the quality of supportiveness, not just the availability of a contact, was highlighted in the measure of crisis support which took account of negative responses. It also stood out in the findings concerning quality of care in childhood and how unsupportive relationships then, as much as in the recent period, could put a woman on a trajectory to experiencing a higher rate of current provoking agents. Further research with frequent re-interviews may or may not establish that reductions in self-evaluation are the mechanism through which such unsupportiveness has its depressogenic effects. But meanwhile it certainly makes intuitive sense to relate quality of supportiveness to the tendency to generalize hopeless feelings: the degree of hope one feels can be expected to vary according to the degree one believes that other people care about one and will put themselves out to help put things right.

Many current therapeutic and educational strategies have such ideas in the forefront, so spelling this out in the context of preventive recommendations may not at first seem particularly original or worthwhile. On looking more closely, however, it becomes apparent that in the terms outlined here these existing provisions will not be adequately preventive. It is not possible for therapists to act like the 'very close others' in the Islington study whose friendship extended beyond the limits of a professional timetable. In other words the quality of professional support may not be supportive enough. Moreover merely telling girls about contraception is unlikely to help those who, without necessarily being aware of it, are hoping to find in motherhood a relationship with all the elements of care of which they themselves have been deprived. One relatively new approach which might be able to bypass some of these shortcomings is the befriending service, which relies on a system of supervised volunteers who befriend vulnerable individuals for a minimum period of nine months. A major advantage is that such services are inexpensive, although the unpaid befrienders themselves need to have an adequate back-up in terms of training and weekly support groups headed by a salaried professional worker. Encouraged to be maximally available, and to participate in enjoyable activities with the befriendee as well as listening and giving advice, the befrienders can often become genuine core contacts as long-standing friends in a way which is made impossible by the frequent rotations of health service personnel. Furthermore, the organization of befriending outside the official system of medical care helps to offset the less fortunate effects upon self-esteem of the labelling process which is part of attending for psychological treatment. A befriendee will thus continue to see her doctor(s) as well as her befriender.

There has not yet been time for a full evaluation of such a scheme, although several pilot studies have had promising conclusions. But what has been especially encouraging is the number of willing volunteer befrienders who have been forthcoming. It is this hitherto unutilized resource of enthusiasm which permits such services to run without any great logistic problems: after the initial training volunteer and befriendee carry on to a large extent on their own. Thus, work by 'Newpin' in South London has suggested that depressive disorder can be reduced among working-class single mothers and women with poor marriages – just the groups which the Islington study identified as most at risk and as benefiting from crisis support by a woman friend (see Pound and Mills 1985; Mills and Pound 1986). 'Homestart', in a four-year trial of volunteer befriending in Leicester, reports considerable improvements in family adjustment and mothers' mental health (Van der Eyken 1982). The therapeutic impact of volunteer counsellors after bereavement had already emerged earlier (see Parkes 1980 for a summary), but other experiments extending the boundaries of existing professional services afford further confirmation of the value of this approach: Elliott and colleagues report the reduced risk of depression after childbirth among first-time mothers offered additional group support (Elliott et al. 1988) while Corney (1987) reports improvement in women's depression measured by the Clinical Interview Schedule (Goldberg *et al.* 1970) after a special social worker intervention involving both 'sustaining and exploring techniques' and practical help. Interestingly, the greatest improvement in Corney's study appeared in the group which might be expected to benefit most from a close friendship according to the finding reported earlier in Islington – women not recently 'let down' but with chronic major marital problems.

Years of discouraging results supplying 'supportive therapy' of the limited kind currently on offer may have imbued the hardened clinician with a scepticism which makes it easy to dismiss these preliminary reports as examples of the woolly-minded benevolence of the layperson. But because they echo some of the finer details of our community survey findings it is more difficult to write off without a further scientific evaluation what might turn out to be a genuinely cost-effective provision. The struggle for worthwhile preventive strategies must also repudiate any overhasty disparagement of 'common sense' based on data of insufficient subtlety to provide an adequate test for the tenets of traditional wisdom. Particularly if the befrienders' training taught them to try to help prevent the reoccurrence of provoking agents, to promote fresh start events and to reduce difficulties, as well as to provide crisis support *after* severe events, there is every reason to expect a substantial reduction in depression among befriendees. It is of great importance, however, that any assessment of the preventive impact of befriending services should be informed by some estimate of the key measures detailed by this theoretical model of depression, since outside factors can always interfere with the impact of such a preventive measure. For example, in the Newpin experiment two of the befrienders left London without telling either their befriendees or the scheme organizer, and both their befriendees then suffered setbacks in depression – just as would be predicted after such an experience of being 'let down'.

The focus upon befriending as a strategy of choice does not, of course, mean that other policies which can affect other variables in the model should be neglected. Thus, while many stressors cannot be prevented, some provoking agents are amenable to outside intervention (for example, evictions and financial crises). Second, attempts to improve self-evaluation in ways other than through core contacts (for example, through cognitive therapy) should clearly not be ignored. Furthermore, the whole topic of physiological vulnerability factors has yet to be integrated into this psychosocial model, which must ultimately become biopsychosocial. Meanwhile the pursuit of a controlled evaluation of befriending could clearly prove worthwhile.

Acknowledgements

The research underlying the vulnerability model was funded by the Medical Research Council and by the Social Science Research Council. We are particularly indebted to Professor J.E. Cooper and Professor J.R.M. Copeland who pioneered the Bedford College Caseness Threshold.

References

Adam, K., Bouckoms, A., and Streiner, D. (1982) 'Parental loss and family stability in attempted suicide', *Archives of General Psychiatry* 39: 1081–5.

Akiskal, H. and McKinney, W., Jr. (1973) 'Depressive disorders: towards a unified hypothesis', *Science* 182: 20–9.

Bebbington, P., Sturt, E., Tennant, C., and Hurry, J. (1984) 'Misfortune and resilience: a community study of women', *Psychological Medicine* 14: 347–64.

Beck, A. (1967) *Depression: Clinical, Experimental and Theoretical Aspects*, London: Staples Press.

Bifulco, A., Brown, G., and Harris, T. (1987) 'Childhood loss of parent and adult psychiatric disorder: the Islington study', *Journal of Affective Disorders* 12: 115–28.

Birtchnell, J. and Kennard, J. (1984) 'Early and current factors associated with poor-quality marriage', *Social Psychiatry* 19: 31–40.

Brown, G. (1974) 'Meaning, measurement and stress of life events', in B.S. Dohrenwend and B.P. Dohrenwend (eds) *Stressful Life Events: Their Nature and Effects*, New York: Wiley.

Brown, G. (1981) 'Aetiological studies and the definition of a case', in J.K. Wing, P. Bebbington, and L. Robins (eds) *What is a Case? The Problem of Definition in Psychiatric Community Surveys*, London: Grant McIntyre.

Brown, G. and Andrews, B. (1985) 'Comparison of Camberwell and Islington intimacy rating', unpublished MS.

Brown, G. and Bifulco, A. (1988b) 'Women, employment and the development of depression', unpublished MS.

Brown, G. and Harris, T. (1978a) *Social Origins of Depression: A Study of Psychiatric Disorder in Women*, London: Tavistock.

Brown, G. and Harris, T. (1978b) 'Social origins of depression: a reply', *Psychological Medicine* 8: 577–88.

Brown, G. and Harris, T. (1986a) 'Stressor, vulnerability and depression: a question of replication', *Psychological Medicine* 16: 739–44.

Brown, G. and Harris, T. (1986b) 'Establishing causal links: the Bedford College studies of depression', in H. Katschnig (ed.) *Life Events and Psychiatric Disorders*, Cambridge: Cambidge University Press.

Brown, G. and Harris, T. (1989) *Life Events and Illness*, New York: Guilford Press.

Brown, G. and Prudo, R. (1981) 'Psychiatric disorder in a rural and an urban population, 1: Aetiology of depression', *Psychological Medicine* 11: 581–99.

Brown, G., Adler, Z., and Bifulco, A. (1988a) 'Life events, difficulties and recovery from chronic depression', *British Journal of Psychiatry* in press.

Brown, G., Bifulco, A., and Harris, T. (1987) 'Life events, vulnerability and onset of depression: some refinements', *British Journal of Psychiatry* 150: 30–42.

Brown, G., Harris, T., and Bifulco, A. (1986a) 'Long-term effect of early loss of parent', in M. Rutter, C. Izard, and P. Read (eds) *Depression in Childhood: Developmental Perspectives*, New York: Guilford Press.

Brown, G., Bifulco, A., Harris, T., and Bridge, L. (1986b) 'Life stress, chronic psychiatric symptoms and vulnerability to clinical depression', *Journal of Affective Disorders* 11: 1–19.

Brown, G., Andrews, B., Harris, T., Adler, Z., and Bridge, L. (1986c) 'Social support, self-esteem and depression', *Psychological Medicine* 16: 813–31.

Campbell, E., Cope, S., and Teasdale, J. (1983) 'Social factors and affective disorder: an investigation of Brown and Harris's model', *British Journal of Psychiatry* 143: 548–53.

Corney, R. (1987) 'Marital problems and treatment outcome in depressed women: a clinical trial of social work intervention', *British Journal of Psychiatry* 151: 652–60.

Costello, C. (1982) 'Social factors associated with depression: a retrospective community study', *Psychological Medicine* 12: 329–39.

Dean, C., Surtees, P., and Sashidharan, S. (1983) 'Comparison of research diagnostic systems in an Edinburgh community sample', *British Journal of Psychiatry* 142: 247–56.

Dohrenwend, B., Shrout, P., Link, B., Martin, J., and Skodol, A. (1986) 'Overview and initial results from a risk-factor study of depression and schizophrenia', reprinted from J.E. Barrett and R.M. Rose (eds) *Mental Disorders in the Community*, New York: Guilford Press.

Elliott, S.A., Sanjack, M., and Leverton, T.J. (in press) 'Parent groups in pregnancy: a preventive intervention for postnatal depression', in B.H. Gottlieb (ed.) *Marshalling Social Support: Formats, Issues, Processes and Effects*, London: Sage.

Everitt, B. and Smith, A. (1979) 'Interaction in contingency tables: a brief discussion of alternative definitions', *Psychological Medicine* 9: 581–3.

Finlay-Jones, R. (1989) 'Anxiety', in G. Brown and T. Harris, *Life Events and Illness*, New York: Guilford Press.

Finlay-Jones, R. and Brown, G. (1981) 'Types of stressful life event and the onset of anxiety and depressive disorders', *Psychological Medicine* 11: 803–15.

Finlay-Jones, R., Brown, G., Duncan-Jones, P., Harris, T., Murphy, E., and Prudo, R. (1980) 'Depression and anxiety in the community: replicating the diagnosis of a case', *Psychological Medicine* 10: 445–54.

Goldberg, D., Cooper, B., Eastwood, M., Kedward, H., and Shepherd, M. (1970) 'A standardized psychiatric interview for use in community surveys', *British Journal of Preventive and Social Medicine* 24: 18–23.

Harris, T., Brown, G., and Bifulco, A. (1986) 'Loss of parent in childhood and adult psychiatric disorder: the Walthamstow Study, 1: the role of lack of adequate parental care', *Psychological Medicine* 16: 641–59.

Harris, T., Brown, G., and Bifulco, A. (1987) 'Loss of parent in childhood and adult psychiatric disorder: the Walthamstow Study, 2: the role of social class and premarital pregnancy', *Psychological Medicine* 17: 163–83.

Harris, T., Adler, Z., Bridge, L., and Brown, G. (1989) 'Instability of indicator variables and replication studies: depression in women and number of children at home', unpublished MS.

Henderson, S., Byrne, D., and Duncan-Jones, P. (1981) *Neurosis and the Social Environment*, London: Academic Press.

Ingham, J., Kreitman, N., Miller, P., Sashidharan, S., and Surtees, P. (1986) 'Self-esteem, vulnerability and psychiatric disorder in the community', *British Journal of Psychiatry* 148: 373–85.

Ingham, J., Kreitman, N., Miller, P. Sashidharan, S., and Surtees, P. (1987) 'Self-appraisal, anxiety and depression in women – a prospective enquiry', *British Journal of Psychiatry* 151: 643–51.

Kennard, J. and Birtchnell, J. (1982) 'The mental health of early mother separated women', *Acta Psychiatrica Scandinavica* 65: 388–402.

Martin, C. (1985) 'Stress in the puerperium', PhD dissertation, University of Manchester.

Miller, P., Ingham, J., Kreitman, N., Surtees, P., and Sashidharan, S. (1987) 'Life events and other factors implicated in onset and in remission of psychiatric illness in women', *Journal of Affective Disorders* 12: 73–88.

Mills, M. and Pound, A. (1986) 'Mechanisms of change', *Changes* 4: 199–203.

Parker, G. (1979) 'Parental characteristics in relation to depressive disorders', *British Journal of Psychiatry* 134: 138–40.

Parker, G. (1981) 'Parental reports of depressives: an investigation of several explanations', *Journal of Affective Disorders* 3: 131–40.

Parker, G. (1983) 'Parental "affectionless control" as an antecedent to adult depression', *Archives of General Psychiatry* 40: 956–60.

Parker, G. and Hadzi-Pavlovic, D. (1984) 'Modification of levels of depression in mother-bereaved women by parental and marital relationships', *Psychological Medicine* 14: 125–35.

Parkes, C.M. (1980) 'Bereavement counselling: does it work?' *British Medical Journal* 281: 3–6.

Parry, G. and Shapiro, D.A. (1986) 'Life events and social support in working-class women: stress buffering or independent effects?', *Archives of General Psychiatry* 43: 315–23.

Paykel, E., Emms, E., Fletcher, J., and Rassaby, E. (1980) 'Life events and social support in puerperal depression', *British Journal of Psychiatry* 136: 339–46.

Pound, A. and Mills, M. (1985) 'A pilot evaluation of Newpin – home-visiting and befriending scheme in South London', *A.C.C.P. Newsletter*, 7 (4).

Rosenberg, M. (1965) *The Measurement of Self-Esteem: Society and the Adolescent Self-Image*, Princeton, NJ: Princeton University Press.

Surtees, P., Sashidharan, S., and Dean, C. (1986) 'Affective disorder amongst women in the general population: a longitudinal study', *British Journal of Psychiatry* 148: 176–86.

Surtees, P., Dean, C., Ingham, J., Kreitman, N., Miller, P., and Sashidharan, S. (1983) 'Psychiatric disorder in women from an Edinburgh Community: associations with demographic factors', *British Journal of Psychiatry* 142: 238–46.

Tennant, C. and Bebbington, P. (1978) 'The social causation of depression: a critique of the work of Brown and his colleagues', *Psychological Medicine* 8: 565–75.

van der Eyken, W. (1982) *Home-Start – A Four-Year Evaluation*, Leicester: Home-start Consultancy.

Wing, J., Cooper, J., and Sartorius, N. (1974) *The Measurement and Classification of Psychiatric Symptoms: An Instruction Manual for the Present State Examination and CATEGO Programme*, London: Cambridge University Press.

Wing, J. and Sturt, E. (1978) *The PSE-ID-CATEGO-System – A Supplementary Manual*, London: Institute of Psychiatry (mimeo).

Chapter fifteen

Unravelling the causes of homelessness – and of its association with mental illness

Ezra Susser, Anne Lovell, and Sarah Conover

In the last decade the reappearance in the United States of widespread homelessness has been coupled with a high visibility of mentally ill homeless persons in urban centres. This apparent association between homelessness and mental illness has stimulated an intense and ongoing debate on the contribution of mental illness to homelessness. Although mentally ill persons were noticeable among the homeless in prior historical periods (Deutsch 1937; Grob 1973; Rothman 1971), the relationship between the two rarely generated public discourse of a similar scale or intensity. Perhaps a historical precedent can be found in the campaign for asylums in the nineteenth century, when many mentally ill persons were housed in jails. That controversy, however, centred on the deplorable treatment of the mentally ill rather than on the causes of homelessness.

As a response to the current debate, epidemiological studies are needed to unravel the causes of the present-day phenomenon of homelessness, and of its association with mental illness. Yet the methodological problems are many, and to give the flavour we focus in this chapter on four types of question, none yet satisfactorily resolved. First, are there unrecognized generation effects that should be explored in reported time trends?; second, how may direct or indirect causal links be established between homelessness and hypothesized risk factors?; third, how should the role of determinants at several levels be treated analytically?; fourth, what are the determinants of homelessness that apply specifically to mentally ill persons? The first three types of question apply to homelessness in the general population as well as among the mentally ill, while the fourth is of particular interest to psychiatrists and psychiatric epidemiologists.

In elaborating these questions, we use sources from the United States, but the discussion is relevant to research on homelessness throughout the industrialized nations. Similarly, while the text adheres to the usual definition of homelessness in the United States – sleeping overnight in a shelter or a public space – the issues are germane to research using other definitions of homelessness.

Recognizing generation effects in the analysis of time trends

When broad social changes – for instance, housing scarcity (Hartman 1986) and unemployment (Hopper and Hamburg 1986) – have been cited as causes of homelessness, little consideration has been given to the nature or duration of the 'lag' time between the occurrence of these changes and the consequent homelessness. Thus, the causes of the recent rise in homelessness tend to be debated in terms of current social change, or 'period' effects. 'Generation' effects are usually overlooked or misunderstood. Often termed 'cohort' effects, generation effects refer to effects of historical change that are expressed after a latency period. At a given point in time, successive generations or 'birth cohorts' carry their own specific history of exposure to prior historical changes, whereas they share with other cohorts exposure to a current or period effect.

What is the presumptive evidence that generation effects should be investigated? First are the age patterns. In New York City municipal shelters for men there has been a major shift in age distribution towards the young as well as a marked increase in the number of men in the shelters. In a landmark study of Skid Row men in New York in the 1960s (Bahr and Caplow 1973), middle-aged and elderly men comprised the predominant group using public shelters and cheap lodgings on Skid Row. By 1985, in a sample of new arrivals to a greatly expanded New York shelter system, 46 per cent of the men were under the age of 30 (Susser and Struening 1988). Such a change in age distribution, associated with the increase in numbers of homeless men, suggests that there could be a generation effect.

Research on homeless men in New York City shelters (Susser *et al.* 1987) in fact supports the plausibility of a generation effect there. Among new arrivals to the men's shelters, almost one-quarter have a history of childhood placement in foster care, group homes, or other special residences. Possibly institutional care in early life influences subsequent residential patterns among young poor men, leading to increased use of institutions such as municipal shelters. If this is the case, a trend toward institutional care for children will be manifested in patterns of adult homelessness with a lag of a decade or more. Comparison data on domiciled men, and data on secular trends in institutional care for children, would be required to show that there is indeed such a generation effect.

A second line of evidence that highlights the need to consider generation effects applies only to the mentally ill. In the 1960s and 1970s the policy of de-institutionalization diminished the use of asylums for long-term stay without developing adequate treatment and residential alternatives (Bassuk and Lamb 1986; Goldman 1983). Between 1955 and 1980 the number of patients in state and county mental hospitals declined from over 500,000 to less than 150,000. The bulk of the drastic decline in census has been attributed to a general reduction in length of hospital stay, although other factors, such as the transfer of elderly patients to nursing homes, played a role too.

It is widely accepted that the policy contributed to homelessness among mentally ill persons (Lamb 1984). Less well-recognized is that there was a lag of perhaps a decade between the trend toward a lower mental hospital census and the trend toward increasing numbers of mentally ill homeless. Although the state and county mental hospital census dropped by about 200,000 between 1960 and 1970, and by a further 150,000 between 1970 and 1975, the mentally ill homeless became highly visible only in the late 1970s. Furthermore, their numbers appear to have increased exponentially in the 1980s, after the absolute decline in hospital census had already levelled off. Thus, the contribution of that policy to homelessness cannot be understood as a simple period effect. One has to search for intervening variables that occurred at a later time point, or postulate a latency period between the policy and its effects on homelessness.

De–institutionalization affected different generations in different ways. Among older, formerly institutionalized patients, many became homeless when the low-income units they rented after hospital discharge in the1960s and 1970s were lost to reconversion or abandonment in the late 1970s and 1980s (Hartman 1986). In their case, homelessness might best be understood as the combined result of a generation effect due to de-institutionalization and a subsequent period effect due to loss of low-income housing.

For younger mentally ill persons, roughly those now under age 40, de-institutionalization in the 1960s and 1970s meant greater barriers to hospital admission, easier discharges, and few community supports. In these cohorts, adoption of community living styles that predispose to homelessness may be partly attributable to exposure to de-institutionalization at a specific stage in the life cycle – young adulthood – as illustrated by an example concerning social roles. For young mentally ill adults in the community, a transition to adult roles in work and social relationships is expected but often cannot be achieved in a normative fashion, especially when jobs are scarce; membership in a drug culture and 'drifting' are then among the few apparent alternatives to the mental patient identity (Pepper et al. 1981; Lamb 1982). They are also risk factors for homelessness. It is worth noting too that generation effects shared with non-mentally ill peers in the community play an important role in shaping patterns of drug use and residential mobility among young patients (Bachrach 1982). Again, generation effects need not be a sufficient cause of homelessness for that cohort; lack of housing, of jobs, and of community supports may be required for their expression as homelessness.

A third line of evidence is demographic. Bachrach (1984) has noted that the younger generations of mentally ill adults derive from the 'baby boom', that is, they were born during a period of high birth rates between 1946 and

1961. As a result, those who develop mental illness in young adulthood are part of an especially large cohort of young mentally ill persons; yet the mental health system has not expanded its capacity to accommodate them. She suggests that this generation effect too has contributed to homelessness.

In spite of these pointers, the role of generation effects in explaining time trends remains largely unexplored. American homelessness studies are rarely based on data gathered at more than one point in time. No survey has covered three time-points, which would be essential to identifying as well as differentiating generation and period effects. Even where adequate data are available they have not been examined within the framework of age-period-generation analysis. For instance, demographic data, including age, have been recorded for homeless men in New York City municipal shelters over the past decade. These data, along with census data, could provide the basis for an age-period-generation analysis.

A potentially useful sample also exists for such an analysis of secular trends for homelessness among the mentally ill. Appleby and Desai (1985) examined all admissions to Illinois State psychiatric facilities from 1971 to 1980, to document time trends for homelessness among mental patients. They found homelessness to be increasing among patients admitted over that decade. Unfortunately, neither secular trends in the age distribution of homelessness among patients nor analysis in terms of birth cohorts were reported by the authors.

The differentiation of age, period, and generation effects is fundamental in analysing the influence of secular trends and age on morbidity, and no less so on homelessness. Nevertheless, to our knowledge there has yet to be a discussion of homelessness framed in terms of age-period-generation analysis. The need for such an approach is underscored by evidence suggesting the occurrence of generation effects as well as period effects.

Establishing causal links between homelessness and hypothesized risk factors

Epidemiologists are familiar with the problems of establishing the direction of causality between illness and hypothesized risk factors, especially in 'case surveys', cross-sectional surveys, and case-control approaches. Unless proper care is taken, attributes that are due to an illness may be misinterpreted as risk factors. To establish the direction of causality, we need to know which came first.

Homelessness may contribute to social isolation, substance abuse, poor physical health, mental illness, adverse life events, and other burdens which, in turn, have been postulated to render people vulnerable to homelessness. For instance, homelessness may diminish one's social network through physical separation, prolonged dependency, and social stigma. Baxter (1987) has illustrated this point with the example of a woman who was too ashamed to contact her family while she was homeless. Upon finding a room in a residence, she regained a sense of pride and sought to re-establish family relationships.

A second example concerns substance abuse. Field research suggests that buying, selling, and using drugs is common in some New York City municipal shelters (Morrissey *et al.* 1985; Gounis and Susser, in press; Barbanell 1988). Because peers significantly influence drug behaviour at least in some age groups (Kandel 1982), young persons with no prior history of extensive drug use may acquire one in the shelters. Other factors, such as accessibility of drugs and demoralization may also influence drug use there.

The first step in differentiating risk factors from consequences of homelessness – establishing a clear temporal sequence – is difficult to apply. In surveys, the usual source of data on homeless people, problems of temporal sequence are magnified by the nature of homelessness and some of its hypothesized risk factors, by a continuing reciprocal relationship between homelessness and these factors, and by the practical limitations to collecting reliable and valid data.

Illustrating a problem integral to the nature of homelessness is that it defies valid definition as an event with clear onset and termination. Thus, the process of becoming homeless often resembles the natural history of an illness with a long prodrome and an insidious onset. Before becoming homeless, in the narrow sense of residing in the streets and other public spaces or in shelters, individuals may experience a long period of residential instability, of moving about between homes of friends or relatives, or between cheap transient lodgings (Barrow *et al.* 1986). When there are only limited options, individuals may for some time be unable to escape from an increasingly adverse situation. It is difficult at some later point to date the onset of the process that results in evident homelessness.

Marking an end to homelessness also presents problems. Becoming housed at a given moment may simply represent a point in a continuing circulation through cheap accommodations, such as welfare hotels and shelters (Barrow *et al.* 1986). In view of these difficulties of definition, some researchers prefer to think in terms of patterns or levels of residential instability, rather than the simple dichotomy 'domicile' or 'no domicile' (Chafetz and Goldfinger 1984).

Further difficulties arise from the nature of some of the hypothesized risk factors and their ongoing interaction with homelessness. For instance, a history of drug abuse is of primary interest as a risk factor. When data are gathered at a single point in time, rather than longitudinally, the relationship between the process of drug involvement and social roles is difficult to elucidate (Kandel 1982). If, as is plausible, drug use postpones marriage, while at the same time an unmarried status contributes to continued drug use, the causal relationships between marital status and drug use are unlikely to be clarified by cross-sectional data. A similar limitation applies to their value in studying the complex interaction between drug use and residential patterns.

In surveys, practical limitations to collecting reliable and valid data hamper the investigation of such complex temporal relationships. Homeless persons themselves are usually the only source of information. Yet, in large shelters, their responses may be affected by lack of privacy at interview and by fears that information will be passed on to shelter authorities. In our New York shelter survey, for instance, more than a third of the respondents with a New York State record of psychiatric hospitalization did not report it at interview (Struening 1987). In parks, streets, and transportation terminals, length of interview is limited by the fact that homeless people are often on the move. In not a few cases respondents' answers are affected by intoxication, paranoia, or other psychiatric symptoms (Struening 1986). These factors limit the reliability and validity that can be achieved with interviews.

It is not surprising, then, that surveys of homeless persons have not been able to establish convincingly that the attributes of homeless persons at the time of the interview resemble their earlier attributes. Date of onset of hypothesized risk factors has rarely been compared with that of homelessness. In our survey in New York, we attempted to do so but for the reasons stated above rarely felt confidence in our results. More experience and a greater attention to timing the onset both of risk factor and of homelessness will be a precondition for causal research.

An analytic problem: determinants at several levels

Homelessness for any individual has determinants at several levels of analysis. An adequate understanding requires an analysis of factors at three levels: 1) the broad societal level, for instance, urban political economy; 2) the intermediate level of family and social network; 3) the level of individual attributes, such as psychiatric disorder.

Most discussions of homelessness fail to acknowledge the role of factors at each of these levels and their interactions. As one example, we noted above that the societal policy of de–institutionalization almost certainly contributed to homelessness among the mentally ill. Prior to the development of asylums, mentally ill persons were often kept in jails, poorhouses, and other adverse circumstances (Deutsch 1937; Grob 1973; Rothman 1971). Since the discharge of most long-term patients from asylums, mentally ill persons have again become evident in large numbers in jails, and also in shelters and among the homeless who sleep rough. Too often then as now the inference is drawn that, in the absence of close supervision and support, mental illness is a sufficient cause for homelessness.

Yet the relationship between de-institutionalization and homelessness is not as simple as implied by the juxtaposition of these well-known facts. We have already pointed out the role of de-institutionalization as a generation effect. We also alluded to its interaction with urban political economy in producing homelessness. In addition, available and effective kin support probably modifies these factors (Susser *et al.* 1987); when such support is present, homelessness is less likely. Finally, we do not know to what extent the mentally ill homeless represent those who would have been long-term patients in asylums in the past; institutionalization and homelessness have different determinants.

For mentally ill persons, as for other sub-groups, the relative importance of factors at each level varies considerably across time, across regions and across communities. When housing becomes scarcer and more costly, this increases the risk that the disability of mental illness will be associated with the handicap of homelessness. When family groups become less cohesive, the same can occur.

A case history illustrates how poverty and schizophrenia can involve individual, family, and community in a circular process. In a poor urban neighbourhood a young man suffering from schizophrenia left his parental home for a nearby shelter after a family quarrel. Underlying his decision was an exacerbation of his psychiatric symptoms, a worsening scarcity of family resources, increasing conflicts with a family that could no longer tolerate his behaviour, and deterioration in formal and informal community supports due to loss of manufacturing employment and outmigration. Each of these factors contributed to the others, and each was changing simultaneously.

When there are multiple levels of causation and none can be held constant, analytic difficulties arise in several areas. This is illustrated in the interpretation of life events data, important in this field. Homelessness may be precipitated by a relatively minor life event that tips a precarious balance involving factors at several levels. In the above example, it would be simplistic to interpret the occurrence of a family quarrel as the 'cause'. Such interpretations can be misleading in the development of preventive strategies, as therapeutic interventions with families of poor schizophrenics suggest (Goldstein and Dyche 1983). The point is to recognize the combination of factors that allowed a family quarrel to precipitate homelessness.

A related problem in interpreting life events arises from the difficulty of dating the start of homelessness, mentioned above. Life events that have a major impact on disability or resources can occur far earlier in time than the point at which a person begins to sleep in the shelters or public spaces. In another case history of a mentally ill person, the death of a caretaking relative was emotionally traumatic, depleted his resources, and initiated a process that resulted in homelessness years later. Before becoming homeless, he had stayed with other relatives and exhausted his remaining savings over an extended period. Unfortunately, such less recent life events, that are of causal significance and independent of the process leading to homelessness, are not easily ascertained in survey interviews, and tend to be unreported.

The consideration of factors at several levels adds complexity to research as well as to policy decisions and public debate. A narrow perspective, however, misleads. In studying the causes of homelessness and designing experimental preventive strategies, we must adopt a framework that allows for a contribution from the broader society, the social group, and the individual.

Identifying determinants of homelessness that apply specifically to mentally ill persons

The homeless in the United States of the 1980s are not a community with history and tradition, like squatters who have migrated from rural to urban areas or like the *clochards* of French literature and lore. Instead, they include individuals who are arbitrarily grouped together for treatment or policy purposes, because their residential histories, at some point in time, include stays in shelters or public spaces. Homeless persons comprise several distinct sub-groups. In New York City, for example, the largest sub-group currently consists of the members of homeless families. Other sub-groups include: 1) persons who suffer from mental disorders; 2) individuals with drug or alcohol problems; and 3) young men and women without job prospects.

Since homelessness has now reached epidemic proportions for many heterogeneous sub-groups, clearly some common causes apply to all these groups. Possibly these stem from a political economy that has recently transformed the housing market and restructured the job market (Hopper *et al.* 1985) or from changes in family structure (Susser *et al.* 1987). Nevertheless, for each sub-group there must also be specific determinants that do not apply to the others. This is suggested by a more detailed examination of time trends. In New York City, mentally ill persons became the most visible (though perhaps not the largest) sub-group in the 1970s (Reich and Siegel 1978). In the 1980s homeless families predominate (Manhattan Borough President's Task Force 1987).

The development of preventive strategies for the mentally ill therefore requires, in addition to research on causes of homelessness common to all groups, identification of factors specific to them. We need to know who among the mentally ill is at greatest risk and why. Research to yield preventive strategies may in fact need to be even more precise, since determinants of homelessness are likely to be different for men and women, for different age groups, and for people with different diagnoses.

Thus, advance in this field will require specification and differentiation of the research questions. One may be concerned with the reasons why so many people, including the mentally ill, are becoming homeless; with the reasons why people who are mentally ill are at higher risk than those who are not, or with why some mentally ill people become homeless, while others do not. Each of these questions represents a different level of analysis, requires a different design and, in particular, a different choice of comparison group.

A general survey of the homeless, even in the rare event that it furnishes comparison data from a community study, is not well suited to identifying variables related specifically to homelessness among the mentally ill. In a community sample selected for comparison to a survey sample, the number of persons with chronic mental disorders such as schizophrenia is too few to permit a comparison of the mentally ill who are homeless with those who are not. Moreover, other attributes, such as substance abuse and a prison record, are more common among the homeless than in most communities and are often found together with mental illness in individual histories. With such surveys it is therefore extremely difficult to control for confounding factors and identify interaction in the analysis.

The case-control study has more potential than the general survey to explain who becomes homeless among the mentally ill. In such studies, one could select a control group appropriate for a specific question. Moreover, a smaller sample size would suffice than in the general survey, and for some research questions cases (homeless persons) and controls (non-homeless persons) could be selected in clinics and other settings where in-depth interviews and longitudinal study are feasible. Thus, one could afford to devote more resources to gathering elusive information about the individual, clarifying temporal sequence for homelessness and risk factors, investigating family systems, and situating individual histories within a broad social context.

A number of variations on this design are possible. For instance, a San Francisco emergency room survey (Chafetz and Goldfinger 1984), comparing patients who were homeless with those who were not, is perhaps best characterized as a 'cross-sectional survey' since homelessness was ascertained by history-taking and was not the basis of sampling for the study. In two studies that have gathered data on psychiatric patients who were homeless and those who were not (Appleby and Desai 1985; Mowbray et al. 1987) the characteristics of the former have been reported without detailed comparison to the latter; hence the design of these studies lies between 'case-survey' and case-control.

It is not surprising that, in terms of indicating specific approaches to prevention of homelessness for the mentally ill, the yield from homelessness research in the United States has so far been modest. This, in spite of the fact that the bulk of research was funded by national or local agencies primarily concerned with mental illness and its treatment. The most common research design has been the general survey of the homeless. We suggest that this is a weak strategy for investigating the determinants of homelessness that apply specifically to mentally ill persons.

Conclusion

This is an important field in which the perspectives of the psychiatric epidemiologist have much to offer. It is also a difficult area, in part because social and health variables are so intertwined, both as causes and as outcomes. The application of epidemiology to a new field often leads to development for epidemiology itself. Here we are likely to refine our ability to grasp the constant interplay between illness, kin relationships, and broad social change, an interplay which is relevant to virtually any epidemiological outcome.

The framework we propose has implications for the design of preventive strategies as well as research. This is well illustrated with the case of mentally ill persons, a vulnerable population. Among the shortcomings of the de-institutionalization process was the implicit premise that the social environment outside the asylum would remain constant. Yet housing scarcity, the evolution of family systems, and other social changes have resulted in an epidemic of homelessness for mentally ill persons. The epidemic could not have been anticipated by experimental studies that compared out-patient care with hospitalization, since they were limited to the social environment prior to the late 1970s.

Our analysis suggests that prevention of homelessness will require community supports that can adapt to the occurrence of generation effects and of change at the societal and family level, as mentally ill persons in the community pass through a full life course. For instance, protected housing must be available, as a buffer against such processes. Protected housing need not always be segregated, and certainly need not be the asylum. It also need not be permanent, but may, rather, be available for varying periods of time as a 'secure base', much as a family system can be in some cultures. Homelessness, a historically specific phenomenon that also affects non-mentally ill persons, should not be used to justify the removal of the mentally ill from community settings on a long-term basis.

The research strategies suggested here may allow us in future to further specify the type of protection needed. Mentally ill persons who differ in age, gender, diagnosis, severity of illness, and other factors can hardly be expected to accommodate to the same preventive programme. We may also be able to target preventive programmes to the sub-groups at greatest risk. Specific programmes, however, must be located within an overall approach. An understanding of broad social processes that contribute to homelessness among non-mentally ill as well as mentally ill persons is required for the overall approach to be valid.

Acknowledgement

We thank the National Alliance for Research on Schizophrenia and Depression for financial support of this work.

References

Appleby, L. and Desai, P.N. (1985) 'Documenting the relationship between homelessness and psychiatric hospitalization', *Hospital and Community Psychiatry* 36 (7): 732–7.

Bachrach L.I. (1982) 'Young adult chronic patients: an analytic review of the literature', *Hospital and Community Psychiatry* 33: 189–97.

Bachrach, L.I. (1984) 'The homeless mentally ill and mental health services: an analytical review of the literature', in H.R. Lamb (ed.) *The Homeless Mentally Ill*, Washington, DC: American Psychiatric Association.

Bahr, H.M. and Caplow, T. (1973) *Old Men Drunk and Sober*, New York: New York University Press.

Barbanell, J. (1988) 'Crack use pervades life in a shelter', *New York Times*, 18 February 1988, P.A1.

Barrow, S., Hellman, F., Plapinger, J., Lovell, A.M., and Struening, E.L. (1986) *Residence Outcomes: Preliminary Findings from an Evaluation of Programs for the Mentally Ill Homeless*, New York: New York State Psychiatric Institute.

Bassuk, E.L. and Lamb, H.R. (1986) 'Homelessness and the implementation of deinstitutionalization', in E.L. Bassuk (ed.) *New Directions for Mental Health Services: The Mental Health Needs of Homeless Persons*, No. 30, San Francisco: Jossey-Bass, pp.7–14.

Baxter, E. (1987) 'The Heights residence', presentation to families and advocates of the mentally ill, New York: Bronx Psychiatric Center, October.

Chafetz, L. and Goldfinger, S.M. (1984) 'Residential instability in a psychiatric emergency setting', *Psychiatric Quarterly* 56(1): 20–34.

Deutsch, A. (1937) *The Mentally Ill in America*, New York: Columbia University Press.

Goldman H. (1983) 'The demography of deinstitutionalization', in L. Bachrach (ed.) *New Directions for Mental Health Services: Deinstitutionalization*, No. 17, San Francisco: Jossey-Bass.

Goldstein, S.J. and Dyche, L. (1983) 'Family therapy of the schizophrenic poor', in W.R. McFarlane (ed.) *Family Therapy in Schizophrenia*, New York: Guilford Press.

Gounis, K. and Susser, E. (in press) '*Shelterization and its implications for mental health services*', in N. Cohen (ed.) *Psychiatry Takes to the Streets*, New York: Guilford Press.

Grob, G.N. (1973) *Mental Institutions in America: Social Policy to 1875*, New York: Free Press.

Hartman, C. (1986) 'The housing part of the homelessness problem', in E.L. Bassuk (ed.) *New Directions in Mental Health: The Mental Health Needs of Homeless Persons*, No. 30, San Francisco: Jossey-Bass, pp.63–85.

Hopper, K. and Hamburg, J. (1986) 'The making of America's homeless: from Skid Row to the new poor, 1945–1984', in R.G. Bratt, C. Hartman, and A. Meyerson (eds) *Critical Perspectives on Housing*, Philadelphia, PA: Temple University Press.

Hopper K., Susser E., and Conover S. (1985) 'Economies of makeshift: deindustrialization and homelessness in New York City', *Urban Anthropology*, 14 (1–3): 183–236.

Kandel D.B. (1982) 'Epidemiological and psychosocial perspectives on adolescent drug use', *Journal of the American Academy of Child Psychiatry* 21(4): 328–47.

Lamb, H.R. (1982) 'Young adult chronic patients: the new drifters', *Hospital and Community Psychiatry* 33: 465–8.

Lamb, H.R. (1984) 'Deinstitutionalization and the homeless mentally ill', in H.R. Lamb (ed.) *The Homeless Mentally Ill*, Washington, DC: American Psychiatric Association.

Manhattan Borough President's Task Force on Housing for Homeless Families (1987) *A Shelter is Not a Home*, New York.

Morrissey, J.P., Dennis, D.L., Gounis, K., and Barrow, S. (1985) *The Development and Utilization of the Queen's Men's Shelter*, Albany, NY: New York State Office of Mental Health; and New York: New York State Psychiatric Institute.

Mowbray, C.T., Johnson, V.S., and Solarz, A. (1987) 'Homelessness in a state hospital population', *Hospital and Community Psychiatry* 38 (8): 880–2.

Pepper, B., Kirshner, M.C., and Ryglewicz, H. (1981) 'The young adult chronic patient: overview of a population', *Hospital and Community Psychiatry* 32(7): 463–9.

Reich, R. and Siegel, L. (1978) 'The emergence of the Bowery as a psychiatric dumping ground', *Psychiatric Quarterly* 50 (3): 191–201.

Rothman D.J. (1971) *The Discovery of the Asylum: Social Order and Disorder in the New Republic*, Boston, Mass.: Little, Brown and Company.

Struening E.L. (1986) *A Study of Residents of the New York City Shelter System*, report to the New York City Department of Mental Health, Mental Retardation and Alcoholism Services. New York: New York State Psychiatric Institute, Epidemiology of Mental Disorders Research Department.

Struening, E.L. (1987) *A Comparison of Evidence for a History of Mental Disorder Derived from Survey and Record System Data*, report to the New York City Department of Mental Health, Mental Retardation and Alcoholism Services, New York: New York State Psychiatric Institute, Epidemiology of Mental Disorders Research Department.

Susser, E. and Struening, E.L. (1987) *First Time Users of the New York City Shelter System*, report to the New York City Department of Mental Health, Mental Retardation, and Alcoholism Services, New York: New York State Psychiatric Institute, Epidemiology of Mental Disorders.

Susser, E., Conover, S., and Struening, E.L. 'Homeless men in New York City shelters: mental health status', submitted for publication.

Susser, E., Conover, S., and Struening, E.L. 'Homelessness and mental illness: epidemiologic aspects', under review.

Susser, E., Struening, E.L., and Conover S. (1987) 'Childhood experiences of homeless men', *American Journal of Psychiatry* 44: 1599–601.

Wallace, R. 'Homelessness, housing destruction and municipal service cuts in New York City: dynamics of a housing famine', under review.

Chapter sixteen

The effects of research interviews on depressive symptoms in the six weeks following reproductive loss

Richard Neugebauer

Introduction

Miscarriage is an unanticipated life event involving physical pain, real and symbolic loss, and subsequent hormonal change. For these reasons, it may prove a powerful psychological and biological risk factor for depression in women and, in turn, for emotional disturbance in their families. Since 15 to 20 per cent of recognized pregnancies end in a miscarriage, the psychiatric impact of this reproductive loss represents an important potential arena for secondary prevention.

Parental psychiatric reactions to reproductive loss have occasioned considerable clinical interest and concern among paediatricians (Elliot and Hein 1978; Jolly 1976; Morris 1976), obstetricians (Leppert and Pahlka 1984), psychiatrists (Cohen *et al.* 1978; Lewis 1976, 1979), and genetic counsellors (Phipps 1981), together with calls for more observational studies in this area and proposals for intervention strategies. Several cohort studies have examined the impact of infant mortality (Benfield *et al.* 1978; Culberg 1972; Kennell *et al.* 1970; Nicol *et al.* 1986), stillbirth (Bourne 1968; Graham *et al.* 1987; Wilson *et al.* 1985; Clarke and Williams 1979), or miscarriage (Seitz and Warrick 1974; Simon *et al.* 1969) on parental, usually maternal, psychiatric status. Unfortunately, design, measurement, and data analytic problems with these early works cloud interpretation of their results. For example, most investigations lack a comparison cohort of subjects unexposed to recent reproductive loss, thereby precluding calculation of relative risks. Few studies attempted to interview subjects at standardized time points following the loss. Rather, the timing of assessments was determined by subjects' availability, with psychological status being first evaluated anywhere from months to years after the event. Investigators assessing psychopathology clinically often left diagnostic criteria unspecified. Finally, threats to the validity of study conclusions posed by potential confounding variables, Type II error arising from limited sample sizes and high non-response rates are rarely considered.

Research aims and methods

We conducted a prospective cohort study of the effects of spontaneous abortion on psychiatric symptoms and disorders among miscarrying women and on behavioural disturbance among their children. This investigation, the Miscarriage and Depression Study, comprises three cohorts: that of the miscarrying women, constituting the exposed group, and two, unexposed comparison groups: pregnant women and women, drawn from the community, who had not been pregnant in the year preceding the interview. Miscarriage was defined as the involuntary termination of an intra-uterine pregnancy prior to twenty-eight weeks' gestation, with the foetus dead on expulsion.

Miscarrying and pregnant women were recruited from the cases and controls, respectively, in another investigation, the Epidemiology of Early Reproductive Loss Study (Kline *et al.* 1977; 1981). The latter was a hospital-based study of environmental and biological risk factors for spontaneous abortion. The Early Reproductive Loss Study drew its cases from all women attending Columbia Presbyterian Medical Center in New York City following a spontaneous abortion. Controls were selected from among women registered for prenatal care at the Medical Center before the twenty-second week of gestation. The interview for cases and controls included questions on sociodemographic variables; obstetric, contraceptive, and medical history; medication and drug use; consumption of alcohol and caffeine-containing beverages and smoking habits.

At the conclusion of the Early Reproductive Loss interview, miscarried and pregnant women were invited to enter the Miscarriage and Depression Study. Eligibility was restricted to English- or Spanish-speaking women over the age of 17, having the use of a telephone either in their own home or in that of a neighbour. Miscarrying women were interviewed by telephone at roughly one to two weeks (Time 1), six to eight weeks (Time 2), and six to eight months (Time 3) after their spontaneous abortion, regarding psychiatric symptoms and characteristics of their pregnancy, miscarriage, and social environment (Neugebauer 1987). Additional socio-demographic data, including income, were also secured. Information on income was obtained using a method from marketing research, known as 'unfolding', which gradually backs subjects into disclosure of their income bracket. Evidence suggests that this method generates reasonably valid responses, while avoiding high refusal rates by female respondents (Locander and Burton 1976). Only 2 per cent of our subjects refused to answer this question.

The woman's psychiatric status was assessed at each time point with several different psychiatric symptom scales developed for use in the general population, namely, the Center for Epidemiologic Studies Depression Scale (CES-D) (Radloff 1977) and scales from the Psychiatric Epidemiology Research Interview (PERI) (Dohrenwend *et al.* 1980). The CES-D is a twenty-item scale, derived from previously validated instruments, that seeks to measure key dimensions of depressive symptomatology. Item coverage includes depressed mood, feelings of guilt, worthlessness, help-lessness, hopelessness, psychomotor retardation, appetite loss, and sleep disturbance. Reliability and validity of the CES-D are well documented and satisfactory (Radloff 1977; Weissman et al. 1977). PERI scales measuring diverse aspects of psychopathology were selected either to supplement the CES-D in areas of special concern, for example, guilt feelings and suicidal ideation, or to introduce additional domains, e.g., anxiety symptoms.

A newly developed scale, the Miscarriage Grief Scale, was piloted in this study. Grounded in attachment theory, it is aimed to explore somatic, affective, and cognitive responses specific to mourning. The instrument focuses on phantom symptoms of pregnancy, the woman's longing to nurture the lost child, and continued mental preparation for the baby's arrival.

At Times 2 and 3, the interview included PERI measures of social functioning at work, in marriage, and as a parent. These scales are expected to serve as valuable ancillary indicators of psychological status.

The six-month contact included the Diagnostic Interview Schedule (DIS-III), a diagnostic evaluation designed to assess psychiatric disorders in the general population (Robins et al. 1981). Parous miscarried women were also administered a brief behaviour checklist with reference to each child in the family between the ages of 3 and 8 years inclusive.

The Epidemiology of Early Reproductive Loss Study interviewed 75 per cent of its miscarrying subjects within one week of spontaneous abortion; most of the remainder were interviewed over the next few weeks. Conse-quently, entry into the Miscarriage and Depression Study was necessarily similarly staggered. A subject's first interview had two parts, each lasting forty-five minutes to one hour, usually administered on separate days. It began by asking the woman about current physical complaints followed by items from the CES-D and the PERI symptom checklists interspersed with sociodemographic questions. Next, we took a history of the woman's pregnancy including her attitudes about being pregnant, awareness of quickening, hearing the heart beat at the time of a doctor's visit, her plans for the arrival of the baby – e.g., decisions about the child's name, purchases and rearrangement of household furniture – and visible bodily changes.

The second part of the interview involved a recapitulation of the events of the miscarriage and the hospital stay. The woman was asked about early warning signs, the physical pain and social circumstances of the miscarriage proper, and the types of support received in hospital.

All interviewers were female. Their training emphasized verbatim reading of items when administering the psychiatric symptom checklists. Greater latitude was allowed with questions chronicling the pregnancy and miscarriage. Here, the interviewers could elaborate a question to clarify its meaning. However, while permitted to offer empathic but brief responses to a distressed woman, the interviewer was instructed to avoid prolonged ad hoc discussion, offering of consolation or advice.

At the conclusion of the first and second parts of the interview, subjects' opinions of and reactions to the interview were solicited. Typically, the subject took this opportunity to thank the interviewer and, through her, the investigators, for their interest in her emotional responses to the miscarriage. Roughly a quarter of the subjects volunteered that they 'felt better' after the interview. Since subjects frequently also commented on the tedium and apparent repetitiveness of some questions, we do not believe that the expressions of appreciation reflected simply subjects' wishes to present socially desirable responses.

Pregnant women were administered a two-part interview, usually within three weeks of recruitment into the Miscarriage and Depression Study. The interview was similar to that for miscarried women but excluded the diagnostic interview and naturally the miscarriage-specific questions.

The community sample was obtained using a method of random digit dialling of telephone numbers, each dialled number being matched to a given miscarried woman's three-digit geographic regional code and three-digit city district code. The remaining four digits composing the telephone number were derived from a computer-generated random number list. These numbers were dialled in turn until we located a household with an eligible woman who was given the full battery of study measures. Eligibility was progressively constrained so as to achieve frequency matching between the miscarried and community women on age (18–24 and then in five-year age intervals thereafter, through age 44), years of education (0–11 years of education, 12, 13–15, 16 and 17+) and preferred language of interview.

Initially we had planned to create close residential matching of community and miscarried women through the use of telephone directories organized by street address (Neugebauer 1987). However, a pilot study established that roughly half of the telephone numbers of the miscarried women and of other residential telephone numbers in the Borough of Manhattan were not listed in the directory specifically at the customer's request. Since a preference for unlisted status may be associated with psychological characteristics of the telephone owner, sampling that was restricted to the universe of listed numbers risked producing biased estimates of psychiatric symptom levels in the community. Therefore, the random digit dialling method, while achieving a less precise residential match, was adopted to improve the likelihood of securing a community sample with a symptom profile more representative of all phone customers.

Women in the community control group were interviewed once, generally within two to six weeks of recruitment. They were assessed regarding psychiatric symptoms and disorders and most other variables of study interest except those specific to miscarriage. The same interviewing methods and much the same interviewers were used for the pregnant and community samples as for the miscarried women.

Midway through the study, when it became evident that participation rates substantially above 70 per cent could not be achieved in the Miscarriage and Depression Study with miscarrying and pregnant women, we introduced a global measure of mood into the Early Reproductive Loss interview to assess whether, at the time of study invitation, uninterviewed subjects differed in this respect from those who were interviewed. This measure is a single-item visual analogue scale (VAMS) developed by Folstein and Luria (1973). The VAMS is an unmarked horizontal line whose left end represents the subject's 'worst mood' and right end, her 'best mood'. The subject is requested to make a mark on the line indicating her present mood-state in relation to these extremes. The test-retest reliability of this measure, with psychiatric and medical patients, is fairly high. It discriminates depressed patients from manic patients, and from psychiatric patients with non-affective disorders. Furthermore, VAMS scores correlate well with measures of depressive symptomatology, e.g., Zung's self-rating depression scale.

The VAMS was added to the Early Reproductive Loss Study booklet and modified, to facilitate score-computation time, by calibrating the line from 1 to 9 from left to right. The test-retest reliability of this modified scale has been shown to be excellent in a sample of medical patients (Neugebauer, unpublished data). In anticipation of similar problems with response rates in the community survey, the same scale, adopted for telephone administration, was incorporated into the screening interview conducted with eligible subjects.

Recruitment of subjects concluded in August of 1987; data processing is in progress. Three hundred and eighty-one miscarried, 307 pregnant, and 302 community women have been successfully interviewed. This report compares the frequency of depressive symptoms in the miscarriage cohort at one and six weeks following reproductive loss with that found in the first two-thirds of the community sample. Although depressive symptoms were assessed with a variety of measures, we limit this report to scores on the CES-D. The twenty CES-D items are scored from 0 to 3, with 0 indicating that the subject had seldom or never experienced the symptom in the past week, and 3 that it was present most or all of the time. Item scores are summed to give totals ranging from 0 to 60.

The tentative nature of the present findings must be emphasized. Field work with the community sample has just concluded, while processing of the miscarriage data is nearing completion. We are, however, cautiously optimistic that our findings will persist in analyses using the completely assembled and processed data set. Given the theme of this volume, we have directed the analyses towards the discovery of possible opportunities for prevention.

Research findings

During the period of linkage of the Epidemiology of Early Reproductive Loss and the Miscarriage and Depression Studies, the former interviewed 77 per cent of women over age 17 attending the Medical Center for a spontaneous abortion. Of the remainder, 10 per cent refused participation; 8 per cent could not be traced after leaving the hospital. The distribution of interviewed and uninterviewed subjects did not differ on race, marital status, or parity. However, interviewed women were slightly older and of greater gestational age at miscarriage than the uninterviewed.

The Miscarriage and Depression Study administered a complete interview to 237 women at Time 1; of these, 199 (84 per cent) could be interviewed again at Time 2. A further 114 women were first interviewed at Time 2, so that the total interviewed at this stage was 313 (Table 16.1). The participation rate at Time 1 was 72 per cent; at Time 2, 71 per cent. Of those not interviewed, two-thirds refused to take part; the remainder could not be reached within the time limits (each approximately two weeks in duration) established for the Time 1 and Time 2 assessments. However, some of these subjects were successfully interviewed at the time of later study assessments.

Table 16.1 Subject entry into the miscarriage and depression study and attrition at one week (Time 1) and six weeks (Time 2) following miscarriage

| | | Interviewed at Time 2: | | Total |
		No	Yes	
Interviewed at Time 1:	Yes	38	199	237
	No	—	114	114
Total		38	313	351

Extensive information is available on those miscarrying women who did not participate in the Miscarriage and Depression Study because all subjects were successfully interviewed in the Early Reproductive Loss Study. Interviewed subjects were remarkably similar to their uninterviewed counterparts at both Time 1 and Time 2 on major sociodemographic characteristics (Table 16.2) and reproductive history variables (Table 16.3). (For parsimony, Table 16.2 and 16.3 present data for subjects considered study-eligible at the two time points combined. However, the results are equivalent when interviewed and uninterviewed subjects are compared at Time 1 and Time 2 separately.)

Roughly one-third of the subjects in each group are White; just over half are aged 25–34; only half received more than a high school education (12+ years) and 65 per cent were married or living with a partner. Over 60 per cent have at least one child. Neither gestational age nor prior experience of a reproductive loss influenced the participation rates. In both groups,

Table 16.2 Distribution of interviewed and uninterviewed miscarrying women (Times 1 and 2 combined) by sociodemographic characteristics

Characteristic	Interviewed (N=351) %	Uninterviewed (N=137) %
Ethnicity		
White	31.0	31.1
Black	22.7	21.5
Hispanic	38.5	38.6
Other	7.8	8.8
Age		
18–24	26.3	26.6
25–34	52.0	55.9
35–44	21.6	17.6
Education in years		
0–11	30.5	30.0
12	23.9	21.6
13–15	22.7	25.1
16	8.0	10.1
17+	14.9	13.2
Marital		
Married/cohabiting	65.8	64.0
Not married	34.2	36.0
Language of ERLS interview		
English	67.8	71.1

Table 16.3 Distribution of interviewed and uninterviewed miscarrying women (Times 1 and 2 combined) by selected reproductive history characteristics

Characteristic	Interviewed (N=351) %	Uninterviewed (N=137) %
Parity		
0	36.6	34.7
1	30.5	34.2
2+	32.8	31.3
Gestational age at time of miscarriage in days		
1–49	6.1	10.1
50–91	54.0	56.6
> 91	39.9	33.3
Prior Reproductive Loss		
0	67.2	66.2
1	20.1	21.1
2+	12.6	12.7

roughly one-third of the women miscarried after the thirteenth week of gestation; 30 per cent had experienced at least one prior loss.

The VAMS scores of miscarrying women first interviewed at Time 1 and of those first interviewed at Time 2 were combined and compared with those of uninterviewed women, after controlling for the difference between interviewed and uninterviewed women in the time elapsed between miscarriage and VAMS administration. The two groups proved indistinguishable on this scale.

Data on the first 209 women in the community control group to participate in the Miscarriage and Depression Study have been computerized. Measures of mood and depressive symptoms (CES-D scores) as well as sociodemographic information (age, years of education, and preferred language) were secured on most eligible women, irrespective of participation status. However, these data, which will permit an evaluation of the comparability of interviewed and uninterviewed community subjects, are not yet available for analysis.

Frequency matching of miscarried and community-control women on age, education, and language of interview was expected to achieve satisfactory comparability of the two groups more generally. However, while the two groups do exhibit a similar ethnic distribution (see Table 16.2 for the ethnic distribution of the interviewed miscarried women), statistically significant differences have emerged on some other sociodemographic and reproductive history variables. Notably, the community-control women have a higher mean income and are more often single and nulliparous than the miscarried. We suspect that some of those contrasts may endure even when the community data set is complete.

The statistical analyses presented below are reported first in terms of two-tailed t-tests for differences in group means. Where the distribution of the two groups differed significantly on variables associated with CES-D scores, for example, on income, the means were also compared after adjusting for such differences using analysis of covariance.

At Time 1, the mean CES-D score of the miscarriage group is substantially greater than that in the community: 23.9 ± 0.81 versus 14.7 ± 0.74 (p<.0001). The adjusted means for the two groups are 23.7 and 15.2, respectively, again a significant difference (p< .0001). Note that a person with a CES-D score of 24 might report experiencing eight symptoms of depression nearly all of the time in the past week, including somatic complaints (e.g., 'did not feel like eating', 'sleep was restless'), depressive ideation ('thought life had been a failure'), and depressive mood ('had crying spells'; 'felt sad'). The sociological significance of this difference in score means is conveyed by comparing the magnitude of the effect of income on CES-D score – one of the more powerful predictors of CES-D scores – with that of miscarriage. In the community cohort the difference in CES-D means between women with incomes below $10,000 per year and those over $25,000 is 5.8, an entirely typical finding (Frerichs et al. 1981). However, at Time 1, the mean CES-D scores of miscarried and community women differ by 9.2 points.

The CES-D has been used as a screening device to identify subjects with an increased likelihood of having a diagnosable depression (Boyd *et al.* 1982), with a score of 16 or greater adopted as the cutpoint (Weissman *et al.* 1977). Using this criterion with the Time 1 scores, 71 per cent of miscarrying women screened positive compared to 40 per cent in the community.

At Time 2 the CES-D mean score in the miscarriage group was 15.6 ± 0.70, compared with 14.7 ± 0.74 in the community control group: a difference no longer statistically significant in unadjusted ($p<.38$) or adjusted (14.9 vs. 15.2, $p<.78$) analyses. Such an apparently marked abatement at six weeks in depressive symptomatology could, however, arise artefactually from a change in the cohort composition by Time 2 or from some effect of the Time 1 interview, rather than as a result of a recuperative process associated with the passage of time since the loss.

That the decline in CES-D means did not arise from a change in cohort composition – for example, by the exit after Time 1 of more depressed women and the entry by Time 2 of less symptomatic subjects – is shown most simply by comparing the CES-D means at Time 1 and Time 2 with the analysis restricted to women interviewed at both time points. In this analysis the CES-D mean of 14.0 ± 0.84 at Time 2 is still decisively lower than the same women's mean at Time 1, $24.7, \pm 0.90$, ($p<.0001$, paired t-test). It is also of interest to note that the thirty-eight women interviewed at Time 1 but not at Time 2 had a lower CES-D mean (19.7) compared to those who could be contacted again at Time 2.

While a change in cohort composition does not account for the lower CES-D mean at Time 2, these analyses invite an alternative explanation; namely, the operation of some effect of the Time 1 interview itself on the scores at Time 2. Subjects may be inclined to report fewer symptoms on retest (despite the fact that the Time 2 CES-D pertained to a different time period) or the Time 1 interview may have proved unintentionally therapeutic. Support for this explanation of some intervention effect emerges from a comparison of Time 2 scores, stratified by subjects' interview status at Time 1. The CES-D Time 2 mean of 14.0 for women seen at Time 1 is significantly different from 18.6, the Time 2 mean for women not previously interviewed (Table 16.4).

Table 16.4 Mean CES-D scores in the miscarriage cohort at Time 2 by Time 1 interview status

	Time 2 Mean (SE)
Time 1 status (N)	
Interviewed at Time 1 (199)	14.0 (0.84)
Not interviewed at Time 1 (114)	18.6 (1.21)

$t=3.20$, df=311,
$p < .002$, t-test, two-tailed

Table 16.5 arrays the mean scores for each component of these cohorts. All paired comparisons reflect statistically significant differences in mean CES-D scores after adjustment. The CES-D mean of 18.6 for the miscarrying women interviewed for the first time at Time 2 is significantly different from the overall Time 1 mean of 23.9 (p<.005) and from the community mean of 14.7 (p<.004). (Much the same results emerged from adjusted analyses: 18.3 versus 24.9 (p<.0001) and 17.8 versus 15.0 (p<.04), respectively.) The CES-D mean of 14.0 of miscarrying women reinterviewed at Time 2 was also significantly lower after adjustment from the mean score for the community: 13.3 vs. 15.3, p<.03.

Table 16.5 Summary of mean CES-D scores for the miscarriage cohort by stage of study entry and for the community sample

		Miscarriage mean at:		Community mean
		Time 1	Time 2	
Interviewed at Time 1:	Yes	23.9	14.0	
				14.7
	No	–	18.6	

See text for statistically significant differences in paired comparisons.

At Time 1, miscarried women are markedly more depressed than a matched group of community women. At Time 2, miscarrying women report significantly fewer symptoms compared to Time 1. If a woman has been interviewed previously about her feelings following the miscarriage, her reported symptom levels at Time 2 are at least as low as those of community women and our results here suggest that they are even significantly lower. On the other hand, women reached for the first time at six weeks post-miscarriage report significantly more symptoms than women in the community, indicating a continuing although diminished effect of reproductive loss with the passage of time.

Discussion

The comparatively low participation rate of eligible miscarrying and community women reflects the increasing difficulty of subject recruitment in the United States and abroad. The extensive use of segments of these populations in social science and medical studies, and the fact that these populations are routinely and systematically canvassed by market researchers on behalf of private industry, doubtless contributes to these rising refusal rates (Steeh *et al.* 1983; Thomsen and Siring 1983).

High non-response rates inevitably raise questions about the representativeness of the interviewed samples and the validity of estimates of depressive symptomatology in the study groups. In the present investigation, extensive data on the sociodemographic characteristics, reproductive history, and mood states of eligible miscarrying women, and similar but somewhat less extensive information on eligible community controls, permit an assessment of representativeness. Analyses to date suggest that miscarrying women successfully interviewed at Time 1 and Time 2 were essentially no different from the uninterviewed women either in objective biosocial and medical characteristics or in their appraisal of their own affective state at the time of their invitation to enter the study. Similar analyses for the community group are pending.

Mindful of these sampling issues and the incompleteness of the data set at this time, we advance several tentative early conclusions. First, compared to the level of depressive symptoms exhibited by women in the community, miscarrying women show a pronounced elevation in depressive symptomatology at one week following reproductive loss. At six weeks, after controlling for the effect of the Time 1 assessment, women are still at markedly increased risk for depressive symptoms. Second, interviewing women at one week after a reproductive loss leads to a marked reduction in reported symptom levels at six weeks. This reduction may represent either a test effect or a therapeutic consequence of the women having an opportunity to review systematically the events of the pregnancy and miscarriage with an individual associated with the Medical Centre. Both processes may be operating here. If a therapeutic effect explains a portion of the observed decline in CES-D scores at Time 2 in miscarrying women interviewed at Time 1, the possibility is raised that a brief intervention within a couple of weeks after miscarriage may substantially reduce a woman's risk of continued depressive symptoms.

Test-retest effects that reduce the volume of reported symptom data in second and later interview waves are widely recognized and have recently proved troublesome in some analyses in the Epidemiologic Catchment Area Studies (Robins 1985). However, early work specifically with the CES-D indicated that such test-retest effects using this instrument should prove negligible (Radloff 1977). While a proper exploration of the potential therapeutic benefits of early counselling of miscarrying women awaits an intervention study, we will devote further attention in analysing these research data to assessing the relative contribution of test-retest and therapeutic effects to our findings.

Analyses will proceed on two levels. The first will scrutinize these Time 1–Time 2 data by examining, for example, whether women who made the most use of the less structured sections of the interview to ventilate their feelings exhibited a greater decrement in symptom levels at Time 2. The second type of analysis will investigate whether a similar phenomenon occurs among those subjects first interviewed at Time 3 compared to those interviewed previously.

Acknowledgements

This investigation is supported by grant MH39581 from the National Institute of Mental Health. The other investigators on this grant are Jennie Kline, Patricia O'Connor, Patrick Shrout, Andrew Skodol, Zena Stein, and Mervyn Susser.

References

Benfield, D.G., Leib, S.A., and Vollman, J.H. (1978) 'Response of parents to neonatal death and parent participation in deciding care', *Pediatrics* 62: 171–7.

Bourne, S. (1968) 'The psychological effects of stillbirths on women and their doctors', *Journal of the Royal College of General Practitioners* 16: 103–12.

Boyd, J., Weissman, M., Thompson, W.D., and Myers, J.K. (1982) 'Screening for depression in a community sample: understanding the discrepancies between depressive symptoms and diagnostic scales', *Archives of General Psychiatry* 39: 1195–200.

Clarke, M. and Williams, A.J. (1979) 'Depression in women after perinatal death', *Lancet* ii: 916–17.

Cohen, L., Zilkha, S., Middleton, J., and O'Donnohue, N. (1978) 'Perinatal mortality: assisting in parental affirmation', *American Journal of Orthopsychiatry* 48: 727–31.

Culberg, J. (1972) 'Mental reactions of women to perinatal death', in *Psychosomatic Medicine in Obstetrics and Gynaecology: Third International Congress*, Basel: Karger.

Dohrenwend, B.S., Shrout, P.E., Egri, G., and Mendelsohn, F.S. (1980) 'Non-specific psychological distress and other dimensions of psychopathology', *Archives of General Psychiatry* 31; 1229–36.

Elliott, B.A. and Hein, H.A. (1978) 'Neonatal death: reflections for physicians', *Pediatrics* 62: 96–100.

Folstein, M.F. and Luria, R. (1973) 'Reliability, validity, and clinical application of the visual analogue mood scale', *Psychological Medicine* 3: 479–86.

Frerichs, R.R., Aneshensel, C.S., and Clark, V.A. (1981) 'Prevalence of depression in Los Angeles County', *American Journal of Epidemiology* 113: 691–9.

Gilson, G.J. (1976) 'Care of the family who has lost a newborn', *Postgraduate Medicine* 60: 67–70.

Graham, A.M., Thompson, S.C., Estrada, M., and Yonekura, M.L. (1987) 'Factors affecting psychological adjustment to fetal death', *American Journal of Obstetrics and Gynecology* 157: 254–7.

Jolly, H. (1976) 'Family reactions to stillbirth', *Proceedings of the Royal Society of Medicine* 69: 835–7.

Kennell, J.H., Slyter, H., and Klaus, M.H. (1970) 'The mourning response of parents to the death of a newborn infant', *New England Journal of Medicine* 13: 344–9.

Kline, J., Shrout, P., Stein, Z., Susser, M., and Warburton, D. (1981) 'Drinking during pregnancy and spontaneous abortion', *Lancet* ii: 176–80.

Kline, J., Stein, Z., Susser, M., and Warburton, D. (1977) 'Smoking: a risk factor for spontaneous abortion', *New England Journal of Medicine* 297: 793–6.

Leppert, P.C. and Pahlka, B. (1984) 'Grieving characteristics after spontaneous abortion: a management approach', *Obstetrics and Gynecology* 64: 119–22.

Lewis, E. (1976) 'The management of stillbirth: coping with an unreality', *Lancet* ii: 619–20.

Lewis, E. (1979) 'Mourning by the family after a stillbirth or neonatal death', *Archives of Diseases of Childhood* 54: 303–6.

Locander, W.B. and Burton, J.P. (1976) 'The effect of question form on gathering income data by telephone', *Journal of Market Research* 8: 189–92.

Morris, D. (1976) 'Parental reaction to perinatal death', *Proceedings of the Royal Society of Medicine* 69: 33–4.

Neugebauer, R. (1987) 'The psychiatric effects of miscarriage: research design and preliminary findings', in B. Cooper (ed.) *Psychiatric Epidemiology: Progress and Prospects*, Baltimore, MD: Johns Hopkins University Press.

Nicol, M.T., Tompkins, J.R., Campbell, N.A., and Syme, G.J. (1986) 'Maternal grieving response after perinatal death', *Medical Journal of Australia* 144: 287–9.

Phillips, S.L. and Fischer, C.S. (1981) 'Measuring social support networks in general populations', in B.S. Dohrenwend and B.P. Dohrenwend (eds) *Stressful Life Events and their Contexts*, New York: Prodist.

Phipps, S. (1981) 'Mourning response and intervention in stillbirth: an alternative genetic counseling approach', *Social Biology* 28: 1–13.

Radloff, L.S. (1977) 'The CES-D Scale: a self-report depression scale for research in the general population', *Applied Psychological Measurement* 1: 385–401.

Robins, L.N. (1985) 'Epidemiology: reflections on testing the validity of psychiatric interviews', *Archives of General Psychiatry* 42: 918–24.

Robins, L.N., Helzer, J.E., Croughan, J., and Ratcliff, K.S. (1981) 'National Institute of Mental Health Diagnostic Interview Schedule: its history, characteristics, and validity', *Archives of General Psychiatry* 38: 381–9.

Seitz, P.M. and Warrick, L.H. (1974) 'Perinatal death: the grieving mother', *American Journal of Nursing* 74: 2028–33.

Simon, N.M., Rothman, D., Goff, J.T., and Senturia, A.G. (1969) 'Psychological factors related to spontaneous and therapeutic abortion', *American Journal of Obstetrics and Gynecology* 104: 799–808.

Steeh, G.H., Groves, R.M., Comment, R., and Hansmire, E. (1983) 'Report on the survey research centre's surveys of consumer attitudes', in W.G. Madow, H. Nisselson, and I. Olkin (eds) *Incomplete Data in Sample Surveys 1*, Proceedings of the Symposium, New York: Academic Press, pp. 173–208.

Thomsen, I.B. and Siring, E. (1983) 'On the causes and effects of nonresponse: Norwegian experiences', in W.G. Madow and I. Olkin (eds) *Incomplete Data in Sample Surveys 3*, Proceedings of the Symposium, New York: Academic Press, pp. 25–55.

Weissman, M., Sholomskas, O., Pottenger, M., Prusoff, B.A., and Locke, B.Z. (1977) 'Assessing depressive symptoms in five psychiatric populations: a validation study', *American Journal of Epidemiology* 106: 203–14.

Wilson, A.L., Witzke, D., Fenton, L.J., and Soule, D. (1985) 'Parental response to perinatal death', *American Journal of Diseases of Childhood* 139: 1235–8.

Part five

Preventive action in mental health and other medical services

Chapter seventeen

Multi-level approaches to the prevention of mental disorders in the community: the Athenian experience

M.G. Madianos, D. Madianou, G. Gournas, and C.N. Stefanis

Introduction

Historically, measures for the prevention of mental disorders have been delineated on three levels, primary, secondary, and tertiary (Caplan 1961, 1964; Bellak 1964; Rae Grant and Rae Grant 1970; Bolman and Westman 1967; Bolman 1968, 1969; Beigel and Levenson 1972).

Primary prevention refers to the elimination of those factors which may cause or contribute to the incidence of mental disease. Consequently, lowering the rates of new psychiatric cases in a population over a certain period of time or reducing the risk for developing a crisis is considered primary prevention (Caplan and Grunebaum 1967; Berlin 1979a).

Secondary prevention involves early referral, diagnosis, and treatment of any person presenting a psychological problem or a specific nosological entity, while tertiary prevention aims to reduce the prevalence of functional impairment and disability in the community due to a long-term course of psychiatric illness (Caplan 1964; Bolman 1968; Berlin 1979b).

Caplan proposed a preventive model based on community mental health care. He defined several principles, the most basic one being that the programme should be comprehensive, comprising primary, secondary, and tertiary prevention in a defined geographic (catchment) area. The concept of preventive psychiatry was officially introduced in the planning of a country-wide network of community mental health centres providing 'services for the prevention or diagnosis of mental illness or care and treatment of mentally ill patients or rehabilitation of such persons' (US House of Representatives 1963).

Prevention was thus envisaged as a community concept, to be achieved by the comprehensive community mental health centres' various activities and programmes, in which providers and consumers co-operate for the promotion of the community's mental health (Caplan 1964; Dunham 1965; Sussex 1979).

Across the Atlantic, in the late-1960s and early-1970s, several European countries gradually reorganized their mental health care delivery systems, by decentralizing their services and incorporating the basic community psychiatry principles (Gittelman 1972; WHO 1973; WHO 1980; Freeman *et al.* 1985; Perris and Kemali 1985).

Greece, a country rapidly changing through migration, urbanization, and industrialization, had until recently a rather traditional mental health care system, based on centralized services with an absence of community-based alternatives to in-patient care (Madianos 1983; Stefanis *et al.* 1986). In 1979 a comprehensive Community Mental Health Centre (CMHC), the first of its kind, was established as a model service, serving two boroughs in the Greater Athens area (Stefanis and Madianos 1983; Stefanis *et al.* 1985).

During the first eighteen months, the mental health needs of the catchment area and the public's attitudes towards mental illness were assessed by conducting systematic surveys (Madianos *et al.* 1985, 1987a, 1987b; Gournas *et al.* 1985). A psychiatric case-register has been established since 1979, primarily based upon data collected through these studies (Madianos and Madianou 1987). The Centre is a preventively oriented service with a broad spectrum of activities (Madianos and Stefanis 1984).

The purpose of this study was, first, to explore the efficacy of CMHC activities in achieving different levels of prevention of mental disorders in the community; second, to readjust our intervention strategies in order to accomplish the required levels of effectiveness. It thus serves as a feedback mechanism for the development of future preventive activities.

Material and methods

The Community Mental Health Centre (CMHC) setting

The CMHC is located in the eastern part of Greater Athens, serving two boroughs with a total population of 86,852 middle-class and lower-class inhabitants (Madianos and Madianou 1987). Its facilities include a walk-in clinic, a follow-up and domiciliary service for all ages, an outreach programme, a day-care and evening social club, a vocational training workshop, and a sheltered workshop.

There is no twenty-four-hour psychiatric emergency service in the CMHC and every case of emergency from the catchment area has to be admitted to the psychiatric emergency unit of Eginition Hospital, a back-up service for the Centre and part of the Athens Central Emergency System. The CMHC outreach programme includes a liaison service with this unit, so that community residents who have contacted the emergency service and are unknown to the CMHC case-register can be contacted by a visiting nurse within one week for purposes of further treatment and care. It should be noted that 90 per cent of these emergencies constitute new episodes and only 10 per cent are relapses.

All services providing extramural care are located in the CMHC and in four satellite clinics, each integrated with local sociomedical agencies. Training, research, and community mental health intervention are parallel activities. The latter includes a wide range of services provided for target population groups (parents; high school students; teachers). The strategies of community mental health intervention in the boroughs of Kessariani and Byron, oriented toward the three levels of prevention, are shown in Table 17.1.

Table 17.1 Strategies of community mental health intervention in the boroughs of Kessariani-Byron, Greater Athens (1979–86)

Target population	Mode of intervention	Goals	Level of prevention
High-risk individuals; persons in crisis	Outreach programme of central emergency unit liaison service	Crisis intervention; problem-solving	Primary
General population; parents; primary and secondary school pupils; teachers	Public mental health educaton programme; lectures; sensitivity group; small-group discussion; neighbourhood mental health committee	To increase awareness in psychosocial issues and ability in early response to mental health problems	Primary
Any community resident in need of treatment or consultation; nursery and elementary school children	Walk-in clinic; follow-up services; domiciliary care; broad spectrum of interventions; screening speech and learning difficulties	Early referral, diagnosis and treatment to modify and treat pathologic behaviour and reorganize support system	Secondary
Any chronic mentally disabled person	Psychosocial rehabilitation unit (day care; vocational programme; social club; co-operative). Group and individual therapeutic activities	To increase social reintegration and occupational adjustment	Tertiary

The aim is to reach high-risk individuals and persons in crisis, at an early stage, for the purpose of intervention as an early response to mental health problems. In addition, any community resident in need of consultation, therapy, or rehabilitation is referred to CMHC services.

Indices of prevention

In order to examine the effects of this service on the prevention of mental disorders, the following indices have been selected.

1. The number of psychiatric emergencies (new episodes) recorded prospectively for an eight-year period from the catchment area served by the CMHC, compared to the emergencies from the neighbouring borough of Zografou (control area), which is not served by a CMHC or any other extramural psychiatric service.

The lack of development of community mental health services in most of Greater Athens provides the opportunity for this comparison. According to Caplan (1964) any decrease in the number of emergencies (new psychiatric episodes) from the catchment area constitutes a primary preventive achievement.

Table 17.2 Demographic characteristics of boroughs of Kessariani-Bryon (catchment area) and Zografou (control area)

	Catchment Area	Control Area
Population[1]	86,852	84,509
% Population of Greater Athens	2.85	2.78
Population density per km^2	8,623	8,103
Sex: Males %	47.53	47.64
Females %	52.47	52.36
% Population $\leqslant$ 15	20.82	22.38
15–34	33.57	36.34
35–64	35.75	33.00
$\geqslant$ 65	9.86	8.28

[1] 1981 population census

The two areas present similar demographic characteristics in terms of total population, proportion of the Greater Athens population, population density, and male–female ratio. Data on the recent socio-economic structure of the two areas are not available, although the 1971 population census showed minor differences in socio-economic distribution, our catchment area being somewhat more economically disadvantaged than the control area. Numbers of psychiatric emergencies in the two areas are compared in the form of proportions, using the chi-square statistic with Yates correction, and of annual age-standardized rates, taking as the standard the Greater Athens population. Supplementary information is related to the proportion of schizophrenic episodes among the total number of emergencies from the two areas during the eight-year period (1978–86). The breakdown by one-year periods (1979–80, etc.) is because the CMHC started its operation on 1 October 1979 so a year is defined as the twelve-month period between 1 October and 30 September.

Psychiatric emergencies from the two areas and the rest of Greater Athens are referred to the twenty-four-hour psychiatric emergency unit of the Eginition Hospital in the city of Athens. This unit is located at an equal distance from each of the two areas. Details about the psychiatric emergency system in Athens have been reported previously (Madianos *et al.* 1984).

2. The proportion of first attendances at the CMHC of adults with a psychiatric illness of under six months duration and no previous contacts with any psychiatric service for this episode.

To the extent that a greater number of such mentally ill individuals are reached by the CMHC system than by the conventional type of service, it provides evidence of a secondary preventive function.

3. The long-term (five-year) effect of CMHC services on relapses, readmissions, global functioning, social adjustment, and family atmosphere of a cohort of thirty-two chronic schizophrenic community residents, compared to another cohort of fifty-four patients with the same clinical and sociodemographic characteristics treated by non-sectorized out-patient psychiatric services by prescription of medication alone.

The statistical analysis compared the difference of mean scores on the Global Assessment Scale (Endicott *et al.* 1976), Community Adjustment Scale (Madianos 1984), and Family Atmosphere Scale (Madianos *et al.* 1987c). The GAS is a widely used instrument, measuring overall functioning combined with psychopathologic status. It has proved to be of high predictive validity. The CAS and FAS are original survey research instruments developed by the first of the present authors, which record quantitative, scaled judgements of the patients' family and community life and functioning, based on information reported by the patient and the family or from other sources. The instruments incorporate twelve and six scales respectively and have shown high internal consistency and validity. This project was an extension of the WHO Collaborative Study of Mental Health Services in Pilot Study Areas (Madianos and Madianou 1987) and its methodology has been described elsewhere (Madianos 1984; Madianos *et al.* 1987c).

4. The incidence of episodes of deviant behaviour ('trouble-making', vandalism, aggression, truancy, and disrespect to teachers or peers).

This was recorded in two high schools of the catchment area before and after completion of a mental health education programme including several aspects of psychosocial issues, delivered for the last three academic periods by CMHC members, and involving teachers, parents, and students. A third high school, in the same area, in which no intervention was carried out, served as a control for comparison of episode rates. Both experimental and control schools are sectorized and cannot take pupils from other parts of the city. Any influence on the incidence of such episodes in the two local high schools after the completion of the intervention programme is considered as a primary preventive function. Each of the three schools had on average 655 pupils with similar sociodemographic characteristics. The intervention programme was addressed to pupils in equal numbers of classrooms and grades.

Research findings

Psychiatric emergencies from the catchment and control area

Of a total of 25,173 emergencies dealt with at the Athens psychiatric emergency unit, Eginition Hospital, in the period 1978–86, 798 (2.89 per cent) came from the CMHC catchment area and 861 (3.42 per cent) from the control area. The annual distribution of the emergencies from the two areas is shown in Table 17.3.

Table 17.3 Psychiatric emergencies from boroughs of Kessariani-Byron (catchment area) and Zografou (control area), 1979–86

Year	Catchment area[1]	Control area	Chi-sq (with Yates correction)	Significance level
1978–1979	76	61	2.15	N.S.
1979–1980	80	71	1.18	N.S.
1980–1981	101	89	2.43	N.S.
1981–1982	127	106	4.75	0.05
1982–1983	71	112	6.71	0.01
1983–1984	84	118	3.62	$0.10>p>0.05$
1984–1985	92	125	3.00	$0.10>p>0.05$
1985–1986	86	179	30.19	0.001

[1]Served by CMHC since 1979

The number of emergencies (new psychiatric episodes) from the catchment area increased from seventy-six in 1978–9 (before the CMHC was established) to 127 cases in the years 1981–2, and then dropped to eighty-six in 1985–6. It should be noted that the initial phase of the CMHC development lasted from October 1979 up to October 1983, when the Centre expanded its services after moving to a new, more spacious building and doubling its personnel. For the same period the number of emergencies from the control area increased constantly from sixty-one cases in 1978–9 up to 179 in 1985–6.

The difference between the numbers of emergencies coming from the two areas under investigation was found to be statistically significant for the period 1981–2, the catchment area producing a higher number of emergencies. A significant proportion of these cases were patients of the CMHC who had been advised to visit the psychiatric emergency unit in the event of a crisis during the night or at the weekend when the centre is closed. The difference was also significant for the last four years, but now in the reverse direction.

When the annual standardized emergency rate per 100,000 population for each area was computed, an increasing trend in emergency rates from the control area was noted, sixty-eight cases per 100,000 being recorded in 1978–9 as against 200 cases per 100,000 in 1985–6 (Table 17.4).

Table 17.4 Annual standardized[1] rates per 100,000 population of psychiatric emergencies from boroughs of Kessariani-Byron (catchment area) and Zografou (control area), 1979–86

Year	Catchment area	Control area
1978–1979	87	68
1979–1980	92	84
1980–1981	116	101
1981–1982	148	127
1982–1983	82	127
1983–1984	97	136
1984–1985	106	141
1985–1986	99	200

[1]Standardized against population of Greater Athens: 3,036,560 (1981)

In the catchment area, in contrast, while a similar trend was noticed during the first years (1978–82), a stable rate of emergencies was observed during the last four years of the study. These years coincide with the development of satellite services, the outreach and community inter-vention programmes. The annual standardized emergency rates per 100,000 population from the two areas are presented in Figure 17.1

A difference was also found with regard to the proportion of acute schizophrenic and other psychotic episodes among the emergencies referred to the psychiatric emergency unit from the two areas. The proportion of acute psychotic episodes from the CMHC catchment area decreased from 31.5 per cent in 1978–9 to 22 per cent in 1985–6, while the proportion from the control area fell only slightly during these years (42.6 per cent–38 per cent).

The first attendances at the CMHC by patients with no previous psychiatric history

A total of 2,580 residents of all ages made first contact with the CMHC ambulatory care facilities between October 1979 and October 1986 and had

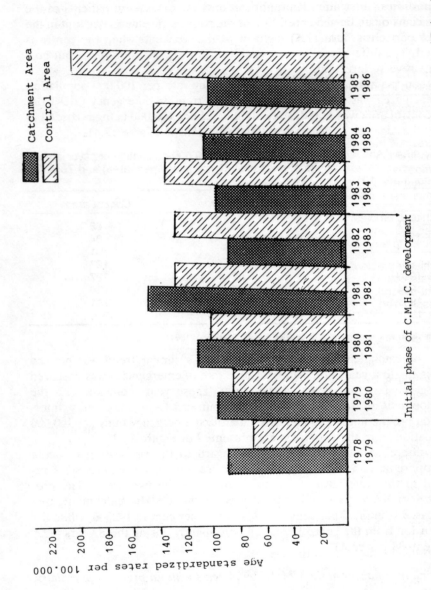

Figure 17.1 Annual age-standardized rates per 100,000 population of psychiatric emergencies from boroughs A and B (catchment area) and C (control area) 1978–86

a total of 21,425 attendances. The proportion of first attendances by adult patients with no previous psychiatric treatment increased from 32.5 per cent in the initial phase 1979–83 to 52 per cent in 1985–6, while the proportion of first attendances by patients previously treated by general physicians or under the care of social workers decreased from 18 per cent to 8.7 per cent (Table 17.5).

Table 17.5 First attendances (%) in the Kessariani-Byron CMHC adult services, according to previous psychiatric history

Psychiatric history	1979–1983	1983–1984	1984–1985	1985–1986
	%	%	%	%
No previous treatment				
Onset within 6 months	11.4	21.4	22.2	25.3
Onset before 6 months or more	21.1	26.8	28.0	26.7
Psychiatric problem treated by a physician or known to a social service	20.9	12.1	9.4	8.7
Psychiatric problem:				
a) treated by a psychiatrist (out-patient)	30.4	29.8	28.6	30.6
b) hospitalized	16.2	9.9	11.8	8.7
Total	100.0	100.0	100.0	100.0
No. of patients	717	320	384	555

Psychiatric disturbances of recent onset constituted 11.4 per cent of the cases with no previous treatment in 1979–83, but increased to 25.3 per cent in 1985–6. It appears that during these years there was a continuous decrease in the average time between the onset of the mental disturbance and the referral of CMHC services. This observation is under further investigation.

Long-term effect of the CMHC on chronic schizophrenic patients

In Table 17.6 the proportion of relapses and readmissions of patients treated by CMHC services and patients treated by non-sectorized services is shown. The decrease in the numbers in both groups during the follow-up period is due to attrition of the samples.

At the time of the second assessment, three years after the initiation of the cohort study, patients treated by the CMHC had suffered fewer relapses and been readmitted much less often than those treated by non-sectorized psychiatric services. Two years later, at the third assessment,

Table 17.6 Relapses and readmissions of chronic schizophrenic patients treated in CMHC and in non-sectorized psychiatric services

	Second assessment (1982)		Third assessment (1984)	
	Patients treated by CMHC	Patients treated by non-sectorized psych. services	Patients treated by CMHC	Patients treated by non-sectorized psych. services
	%	%	%	%
Relapse without admission	12.6	5.2	31.0	31.8
Relapse and readmission	34.3	81.8	6.9	53.6
No relapse	53.1	13.0	62.1	14.6
Total	100.0	100.0	100.0	100.0
No. of patients	32	54	29	44

$\chi^2=19.78$; $df = 2$; $p < 0.001$. $\chi^2=22.0$; $df = 2$; $p < 0.001$

these differences were found to have been maintained. It has to be noted that relapses before the second assessment were not included in the third assessment.

The differences between patients treated by CMHC services and patients treated by non-sectorized services on mean scores for the three basic scales, measuring global functioning, social adjustment, and family atmosphere, were also found to be significant at the time of the third follow-up assessment (Table 17.7)

Table 17.7 Mean scores on three scales of chronic schizophrenic patients treated in CMHC and in other non-sectorized psychiatric services: third assessment (1984)

Scales	Patients treated by CMHC (n=29)	Patients treated by non-sectorized psych. services (n=41)	t-test	Significance level
GAS[1]	48.25 (1.14)[4]	40.94 (1.05)	3.63	0.001
GAS[2]	24.06 (0.97)	31.15 (1.30)	4.40	0.001
FAS[3]	11.10 (0.62)	13.83 (0.85)	2.60	0.05

[1] Global Assessment Scale
[2] Community Adjustment Scale
[3] Family Atmosphere Scale
[4] Numbers in parentheses are standard errors

Table 17.8 Mental health education in experimental and control high schools: episodes of deviant behaviour before and after the completion of the intervention and total number of days out of school for pupils banned from school attendance

| | Experimental high schools | | | | Control high school | | | |
| | A | | B | | A | | B | |
	Episodes	Days out of school	Episodes	Days out of school	Episodes	Days out of school	Episodes	Days out of school
First high school	24(36)[1]	32	7(10)[1]	16	19(53)[1]	139	24(69)	203
Second high school	21(48)[1]	127	5(13)[1]	27				

A Before the initiation of the intervention
B After the completion of the intervention
[1] Numbers in parentheses represent numbers of pupils involved in episodes of deviant behaviour in school.

Mental health education in high schools

The results of a mental health education programme in two local high schools, as measured by the frequencies of deviant behaviour among the pupils, are presented in Table 17.8

A decrease in the numbers of episodes of truancy, 'trouble-making', disrespect shown to teachers and peers, vandalism, or aggression, the number of pupils involved, and the total number of pupil-days lost by banning from school was observed in both 'experimental' high schools during the course of the programme, compared to corresponding data for the three-year period before its initiation. On the other hand, an increase was observed in the numbers of episodes, pupils involved, and days banned from attendance at the control high school during the same period.

Discussion and conclusion

A number of different outcome measures indicate the effectiveness of CMHC services and programmes in preventing or alleviating various mental health problems, including psychiatric emergencies, relapses and readmissions, chronic schizophrenic illness and related disability, and, lastly, deviant behaviour manifestation in schools.

Prevention of psychiatric emergencies

The eight-year study of psychiatric emergencies, new acute episodes, and crises in the catchment area has documented the filter effect of CMHC services on the pathway to the psychiatric emergency unit and to the mental hospital of mentally disturbed individuals in the community, by means of early intervention and by providing treatment and rehabilitation facilities to persons with chronic mental illness.

This might explain the decrease in the proportion of acute schizophrenic episodes from the catchment area during the last year of the study. It was in 1983, when the number of emergencies from the catchment area decreased for the first time, that the CMHC expanded its services, intensifying the efforts to develop outreach programmes and community intervention.

At the same time an upward trend in psychiatric emergencies was observed in the control borough although its residents are economically somewhat better placed than those of the CMHC catchment area.

Several investigators have studied the factors influencing the utilization of community mental health services, but very few were able to demonstrate a preventive effect in terms of selected outcome variables (Tischler *et al.* 1985; Jacobson *et al.* 1978; Häfner and Klug 1980, 1982; Lavik 1983; Hutton 1985; Tansella *et al.* 1986). Others have described the role of crisis intervention centres in the prevention of mental health impairment and disability (De Smit 1972; Decker and Stubblebine 1972). Lechner and Danzinger (1984) compared hospitalization rates in a sector with a community mental health service to that in a control area not serviced by a CMHC, where the number of hospitalized patients increased over a period of three years. According to Cooper (1979), community-based crisis intervention centres in some European countries have produced data that seem likely to prove that they can reduce mental hospital admission rates over a period of time. It seems, therefore, that an increasing number of recent studies on the prevention of crises and hospitalizations by community-based services are showing that greater emphasis should be placed on this type of psychiatric service.

In Greece, the need to develop comprehensive twenty-four-hour psychiatric emergency services in urban areas is one of great importance.

Reaching individuals with a history of prolonged mental illness

Our data also provide some evidence to suggest that the Community Mental Health Centre is serving to reduce the distance of the mentally sick individual and his family from the locus of care. In this effort, community resources have been utilized directly according to their importance for the early recognition of psychopathology and for referral to a treatment agency. Community resources in our case include key persons (pharmacists, practising physicians, priests, and local authorities) as well as community organizations and agencies. The preliminary finding of a reduction in the time between onset of psychiatric manifestations and referral to the CMHC is important because it suggests an increased willingness, on the part of the patient and his family, to overcome the fear of stigma and to seek psychiatric help.

Prevention of chronic mental illness concomitants

The cohort study of chronic schizophrenic community residents over a five-year period has indicated the beneficial effects of CMHC services on a number of outcome variables (numbers of relapses and readmissions; ratings of global functioning, social adjustment, and family atmosphere) for those patients treated by the centre. These findings agree with those reported by some other workers (Grad and Sainsbury 1968; Häfner and Klug 1982). Chronic psychiatric patients receive a wide range of services, including medication, supportive psychotherapy, social case-work, family intervention, and, in some cases of isolated patients, social support reorganization (Stefanis et al. 1986).

Prevention of episodes of deviant behaviour in schools

Adolescents manifesting deviant behaviour, together with the frequent over-reaction of teachers or family members, give rise in many instances to a real crisis in the school environment. Community mental health professionals were called upon several times by school authorities for consultation on these issues. Finally, a structured mental health education programme was set up in two selected high schools to introduce new concepts and healthier patterns of communication among teachers, parents, and students.

The preliminary findings from this primary prevention programme suggested that indirect approaches of this kind may be effective over a period of time in reducing psychosocial crises, might produce observable results, and encourage the development of similar programmes for other target populations.

In conclusion, over the past decade a comprehensive community mental health service has been evaluated in terms of its preventive effectiveness on a number of outcome variables. The Byron-Kessariani Community Mental Health Centre in Greater Athens is an example of a comprehensive community-based service offering a wide range of facilities. The findings reported here illustrate the impact of these activities on the local community, are encouraging for the achievement of a multi-level prevention of mental disorders in the general population and suggest starting points for further investigation.

References

Beigel, A. and Levenson, A. (1972) *The Community Mental Health Center: Strategies and Programmes*, New York: Basic Books.
Bellak, L. (1964) *Handbook of Community Psychiatry and Community Mental Health*, New York: Grune & Stratton.
Berlin, I. (1979a) 'Primary prevention', in I. Berlin and L. Stone (eds) *Basic Handbook of Child Psychiatry, 4: Prevention and Current Issues*, New York: Basic Books, pp. 14–16.
Berlin, I. (1979b) 'Secondary prevention', in I. Berlin and L. Stone (eds) *Basic Handbook of Child Psychiatry, 4: Prevention and Current Issues*, New York: Basic Books, pp. 186–7.
Bolman, W.M. (1968) 'Preventive psychiatry for the family: theory approaches and programmes', *American Journal of Psychiatry* 125: 458–72.
Bolman, W.M. (1969) 'Toward realizing the prevention of mental illness', in L. Bellak and H.H. Barten (eds) *Progress in Community Mental Health 1*, New York: Grune & Stratton, pp. 203–31.
Bolman, W.M. and Westman, J.C. (1967) 'Prevention of mental disorder: an overview of current programmes', *American Journal of Psychiatry* 123: 1058–68.
Bower, E.M. (1961) 'Primary prevention in a school setting', in G. Caplan (ed.) *Prevention of Mental Disorders in Children*, New York: Basic Books, pp. 353–78.
Caplan, G. (1961) *Prevention of Mental Disorders in Children*, New York: Basic Books.

Caplan, G. (1964) *Principles of Preventive Psychiatry*, New York: Basic Books.

Caplan, G. and Bolman, W.M. (1967) 'Perspectives on primary prevention', *Archives of General Psychiatry* 17: 331–46.

Caplan, G. and Grunebaum, H. (1967) 'Perspectives on primary prevention: a review', *Archives of General Psychiatry* 17: 33–41.

Cooper, J. (1979) *Crisis Admission Units and Emergency Psychiatric Services*, Copenhagen: World Health Organization Regional Office for Europe.

Decker, J.B. and Stubblebine, J.M. (1972) 'Crisis intervention and prevention of psychiatric disability: a follow-up study', *American Journal of Psychiatry* 129: 725–9.

De Smit, N.W. (1972) 'Crisis intervention and crisis centers: their possible relevance for community psychiatry and mental health care', *Psychiatria, Neurologia, Neurochirurgia* 75: 299–301.

Dunham, W. (1965) 'Community psychiatry: the newest therapeutic bandwagon', *Archives of General Psychiatry* 12: 303–13.

Endicott, J., Spitzer, R., Fleiss, J., and Cohen, J. (1976) 'The Global Assessment Scale: a procedure for measuring overall severity of psychiatric disturbance', *Archives of General Psychiatry* 33: 766–71.

Freeman, H., Fryers, T., and Henderson, J. (1985) *Mental Health Services in Europe: 10 Years On*, Copenhagen, WHO Regional Office for Europe.

Gittelman, M. (1972) 'Sectorization: the quiet revolution in European mental health care', *American Journal of Orthopsychiatry* 42: 159–65.

Gournas, G., Madianos, M., and Stefanis, C. (1985) 'Prevalence of depression and depressive symptoms among elderly in two Athenian communities', presented at the Symposium on Affective Disorders, WPA, Athens, Greece.

Grad, J.C. and Sainsbury, P. (1968) 'The effects that patients have on their families in a community care service: a two year follow-up', *British Journal of Psychiatry* 114: 265–9.

Häfner, H. and Klug, J. (1980) 'First evaluation of the Mannheim Community mental health service', in E. Strömgren (ed.) 'Epidemiological research as a basis for organization of extramural psychiatry', *Acta Psychiatrica Scandinavica*, supplement 285, 62: 68–78.

Häfner, H. and Klug, J. (1982) 'The impact of an expanding community mental health service on patterns of bed usage: evaluation of a four-year period of implementation', *Psychological Medicine* 12: 177–90.

Hutton, F. (1985) 'Self-referrals to a community mental health center: a three-year study', *British Journal of Psychiatry* 147: 540–4.

Jacobson, A.M., Regier, D.A., and Burns, B.J. (1978) 'Factors relating to the use of mental health services in a neighbourhood health center', *Public Health Reports* 93: 232–9.

Lavik, N.J. (1983) 'Utilization of mental health services over a given period', *Acta Psychiatrica Scandinavica* 67: 404–13.

Lechner, H. and Danzinger, R. (1984) 'Experiences with a community mental health center in the rehabilitation of psychiatric patients in Graz', in V. Hudolin (ed.) *Social Psychiatry*, New York: Plenum, pp. 639–47.

Madianos, M. (1983) 'Mental illness and mental health care in Greece', *Public Health Review* 11: 73–93.

Madianos, M. (1984) 'The prognosis of the course of chronic schizophrenia: a prospective longitudinal study', Associate Professorship Dissertation, University of Athens Medical School.

Madianos, M. and Madianou, D. (1987) 'Athens, Greece', in R. Giel, J.U. Hannibal, J. Henderson, and G.H.M.M. ten Horn (eds) *Mental Health Services* in Pilot Study Areas: Report on a European Study, Copenhagen: WHO Regional Office for Europe, pp. 323–37.

Madianos, M. and Stefanis, C. (1984) 'Developmental issues and intervention strategies in a community mental health center in Greece', in V. Hudolin (ed.) *Social Psychiatry*, New York: Plenum, pp. 283–90.

Madianos, M., Lykouras, E. and Stefanis, C. (1984) 'Evaluation of psychiatric emergencies in Greater Athens', in V. Hudolin (ed.) *Social Psychiatry*, New York: Plenum, pp. 349–60.

Madianos, M., Vlachonikolis, I., Madianou, D., and Stefanis, C. (1985) 'Prevalence of psychological disorders in Athens area: prediction of causal factors', *Acta Psychiatrica Scandinavica* 71: 479–87.

Madianos, M., Madianou, D., Vlachonikolis, I., and Stefanis C. (1987a) 'Attitudes towards mental illness in the Athens area: implications for community mental intervention', *Acta Psychiatrica Scandinavica* 75: 158–65.

Madianos, M., Stefanis, C., and Madianou, D. (1987b) 'Prevalence of mental disorders and utilization of mental health services in two areas of Greater Athens', in B. Cooper (ed.) *Psychiatric Epidemiology: Progress and Prospects*, London: Croom Helm, pp. 372–86.

Madianos, M., Gournas, G., Tomaras, V., Kapsali, A., and Stefanis, C. (1987c) 'Family atmosphere on the course of chronic schizophrenia treated in a Community Mental Health Center: a prospective longitudinal study', in C. Stefanis and A. Rabavilas (eds) *Schizophrenia: Recent Biosocial Developments*, New York: Human Sciences Press, pp. 246–56.

Perris, C. and Kemali, D. (1985) 'Focus on the Italian psychiatric reform', *Acta Psychiatrica Scandinavica* 71, supplement 316.

Rae Grant, Q. and Rae Grant, N. (1970) 'Preventive care', in H. Grunebaum (ed.) *The Practice of Community Mental Health*, Boston, Mass: Little, Brown and Company, pp. 247–76.

Stefanis, C. and Madianos, M. (1983) 'University mental hospital and community mental health center: competing or complementary services', in J.J. Lopez Ibor Jnr, J. Saiz, and J.M. Lopez Ibor (eds) *General Hospital Psychiatry*, Amsterdam: Elsevier, pp. 57–63.

Stefanis, C., Madianos, M., Madianou, D. and Kounalaki, A. (1985) 'The first community mental health center in Greece: three years assessment of an experiment', in P. Pichot, P. Berner, R. Wolf, and K. Thatt (eds) *Psychiatry: The State of the Art, 7: Epidemiology and Community Psychiatry*, New York: Plenum, pp. 313–19.

Stefanis, C., Madianos, M., and Gittelman, M. (1986) 'Recent developments in the care, treatment and rehabilitation of the chronic mentally ill in Greece', *Hospital and Community Psychiatry* 37: 1041–4.

Sussex, J. (1979) 'The role of the community in primary, secondary and tertiary prevention', in I. Berlin and L. Stone (eds) *Basic Handbook of Child Psychiatry 4: Prevention and Current Issues*, New York: Basic Books, pp. 312–26.

Tansella, M., Micciolo, R., Balestrieri, M., and Gavioli, I. (1986) 'High and long-term users of the mental health services: a case-register study in Italy', *Social Psychiatry* 21: 96–103.

Tischler, G.L., Heinisz, J.E., Myers, J.K., and Boswell, P.C. (1975) 'Utilization of mental health services, II: mediators of service allocation', *Archives of General Psychiatry* 32: 416–18.

United States House of Representatives #3688, 88th Congress, First Session, 1963 'A bill to provide for assistance in the construction and initial operation of community mental health centers and for other purposes'.

World Health Organization (1973) *The Development of Comprehensive Mental Health Services in the Community*, Copenhagen: WHO Regional Office for Europe.

World Health Organization (1980) *Changing Patterns in Mental Health Care,* Copenhagen: WHO Regional Office for Europe.

Chapter eighteen

Preventive aspects of mental health policy in the Netherlands

O.H. Brook

Introduction

During the past two decades Dutch mental health care has been under-going an extensive revision involving the entire range of mental health services. This revision is characterized by attempts to increase continuity of care and to decrease admissions to mental hospitals, by a stronger emphasis on the role of primary care, by increasing the provision and diversity of non-residential services, and by reducing the number of beds in mental hospitals.

As in some other western countries, the Dutch government is following a de-institutionalization policy, directed at reducing the capacity and size of mental hospitals and preventing clinical admissions by stimulating out-patient and day-patient care.

In this period the influence of local government in planning and financing mental health care services has been strengthened by new legislation. Decentralized planning with regionalization, echelonization, i.e., grouping mental health services into sectors, and increased consumer participation were the concepts underlying these governmental plans (Ministry of Welfare, Health and Cultural Affairs 1974). The Health Care Tariffs Act and the Health Care Facilities Act of 1982 are the main tools which the government has passed in order to accomplish its goals. Besides prevention of hospital admissions, these goals include a reduction of mental hospital beds from 1.5 to 1.1. per 1,000 of the population, their replacement by places in sheltered homes, reinforcement of out-patient care, a run-down of renovation costs for existing mental hospitals, and, last but not least, cost control (Ministry of Welfare, Health and Cultural Affairs 1984).

However, the Dutch Inspectorate of Mental Health has some doubts about whether all these changes will improve the quality of care, especially that for psychiatric in-patients (Brook 1987a; Inspectorate of Mental Health 1987). Giel has warned of a real risk that in the near future people with chronic mental illness will fall victim to a mental health policy which, he argues, is based on a confused blend of enlightened ideas and misconceptions (Giel 1984). According to Giel, the bureaucratic needs of planners and mental health service administrators are taking precedence over the needs of patients and their relatives, while mental health workers are insufficiently aware of the social impairments and disabilities of their patients because these are not systematically assessed.

This article is designed to analyse the discrepancy between what Kiesler has described as '*de jure*' and '*de facto*' policies (Kiesler 1982). The *de jure* policy is that which the government implements legislatively in the name of mental health. The *de facto* policy is that embodied in the changes which actually occur, regardless of official goals or intention. Special attention will be paid in this context to the issue of prevention in mental health policy.

Prevention in mental health policy

Public health practitioners classify preventive activities as primary, secondary, and tertiary, and these terms have been adopted by proponents of preventive psychiatry, of whom Caplan is one of the best known. According to Caplan, the term 'preventive psychiatry' refers to the body of professional knowledge, both theoretical and practical, which may be utilized to plan and carry out programmes for reducing:

1. the incidence of all types of mental disorders in a community ('primary prevention');
2. the duration of a significant number of those disorders which do occur ('secondary prevention');
3. the long-term impairment which may result from those disorders ('tertiary prevention').

This body of knowledge, according to Caplan, is closely related to the main part of psychiatry, being based on an understanding of the nature and manifestations of mentally disordered behaviour in individuals and on traditional theory and practice in the psychiatric treatment and rehabilitation of patients (Caplan 1964).

At present, the prevalence of mental disorders and the resulting chronic impairments appear to be increasing throughout the world as a result of demographic trends: a development described by Kramer as the rising pandemic of mental disorders and associated chronic diseases and disabilities (Kramer 1980). Kramer emphasizes that two mechanisms are responsible for this situation. One is the large relative increase in the number of persons in age groups with a high risk for developing these conditions, which increases crude prevalence ratios. The other is the increase in average duration of chronic diseases resulting from the successful application of techniques for arresting their fatal complications and prolonging the lives of affected persons.

This raises the age-specific prevalence ratios. In the absence of effective psychiatric techniques or therapies for reducing incidence, the prevalence of such diseases will continue to increase.

In 1984 the Dutch government announced a new policy in mental health, according to which the main focus of attention is to shift gradually from health service structures to the health status and conditions of the population. Until then the emphasis in the Dutch health policy had been on services and on resources. Awareness of the pandemic of mental disorders, the conviction of the government that the expansion of services and efforts towards cost-control had not resulted in improvement in the health of the population, and, finally, the economic recession which forced the need to establish priorities were the main reasons for a new mental health policy, designed to emphasize prevention and alternatives to hospital care. In 1984 this new policy was announced in the *Memorandum on Mental Health* (Ministry of Welfare, Health and Cultural Affairs 1984).

Actually, prevention of mental illness and reduction of the in-patient capacity of mental hospitals in favour of out-patient care and treatment were already the main goals specified in previous governmental reports. Using data from the National Psychiatric Inpatient Case Register (PIGG) these stated aims of government can be compared with the actual developments in the period 1970–84 (Inspectorate of Mental Health 1986). These data, which indicate a notable gap between the *de jure* policy and *de facto* situation, ought to be a warning for the relevant governmental policy and decision-makers: setting goals often turns out to be a matter of wishful thinking (Patton 1977).

In this article the term primary prevention refers to all those activities aimed at the prevention and reduction of the incidence of mental disorders in the population. Secondary prevention refers to the early recognition and treatment of mental disorders and tertiary prevention to activities concerning the reduction or containment of illness-associated chronic disability and handicap of psychiatric in-patients. Reducing disability could lead to shorter hospital stay and reduced readmission rates, which are the main governmental aims.

Tertiary prevention

The Dutch *de jure* policy for preventing chronicity concentrated on prevention of admissions and on shortening the length of treatment and stay in mental hospitals. *De jure* policy in the years 1970–84 can be described as one of de-institutionalization linked with extramuralization (Dekker 1983). Parameters such as size of institutions, numbers of in-patient days, admissions, readmissions, and admitted patients and the

274

Table 18.1 Numbers of admissions (including readmissions), readmissions, patients with only one admission within the same year and 'revolving door' patients in the period 1970–84; in absolute numbers and index figures (in brackets)

Admission year	Total number of admissions, including readmissions		Number of readmissions		Number of patients with one admission		Number of patients with two or more admissions	
1970	12,829	(100)	1,559	(100)	9,894	(100)	1,376	(100)
1971	13,671	(107)	2,089	(134)	9,815	(99)	1,767	(128)
1972	14,882	(116)	2,404	(154)	10,552	(107)	1,926	(140)
1973	16,288	(127)	3,011	(193)	10,951	(111)	2,326	(169)
1974	17,467	(136)	3,500	(225)	11,297	(114)	2,670	(194)
1975	18,534	(144)	3,418	(219)	12,445	(126)	2,671	(194)
1976	19,347	(151)	3,747	(240)	12,667	(128)	2,933	(213)
1977	19,321	(151)	3,740	(240)	12,685	(128)	2,896	(210)
1978	18,672	(146)	2,848	(183)	13,537	(137)	2,247	(163)
1979	19,280	(151)	3,078	(197)	13,813	(140)	2,387	(173)
1980	20,163	(157)	3,306	(212)	14,348	(145)	2,508	(182)
1981	20,663	(161)	3,523	(226)	14,416	(146)	2,624	(195)
1982	22,466	(175)	3,902	(250)	15,588	(158)	2,967	(216)
1983	24,781	(193)	4,564	(293)	16,842	(170)	3,375	(245)
1984	24,723	(193)	4,845	(311)	16,294	(165)	3,584	(260)

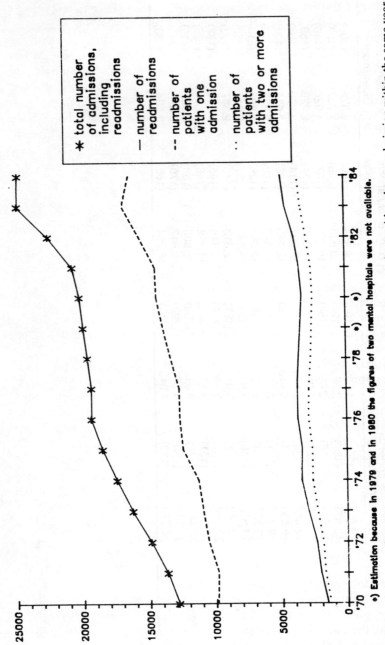

Figure 18.1 Numbers of admissions (including readmissions), readmissions, patients with only one admission within the same year and 'revolving door' patients in the period 1970–84. In absolute numbers

Legend:
* total number of admissions, including readmissions
— number of readmissions
-- number of patients with one admission
... number of patients with two or more admissions

•) Estimation because in 1979 and in 1980 the figures of two mental hospitals were not available.

mean duration of stay specified by age and diagnosis may indicate the effectiveness of this *de jure* policy to a certain extent (Haveman 1986).

There was indeed a slight decrease in the mean number of patients in each mental hospital from 727 in 1975 to 655 in 1983. Yet the size and the overall capacity of the bigger mental hospitals remained the same. Moreover, de-concentration of some of the functions of mental hospitals and transfer of beds and patients to protective living environments, nursing homes, half-way homes, or institutions for the mentally retarded can hardly be regarded as a de-institutionalization policy but rather as one of change from one form of institution to another, i.e., trans-institutionalization.

In-patient days, 'revolving door', and 'new long-stay' patients

As regards the index in-patient days, figures published by PIGG show that for stays of less than one year, the mean duration of stay decreased from 4.1 months in 1970 to 3.4 months in 1984. In addition to this decline there was an increase in the proportion of short-stay patients. In 1970 45 per cent of the patients were discharged within three months and 68 per cent within six months, whereas in 1984 these percentages were 63 per cent and 76 per cent respectively.

Yet shorter in-patient stay was counterbalanced by an increase in the number of patients admitted, including the 'revolving door' patients. This tendency is illustrated in Table 18.1 and in Figures 18.1 and 18.2.

The Dutch case-register studies of Haveman and Brook show that these 'revolving door' patients tend to be in the younger age groups, to be single, and to be significantly more often diagnosed as cases of schizophrenia, personality disorder, or drug dependence (Haveman 1980; Brook 1984).

It appears that the long-stay schizophrenic of the 1950s has become the 'revolving door' patient of the 1980s. This conclusion supposes no dramatic change in types of impairment or in the effectiveness of treatment. If this is true, the governmental *de jure* policy of preventing or postponing admissions to mental hospitals has been counterbalanced by a change in the admission and discharge policy of the mental hospitals. In addition to the phenomenon of the 'revolving door' there has been, since the end of the 1970s, no further decrease in patients with a stay of from one to five years: the 'new long-stay' population. This is shown in figures 18.3 and 18.4 and in Table 18.2.

Although the number of old long-stay patients (stay of five years or more) is constantly slowly decreasing because of death, the size of the total long-stay population remained the same because of the 'new' long-stay patients. At the end of 1984 63 per cent of the in-patients were long-stay patients (Brook 1987a).

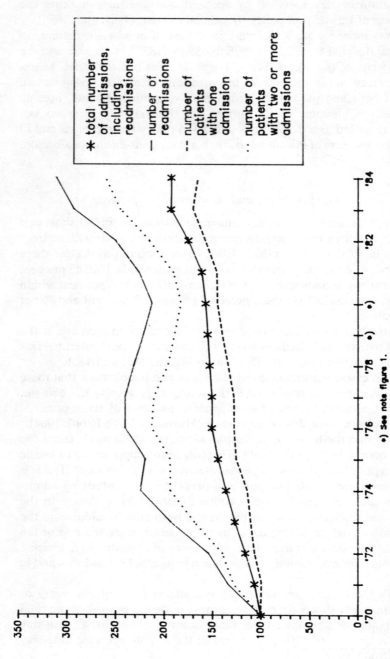

Figure 18.2 Numbers of admissions (including readmissions), readmissions, patients with only one admission and 'revolving door' patients in the period 1970–84. In index figures (1970 = 100)

*) See note figure 1.

* estimation because in 1979 and in 1980 the figures of two mental hospitals were not available.

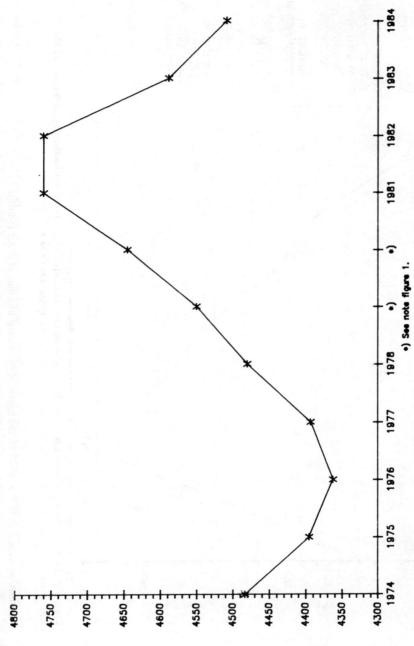

Figure 18.3 'New long-stay' population in Dutch mental hospitals in the period 1971–84. In absolute numbers

•) See note figure 1.

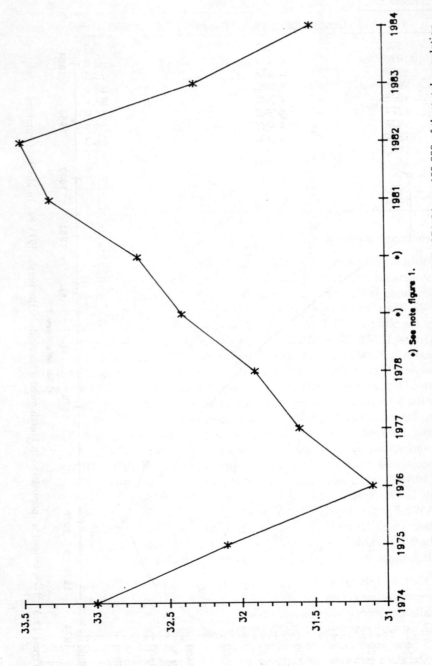

Figure 18.4 'New long-stay' population in Dutch mental hospitals in the period 1974–84 per 100,000 of the total population

Table 18.2 'New' long-stay population in Dutch mental hospitals, in absolute numbers and per 100,000 of the population

Year	Continuous stay of 1–5 years	Per 100,000 of the population
1972	4,860	36.3
1973	4,573	33.9
1974	4,483	33.0
1975	4,395	32.1
1976	4,362	31.1
1977	4,393	31.6
1978	4,483	31.9
1979	4,564	32.3
1980	4,645	32.7
1981	4,760	33.3
1982	4,760	33.5
1983	4,588	32.3
1984	4,508	31.5

Secondary prevention

Political and social pressures in the 1970s resulted in an amalgamation of the several autonomous facilities for ambulatory mental health care into Regional Institutes for Ambulatory Mental Health Care (RIAGG) in 1982. The concept of the RIAGG was already laid down in the *Memorandum on the Structure of Health Care* (Ministry of Welfare, Health and Cultural Affairs 1974). This Memorandum described a geared system of mental health care by means of echelonization and regionalization: admittance to the next higher echelon in a region is made dependent upon referral from a lower and less specialized level of care. Not only was a crucial role assigned to the RIAGGs in this referral system; they were also intended to promote the hoped-for expenditure cuts and shift to extramural care. The underlying idea was that the RIAGG would function on the one hand as a counterpoise to intramural care, and on the other hand as a centre for specialized treatment to which the first echelon could refer their patients.

In 1982 as a result of a ministerial decree to finance the RIAGG out of the funds of the General Insurance for Exceptional Medical Expenses (AWBZ), the services of the RIAGG became available to all Dutch citizens and accessible free of charge after referral by a general practitioner. The Netherlands has been divided into sixty regions of 150,000 to 300,000 inhabitants, in each of which a RIAGG is responsible *de jure* for:

1. short-term psychosocial aid: guidance and advice, crisis intervention, social psychiatry and psychotherapy; in addition, an emergency service is available twenty-four hours a day;
2. consultation, particularly for the agencies of the first echelon;
3. long-term guidance and/or treatment, to prevent premature referrals to the third echelon, and after-care of discharged psychiatric patients;

4. preventive activities, including development of health education and promotion programmes and preventive projects aimed at groups at risk, as well as advising and informing workers of the first echelon.

What are the results of this policy to date? As mentioned before, the concept of echelonization should lead to fewer referrals to the mental hospitals by the first and the second echelon and as a consequence to fewer admissions. We have already shown, however, that the number of admissions increased in the period 1970–84.

As to referrals, the figures published by PIGG show that admissions following referral by a general practitioner increased from 20 per cent in 1974 to 28 per cent in 1978 and then decreased to 20 per cent by 1984, while those by private psychiatrists went down from 10 per cent in 1974 to 3 per cent in 1984. Admissions to mental hospitals following referral by a RIAGG fell from 46 per cent in 1974 to 34 per cent in 1984. Admissions after a referral from out-patient clinics of mental hospitals increased from 8 per cent in 1974 to 14 per cent in 1984. This is shown in Figures 18.5 and 18.6.

Thus, in total the percentage of referrals and admissions of patients to mental hospitals by the first echelon remained unchanged at 30 per cent, while those by the second echelon decreased slightly from 54 per cent to 48 per cent. In addition, there are indications that the RIAGGs are increasingly referring patients with severe psychiatric disorders and aggressive behaviour to the mental hospitals. To some extent this too may have contributed to the growth of the new long-stay population and the 'revolving door' phenomenon.

As to the latter, after-care of discharged psychiatric patients and prevention of readmission is one of the tasks of the RIAGG. In the Netherlands during the past few years the RIAGGs have been allowed to grow each year by 4 per cent because they are supposed to prevent hospital admission and therefore decrease the utilization of psychiatric beds. This policy includes the prevention of readmissions by means of intensive after-care.

Using figures from a Dutch area case-register, Ten Horn showed that of a cohort of 795 discharged psychiatric patients, 47 per cent did not receive any form of after-care (Ten Horn 1982). Of the 53 per cent who were seen by an in-patient or out-patient service, only 26 per cent received after-care from the RIAGG.

In the first twelve weeks following discharge 161 patients were re-admitted and 121 were later readmitted. The rate of readmissions during the first year was 38 per cent. Another important finding was that intensive after-care appeared to delay readmission, especially of those psychotic patients who already had a relatively good prognosis.

Ten Horn concluded that so far none of the out-patient services,

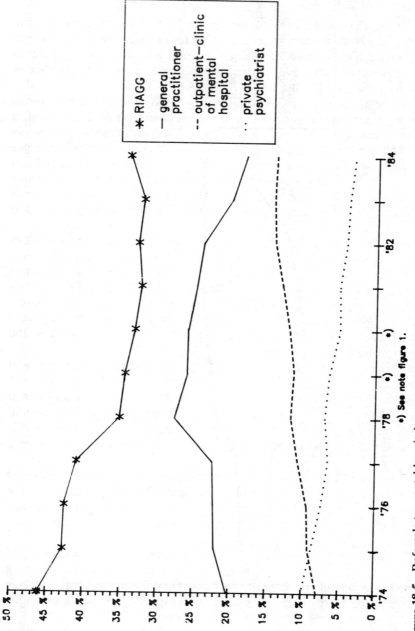

Figure 18.5 Referrals to mental hospitals as a percentage of total number of admissions in the period 1974–84

*) See note figure 1.

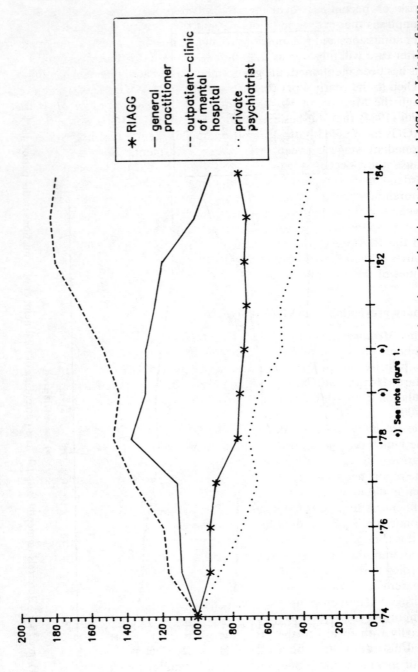

Figure 18.6 Referrals to mental hospitals as a percentage of total number of admissions in the period 1974–84. In index figures (1974 = 100)

including the RIAGG, pay special attention to those patients who are at risk of becoming 'revolving door' cases. She also questioned the assumptions that extension of out-patient services will necessarily lead to fewer admissions and readmissions to mental hospitals and that the quality of after-care will improve as the number of out-patient services grows.

As has been mentioned, the government has created financial conditions attached to the yearly 4 per cent growth of the RIAGGs. This is true even though the Ministry of Health admitted in its *Memorandum of Mental Health* (1984) that the basic assumption of the RIAGG is not valid: the RIAGGs have failed both as an alternative to mental hospitals and as an intermediate stage between primary care and mental hospitals, possibly because they occupy themselves too much with psychosocial ('light') disorders and too little with psychiatric ('heavy') cases. In this memorandum proposals were made for a closer organizational relationship between social psychiatry, out-patient psychiatry, and clinical psychiatry. It was proposed that minor psychiatric disorders should be transferred from the RIAGG to the first echelon of care and the social psychiatric activities of the RIAGG should be linked with out-patient and day-patient facilities of the mental hospitals on behalf of the 'heavy' cases.

Primary prevention in the future and 'facet' policy

In the *Memorandum on Health Care* and more recently in a policy document, the so-called *Health 2000 Report*, the government has given a high priority to primary prevention of mental illness (Ministry of Welfare, Health and Cultural Affairs 1986). This report is a response to stimulation from WHO, as part of their international campaign Health For All 2000.

The *Health 2000 Report* describes the development of the health status of the Dutch population from the mid-1950s and tries by means of health scenarios to foretell the health status by the year 2000.

The report begins with a postulate that, in any given period, the pattern of major diseases, as well as major changes in the pattern of diseases, is influenced to a great extent by demographic developments, socio-economic conditions, and patterns of lifestyle.

In this context, reference is made to social-cultural conditions which will have an important impact on the population's future mental health status. According to this scenario, the increase in divorces, the growing number of one-parent families, long-term unemployment, and the abuse of alcohol and drugs will influence this development unfavourably. This starting point has important consequences for policy making in the area of mental health, especially with regard to the prevention of mental disorders: preventing mental disorder cannot be achieved by policy makers or workers in the field of mental health alone, but requires simultaneous measures in the areas of housing, employment, and social work. Therefore, the *Health 2000 Report* recommends collaboration between several departments in developing mental health prevention programmes. In the Netherlands this is called 'facet' policy. Already in 1964 this idea was introduced by Caplan. He pleaded for a comprehensive approach because he believed that collaboration of psychiatrists with other community workers and a resulting improvement in community programmes in the field of general health care, welfare, education, and urban renewal could not only reduce the vunerability of the population to mental disorder but also improve the care and rehabilitation of those who do become mentally ill (Caplan 1964).

As already stated, the *Health 2000 Report* announces a shift of focus in the Dutch mental health policy from mental health services, care, and resources to health promotion, health conditions, and prevention. Accordingly, a national plan is to be developed whose main objectives will be:

1. stimulation of research (within an international framework);
2. improvement of the diagnostic capability of general practitioners (early detection);
3. improvement of crisis-intervention services and first-admission care in order to prevent chronicity.

As a consequence of this new health policy the focus of research funded by the government will also change from health service structures to disease prevention, health promotion, patterns of lifestyle, and environmental contexts of health. In research policy high priority will be given to psychiatric epidemiology, especially to population-based studies of psychiatric morbidity in the community. These, together with evaluative studies, will be necessary to supply governmental policy makers with the data needed in order to correct faulty developments.

High priority will also be given to psychiatric case registers and in the near future to the development of regional information service systems. In this context it is important to take note of the distinction made in the *Memorandum on Mental Health* between psychiatric illness and psychosocial problems. The latter are to be excluded from psychiatric specialist care and should be treated in the primary health sector. This distinction has led to several discussions about the definitions of mental illness and emotional distress and whether or not such a distinction can be made and maintained in practice. In fact, this debate deals with the problem of the boundaries of mental health and is therefore crucial for the development of primary mental health preventive programmes. If such a distinction really can be upheld, as a consequence this would mean the development of programmes aimed at preventing diagnosable mental illness, and of programmes aimed at prevention of unhappiness or social incompetence. In this case the latter group may well demand attention and support from mental health professionals, but primarily as concerned citizens and not as scientific experts.

According to the government, the distinction between psychiatric disorders and psychosocial problems can and should be made. The starting point of its mental health scenario is that sociocultural factors will have an important impact on the future mental health situation and hence the call for a 'facet' policy. This 'facet' policy stresses the integration of mental health into general education programmes and demands more attention and service capacity of the RIAGG for the prevention of serious psychiatric disorders. The philosophy behind this new policy of mental health prevention is that a holistic approach to health in the primary care sector will be more effective in reducing illness and disability and will therefore reduce the need for specialist professional health care. In addition, the government is attempting to reduce costs in mental health care by promoting so-called 'mantle care', that is, self-help, care by the nearest relatives, and care by voluntary organizations. Furthermore, it has been recommended that fees be charged for care or services that were free of charge before.

Discussion

In sum, cost-containment and rationalization of expenditures, together with structural reform in terms of system cohesion and co-ordination, constitute the incentives underlying the new Dutch mental health policy and the goals set for the year 2000. However, there are several reasons to pose questions about the *de jure* policy, its underlying axioms, and its strategies of implementation.

First of all, the appeal for self-help and 'mantle care' seems hardly realistic at a time of increase in divorces, broken families, one-parent families, and small and unstable social networks. Moreover, health promotion and health education campaigns tend to emphasize health as an important value. These two factors may stimulate the need for and use of professional help in the primary care sector and of specialist mental health care in the second and third echelons. In other words, effective preventive programmes may well increase costs in mental health care.

Second, the long-term policy of the *Health 2000 Report* seems over-ambitious in view of the *de facto* situation. In practice the government follows a short-term policy of budgeting for one to four years ahead, because planning does not depend on a broad vision but rather on the available financial resources, and these are shrinking as a result of economic stagnation and recession. Since the *Health 2000 Report* contains no cost estimates, it is in fact more a discussion paper than a policy memorandum.

Third, the *Health 2000 Report* used three types of information to predict the population's future mental health status: namely, mortality figures, sociodemographic projections, and statistics of mental health care agencies. The reason for this is a pragmatic one: no other figures are available.

Van Lieshout has pointed out that the limitation to these three parameters has led to some very odd statements in the report, for example: 'As to the development in morbidity of serious psychological problems or mental illnesses, no change is to be expected because of insufficient knowledge about the etiology and pathology of serious psychological disorders at this moment'. 'What is unknown, will not change', is one of the odd unspoken assumptions on which the policy of the *Health 2000 Report* is built (Van Lieshout 1987).

Fourth, in pronouncing the 'facet' policy in the area of mental health, the *Health 2000 Report* alters the policy of prevention based on the public health model and presents a prevention model based on the philosophy of equity. 'Facet' policy tries to create optimal conditions in which each citizen will be able to develop his or her personality in harmony and as a result be protected against diseases, psychosocial problems, and disorders. This is a praiseworthy ambition but there are some dangers to take account of. The 'equity' preventive model starts from the assumption that a relationship exists between societal factors and mental illness. However, recent research indicates that major mental illness is probably in large part genetically determined and due to organic factors and therefore probably not preventable and, at most, only modifiable.

Even that it can be modified is questioned and there is little scientific or epidemiological evidence one way or another. If it is granted that there is such a causal relationship, it remains to be demonstrated that the preventive efforts proposed will actually effectively change the occurrence of mental illness. If such activities fall outside the jurisdiction of mental health professionals, then it is appropriate to call on the 'facet' policy.

Another danger is the confusion of moral and scientific issues: what seems morally right, need not be scientifically correct. Quality of life or care refers to a body of values, ideas, and interests that differ in time and from place to place (Brook 1987b). Hence, the public standards used to indicate quality are dynamic and contain an implicit appraisal, whereas scientific standards are objective, universal, changeable in time, and shared by a scientific forum. Much of the discussion and debate over prevention is related to the fact that decisions about preventive programmes are taken by political decision makers whose ideologies influence the programmes, when, in fact, these should be based on the results of basic and applied scientific research.

Finally, there is a danger that overestimation of the benefits of primary preventive activities may have negative consequences for the care of psychiatric in-patients. To date there is no evidence that preventive measures in the primary and secondary echelons of care lead to fewer hospital admissions. Yet there is a governmental policy of strengthening these two echelons by diverting funds from the budgets of the mental hospitals. If this policy continues, the care provided for psychiatric patients will become insufficient in the near future: a good quality of psychiatric care that is *de jure* guaranteed, but financially, *de facto*, cannot be realized.

References

Brook, O.H. (1984) 'Heropnemingen in de Algemene Psychiatrische Ziekenhuizen', *Tijdschrift voor Psychiatrie* 7: 500–25.

Brook, O.H. (1987a) 'New long-stay patients in the Dutch mental hospitals', in B. Cooper (ed.) *Psychiatric Epidemiology: Progress and Prospects*, Baltimore, MD: Johns Hopkins Press, pp. 352–60.

Brook, O.H. (1987b) 'Supervision of mental health care in the Netherlands', *European Archives of Psychiatry and Neurological Science*, 236 (6): 364–8.

Caplan, G. (1964) *Principles of Preventive Psychiatry*, London: Tavistock.

Dekker, E. (1983) 'Het gedwongen samengaan van overheid en geestelijke gezondheidszorg', *Maandblad Geestelijke Volksgezondheid* 4: 372–82.

Giel, R. (1984) 'Onze moeite met moeilijke mensen', *Tijdschrift voor Psychiatrie* 26: 244–61.

Giel, R. (1986) 'Care of chronic mental patients in the Netherlands', *Social Psychiatry* 1: 25–32.

Haveman, M.J. (1980) 'De frequent opgenomen psychiatrische patient', *Tijdschrift voor Psychiatrie* 22: 199–208.

Haveman, M.J. (1986) 'Dehospitalization of psychiatric care in the Netherlands', *Acta Psychiatrica Scandinavica* 73: 456–63.

Inspectorate of Mental Health (1986) *Algemene Psychiatrische Ziekenhuizen, 1984*, The Hague/Rijswijk.

Inspectorate of Mental Health (1987) *Annual Report 1986*, The Hague/Rijswijk.

Kiesler, C.A. (1982) 'Public and professional myths about mental hospitalization', *American Psychologist* 37: 1323–39.

Kramer, M. (1980) 'The rising pandemic of mental disorders and associated chronic diseases and disabilities', in E. Strömgren, A. Dupont, and J.A. Nielsen (eds) (1980) *Epidemiological Research as Basis for the Organization of Extramural Psychiatry*, Copenhagen: Munksgaard.

Ministry of Health, Welfare and Cultural Affairs (1974) *Memorandum on the Structure of Health Care*, The Hague.

Ministry of Health, Welfare and Cultural Affairs (1984) *Memorandum on Mental Health*, The Hague.

Ministry of Health, Welfare and Cultural Affairs (1986) *Health 2000 Report*, The Hague.

Patton, M.G. (1977) *Utilization-Focused Evaluation*, Beverly Hills, Ca: Sage Publications.

Ten Horn, G.H.M.M. (1982) *Nazorg Geeft Kopzorg*, Groningen: University Press.

Van Lieshout, P. (1987) 'Mental health care in the year 2000', in *The Health Report 2000 discussed*, Samsom Stafleu, Alphen a/d Rijn, pp. 135–42.

Chapter nineteen

Completed suicides by patients in medical services

Jan Beskow

Introduction

The numbers of suicides committed by patients on psychiatric wards in Sweden have increased in absolute numbers since the early 1930s (Beskow *et al.* 1983; Perris *et al.* 1980; Socialstyrelsen 1985–7), as they have also done in other western countries (Barner-Rasmussen *et al.* 1986; Ernst 1979; Farberow *et al.* 1971; Hessö 1977; Modestin 1982; Niskanen *et al.* 1974). The psychiatric in-patient unit has in fact the highest concentration of help-seeking persons who will later commit suicide. At the same time, these units also have the largest numbers of personnel who are trained to analyse the problems of such persons and to offer them help. The psychiatric in-patient unit must, therefore, be a focal point for suicide prevention and at the same time a working place for developing concepts and methods in this field. In recent years many authors have reported on the study of these problems and tried to point to possibilities for prevention (Armbruster 1986; Barner-Rasmussen 1986; Crammer 1984; Foerster and Gill 1987; Fujimori and Sakaguchi 1986; Langley and Bayatti 1984; Lönnqvist *et al.* 1974; Modestin 1986, 1987).

In general, there are about ten times as many suicidal attempts as suicides, and about ten times as many persons with serious suicidal ideas as there are suicide attempts in any one year. The epidemiological model of many suicide-prone persons, distributed more or less randomly in the population and reacting with suicidal behaviour to stress situations, may thus have its merits as a complement to the clinical model of an individual suicidal 'process', running from the first serious suicidal idea to the completed act.

The individual approach commonly adopted in research thus needs to be augmented by a field theory approach which places the individual within the context of his social environment. The study of another category of life-endangering events – traffic accidents – did not result in knowledge capable of lowering the mortality rate until the researchers adopted this point of view (Waller 1980). May it perhaps have some merits also for suicidology?

A research project is being undertaken by the author, whose main aims are to describe suicides among patients in medical services in Sweden and to identify suicide-provoking situations and possibilities for prevention.

Methods

Data are collected from three sources:

1. national mortality statistics, 1976–85;
2. linkage of psychiatric care statistics with mortality statistics for the years 1978 and 1983, the only years during the past decade for which the former data are so far available;
3. medical records concerning reported suicides in medical care services, 1983–5.

Since 1983 there has been a *general* obligation to report to the National Board of Health and Welfare all completed suicides which have occurred in or in near relation to medical care: i.e., suicides committed by in-patients and those committed by out-patients in locations designated for health and medical care.

During the years 1983 and 1984 there was also a *limited* obligation to report cases of suicide in all types of medical out-patient care, but only if a relationship between the out-patient care and the act could be suspected. In order to clarify the situation, this requirement has been supplemented since 1 January 1985 by a *general* obligation to report suicides committed by patients discharged on trial from psychiatric in-patient care, as well as those committed by former patients within one month of discharge from an in-patient unit.

Suicides (E 950–959) and 'injuries undetermined whether accidentally or purposely inflicted' (E 980–989) are combined. There are two reasons for this. The relative proportion of the latter group is very high in Sweden: 27 per cent in the decade 1976–85. About 70 per cent of such cases have been estimated to be probably completed suicides (Hörte 1983). The same proportion of each group, about 50 per cent, has received treatment as psychiatric patients. A positive consequence of combining the categories is also that the total number of cases is larger and this makes possible a more detailed breakdown of the data.

For reasons of confidentiality, the psychiatric care statistics in Sweden are based on discharges and not on persons. The number of persons discharged at least once during a year can, however, be calculated in an indirect way. The total number of patients in hospital at the end of the year, together with the number of persons discharged during the year can only be roughly estimated. For 1978 it is estimated at about 100,000 and for 1983 at about 90,000 patients.

Care was taken to ensure complete coverage of the cases of suicide.

Some patients are transferred to an intensive care unit following suicide attempts, and may subsequently die there. Others who commit suicide while on leave from hospital, or after leaving the unit without permission, may be retrospectively discharged a day before the suicide and are thus not officially registered as having committed suicide while in care. For these reasons I have in some calculations included both in-patients and persons who committed suicide within seven days following discharge.

Both quantitative and qualitative analyses have been undertaken. The latter are undertaken by means of a technique of 'psychological autopsy', modified for application to medical records (Beskow 1987). It consists of a systematic review and interpretation of the records, aimed at giving as comprehensive and accurate as possible a picture of the psychiatric disorder and the suicidal process. I have analysed the texts using three different perspectives – those of the suicidologist, the psychiatrist, and the medical administrator – often also complemented by the viewpoints of the ward nursing staff, the family, and the patient himself. Many of the psychiatric records were very informative, while others were of lower quality. In records from non-psychiatric units, data necessary to assess psychiatric symptoms and suicidal behaviour were often scanty, sometimes totally absent indeed. The study findings must be appraised against these limitations.

The aim of the study has been to identify possible preventive measures. A special reference group of highly qualified psychiatric colleagues has scrutinized the analyses and conclusions in detail. The suggestions for possible preventive action obtained by this procedure must be further evaluated before any of them can be introduced into training or clinical practice.

Research findings

National mortality statistics, 1976–85

In Sweden during the years 1976–85, there was an annual mean of 1,587 completed suicides (E950–959) and 582 'undetermined' deaths (E980–989), i.e., 2,169 deaths combined. In the year 1976 there were 2,121 and in the year 1985 there were 2,068. There was thus no over-all tendency for the suicide rate to increase or decrease during this decade.

Psychiatric patients: case-register studies 1978 and 1983

The number of suicides and 'undetermined' deaths by psychiatric in-patients, on the wards or within seven days of discharge, was 155 in the year 1978, i.e., 7 per cent of all suicides in the country in that year. In 1979 the number of cases reached a peak of 218 (9.1 per cent of all suicides), but

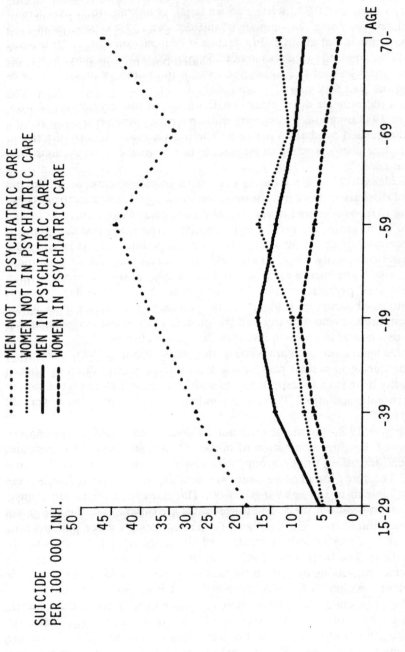

Figure 19.1 Suicide in Sweden per 100,000 inhabitants, 15+ years of age, 1983 (N = 2,083).

by 1983 the number had fallen to 148 (7.1 per cent of all suicides). Unfortunately, we do not know the numbers of suicides for the years between 1978 and 1983, neither do we know exactly the total numbers of psychiatric patients. The number of suicides per 100,000 patients in 1983 can be estimated at about 163: a decline in comparison with 1979, but not with 1978, when the rate was about 155 per 100,000. This may, however, be the first sign that the steady increase in the numbers of such suicides during the past fifty years has been halted.

The total number of psychiatric patients in the country decreased from 1978 to 1983 by about 9 per cent, while over the same period the suicide rate diminished by about 4 per cent. There is thus no evidence of a rise in suicide rate corresponding to a decrease in the numbers in psychiatric in-patient care.

Suicides which occurred during psychiatric in-patient care, or within one year of discharge from care, showed a different age distribution from those among persons who had never received such care (Figure 19.1).

The latter group showed for both sexes the typical age distribution with an increase up to 50–59 years and then a levelling off. However, the decrease commonly found among elderly women was not so prominent here, possibly because a relatively high proportion of suicide-prone women had received psychiatric care. The ratio of psychiatric patients to persons with no psychiatric care is highest in the younger age groups, especially for women, among whom nearly half the persons who committed suicide had been psychiatric in-patients less than one year beforehand.

Males aged over 14 years who, in the years 1978 and 1983, committed suicide during in-patient care or less than one year after discharge had a mortality from suicide respectively 19 and 23 times as high as that of men in the general population. The corresponding multiples for women were 38 and 41.

In Figure 19.2, the suicide rates among discharged psychiatric patients in the year following termination of in-patient care are plotted for men and women, according to age group, with respect to the two years 1978 and 1983. The rates for the two years are similar, each showing a relatively stable plateau in the age range 30–69. The rates for women are slightly lower than those for men. The lowest rates are observed in the age group 70 years and above. The number of suicides among former patients thus appears to be essentially a function of the number of patients who are discharged. The frequency of suicide in the highest age groups is less than expected, suggesting that, from the point of view of suicide prevention, it is the elderly patients who have benefited most from psychiatric care.

When the diagnostic distribution for patients who committed suicide as in-patients in 1983 was compared with that for all psychiatric in-patients, the most striking findings were the low number of alcoholics (11 per cent compared with 30 per cent) and the relatively high numbers with

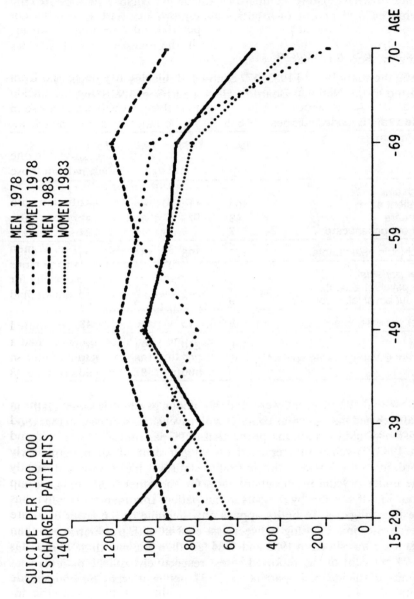

Figure 19.2 Suicide less than one year after discharge related to discharged patients (1978 n = 619, 1983 n = 611)

schizophrenia (12 per cent compared with 9 per cent), affective psychosis (14 per cent compared with 8 per cent) and neurosis (23 per cent compared with 16 per cent). When patients who committed suicide within one year of hospital discharge were compared with all psychiatric in-patients, the differences in diagnostic distribution were much less marked.

Reported cases in psychiatric care

During the years 1983 to 1985, 572 completed suicides in medical care were reported to the National Board of Health and Social Welfare.

Table 19.1 Reported suicides, 1983–5

	1983	1984	1985	Total for 3-year period	%
Psychiatric patients					
In-patient care	100	116	92	308	54
After-care	43	73	81	197	34
Only out-patient care	7	6	11	24	5
Psychiatric patient, total	150	195	184	529	92
Other patients					
With psychiatric contact	9	7	4	20	4
Without psychiatric contact	9	8	6	23	4
Other patients, total	18	15	10	43	8
Total	168	210	194	572	100
Thereof with psychiatric contact	159	202	188	549	
%	95	96	97	96	

Of this total, 92 per cent were patients under psychiatric care. Half the remainder had had previous contacts with psychiatric services, so that their inclusion would increase the proportion to 96 per cent.

In 1983, psychiatrists reported on 93 per cent of all patients who, according to the linkage with mortality statistics, had committed suicide while under psychiatric in-patient care. On the other hand, only a small proportion of suicides by patients in out-patient treatment were reported, since the obligation to notify applies only in some of the latter cases. In general, the time elapsing between last contact with psychiatric care and the suicide was short: in 1983 and 1984 less than one month in 93 per cent and 94 per cent of the reported cases, respectively. Of the patients who committed suicide in in-patient care, 37 per cent were on compulsory orders.

Most of the 308 patients recorded as psychiatric in-patients had actually left the wards before committing suicide. Of these patients 147 (48 per cent) committed suicide while on leave or during a stay outside the ward on their own responsibility. Seventy-nine patients (26 per cent) had left the ward without permission, while a further thirteen (4 per cent) killed themselves off the ward but in the hospital or hospital grounds. Only the remaining sixty-nine patients (22 per cent) committed suicide on the ward: twenty-nine in 1983, twenty-five in 1984 and fifteen in 1985. This declining tendency may have been an effect of the increased discussion and awareness of suicide prevention in psychiatry during recent years. Over the same period, however, the number of suicides within one week of hospital discharge increased.

Age   The age distribution for patients who committed suicide while in out-patient care (Figure 19.3A) shows a displacement towards the younger age groups when compared with all patients in in-patient care (Figure 19.3D). This shift was more pronounced for patients who had left the wards before committing suicide (Figure 19.3B). Patients who killed themselves on the wards had a different age distribution (Figure 19.3C), with peaks in the age groups 20–29 and 60–69 years. This observation, if confirmed in other investigations, underlines the importance of designing suicide preventive measures differently for different age groups.

Suicide methods   The distribution of the different suicide methods was about the same for psychiatric out-patients as for suicide in the general population (Table 19.2), apart from a small relative excess of deaths by hanging.

The psychiatric patients did not tend to use drugs more than other persons who committed suicide. Patients who had left hospital shortly before their suicide used drugs less often and 'other methods' more often than other persons who committed suicide. The high figure of 51 per cent for 'other methods' is due to the large number of suicides through jumping in front of trains or cars (22 per cent), which contrasts with only 5 per cent among persons in in-patient care. Train and car deaths are rapid methods used in impulsive suicide, or when the individual acts quickly for some other reason.

Sub-groups   The qualitative study was restricted to a detailed analysis of six suicidal processes, to be reported separately (Beskow 1987), and shorter analyses of twenty-three of the twenty-five suicides in in-patient psychiatric care in the year 1984. The remaining two patients in this group had been living in nursing homes and little information was available about them. The research aim was to find combinations of individual psychiatric and other risk factors for suicide. The following tentative sub-groups are the result of this attempt:

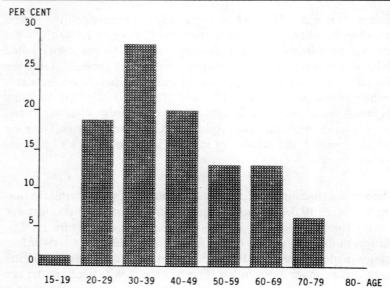

Figure 19.3A

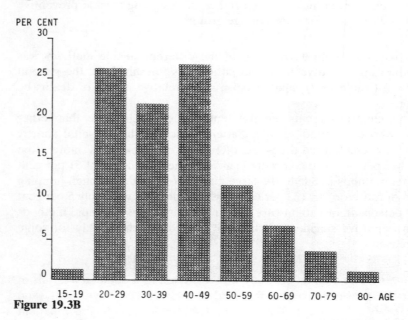

Figure 19.3B

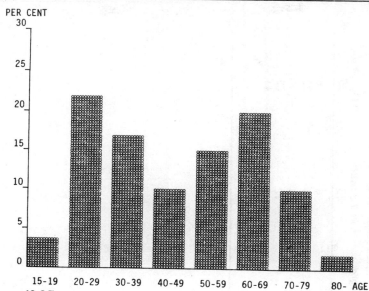

Figure 19.3C

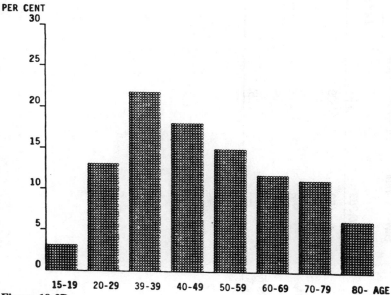

Figure 19.3D

Figure 19.3 Reported suicide in psychiatric care 1983–5 (N = 529) compared with discharged patients 1983, 15+ years of age (N = 64,343)
A Out-patient care (n = 221)
B In-patient care, left the ward (n = 239)
C In-patient care, on the ward (n = 69)
D Discharged psychiatric patients 1983 (N = 64,343)

299

Table 19.2 Suicide methods, 1983–5 (percentages)

Suicide methods	Sweden total	Out-patient care	Psychiatric clinics In-patient care		Somatic clinics
			Left the ward	In the ward	In the ward
N/n	6,363	221	243	65	35
Poisoning	32	29	14	6	6
Hanging	24	30	25	74	20
Jumping from high places	5	5	9	12	63
Other methods	40	35	51	8	11
Thereof: jumping in front of train or car	–	(5)	(22)		

1. young women with severe personality disorder and a history of previous suicidal attempts, who had been in in-patient psychiatric care – one repeatedly and one continuously for many years – and who committed suicide in one of many critical episodes in their relationship with the psychiatric services (n = 2);

2. young men and women with chronic or relapsing psychoses, who killed themselves after being readmitted to psychiatric care (n = 3);

3. young chronic schizophrenic patients who committed suicide during a critical phase in the rehabilitation process (n = 4);

4. middle-aged women with a differential diagnosis lying between melancholia and neurotic disorder, and with problems in their primary group, which made them feel that the way out of hospital was closed to them (n = 3);

5. middle-aged men with depression and psychosocial problems (n = 3);

6. elderly men with melancholia (n = 3);

7. elderly alcoholic men with organic mental impairments and difficulties in the primary group, who also felt that the way out of hospital was closed (n = 3);

8. an elderly man with a hypochondriacal neurosis (or possibly agitated depression) and a young man with an unspecified depressive illness, neither of whom could be grouped elsewhere (n = 2).

It may be noted that only one patient corresponded to the commonest stereotype of the suicidal patient: the person with melancholia who relapses and becomes intractably depressed leading to chronic deterioration.

Reported cases in hospital medical or surgical units

Only forty-three cases of suicide while under general hospital care were reported. Of these, four were in out-patient care at the time, four had been discharged from hospital shortly beforehand, and thirty-five had committed suicide on the hospital wards. The first two groups are probably greatly under-represented, and indeed the number of suicides on general hospital wards may also be much under-reported. A drop-out analysis, however, has not been possible for practical reasons, the reported cases being drawn from the whole of Sweden. The analysis of these data is therefore very tentative, and only a few basic findings are presented here.

Patients who committed suicide on the wards tended to have a two-peak age distribution, like the corresponding group of psychiatric patients. The main peak was in the age group 60 years and above; the lesser one in the group below 30 years of age.

As can be seen from Table 19.2, the distribution according to suicide method differs from that manifested by patients who killed themselves on the psychiatric wards, and shows a large relative excess of cases of jumping from high buildings. This is partly explained by the fact that the medical and surgical wards are often situated in high buildings with windows which can be opened and have no security glass. Perhaps more remarkable is the low number of hangings, although this is a method relatively easy to undertake in the general hospital setting.

Sub-groups The qualitative analysis indicated that those patients who committed suicide on general hospital wards could be divided provisionally into three sub-groups:

1. elderly patients with physical diseases who were near to death; they had incurable diseases with restricted possibilities for symptomatic relief (n = 9);
2. elderly persons with psychiatric disorders, mostly depression (n = 10);
3. young persons, predominantly with psychiatric disorders (n = 8): four of these had been admitted following a suicidal attempt or an accident; one had been admitted to a physical rehabilitation department because of chronic psychiatric disability; one patient with an anxiety neurosis, who was pregnant, was admitted to an obstetric unit; only two of these eight patients had physical diseases, in each case combined with a psychiatric disorder.

For the remaining eight patients, the available information was too scanty to permit any attempt at classification.

Discussion

The aim of this study was to obtain a general description of suicides committed in near relation to medical services, and to try to identify possible approaches to prevention. The study was based on annual mortality statistics for Sweden 1976–85, linkage with psychiatric care statistics for the years 1978 and 1983, and medical records on reported suicides in hospital care. Interpretation of the findings is limited by the variable quality of the data base. The project is reported more fully elsewhere in Swedish (Beskow 1987).

The data indicate that suicides among psychiatric in-patients increased gradually to a peak of 218 cases in the year 1979. The only more recent figure which is available from the mortality statistics, that for 1983, suggests a drop to 148 cases. The numbers of cases reported to the National Board of Health and Welfare for the years 1983–5 also fail to show any recent increase. The trend towards increasing rates seems, therefore, to have been halted.

Numbers of suicides on psychiatric wards are relatively small: on average twenty-three annually in the period 1983–5, or about 1 per cent of all suicides in the country. Moreover, during these three years there was an apparent decrease in the numbers, from twenty-nine to twenty-five to fifteen. This may have been a consequence of the circulation by the National Board of Health and Welfare of information on suicide prevention in psychiatric units. Probably, however, some patients killed themselves immediately after discharge from hospital.

Some findings concerning the distribution of cases are of interest for further research. The age distribution for patients who killed themselves on psychiatric wards, and also for suicides committed on other types of hospital ward, shows two peaks. In the age range 30–69 years, the number of suicides within one year of discharge is related to the number of discharges. This, however, is not true for elderly patients, for whom psychiatric care seems more effective as a protection against suicide than it is for those under 70 years.

The excess mortality among psychiatric patients was much more pronounced for women than for men. One reason may be the much higher suicide rate for men in the general population, and another the higher proportion of potentially suicidal women who seek psychiatric help for their problems (cf. Figure 19.1).

It is possible here to give only a few tentative suggestions for suicide prevention measures, based on the qualitative part of the study. The evidence of the records suggests that failures and shortcomings of psychiatric care often arise less from lack of knowledge than from difficulties in applying well-known principles of care, for example, in the assessment and management of depressive states. Often it seems to be not so much his illness that is intolerable for the patient as certain resulting situations which are perceived as crise. Informing a depressed patient that he is to be transferred next day to a psychiatric ward; taking back into hospital care a schizophrenic patient after a long period in the community; planned discharge from hospital when the prospects for successful rehabilitation and achievement of a normal lifestyle in the community appear doubtful: these are all types of situation that require special attention and alertness from the point of view of suicide prevention.

In the hospital records there was in general a lack of analysis of the suicidal behaviour and predicaments of individual patients. The proper time for such an analysis is when a patient is admitted for a psychiatric disorder complicated by suicidal ideas or following a suicidal attempt. One goal of such an analysis is to identify the patient's motives and any possible suicide-provoking – but also suicide-preventive – factors in his or her surroundings. Such an analysis provides the basis for an individually tailored suicide prevention strategy. As a rule, the psychosocial problems which underlie the patient's suicidal behaviour or tendencies, and his or her capacity for solving them, with or without support, must be kept at the focus of attention. Suicidal behaviour should be the focus of interest only as much as is necessary for the prevention of further suicidal acts. An additional way of augmenting our knowledge of suicide in the medical setting is by undertaking 'psychological autopsies' following completed suicides which have occurred while under hospital treatment.

Suicidal behaviour is a complex phenomenon, and its scientific study has as yet only a short history. There are grounds for hoping that the advance of knowledge will present new possibilities for reduction of the rates of suicidal acts both in the general population and among psychiatric patients.

References

Armbruster, B. (1986) 'Suizide während der stationären psychiatrischen Behandlung', *Nervenarzt* 57: 511–16.

Barner-Rasmussen, P. (1986) 'Suicide in psychiatric patients in Denmark, 1971–1981, II: hospital utilization and risk groups', *Acta Psychiatrica Scandinavica* 73: 449–55.

Barner-Rasmussen, P., Dupont, A., and Bille, H. (1986) 'Suicide in psychiatric patients in Denmark, 1971–81, I: demographic and diagnostic description', *Acta Psychiatrica Scandinavica* 73: 441–8.

Beskow, J. (1987) *Självmord i sjukvärden. Del I: Sex individuella suicidala analyser. Del II: Anmälningar 1983–1985*, Stockholm: Socialstyrelsen, manuscript.

Beskow, J., Runeson, B., and Andrén, A. (1983) 'Självmord bland patienter i sluten psykiatrisk värd', *Socialmedicinsk Tidskrift* 60: 156–66.

Crammer, J.L. (1984) 'The special characteristics of suicide in hospital in-patients', *British Journal of Psychiatry* 145: 460–76.

Ernst, K. (1979) 'Die Zunahme der Suizide in den Psychiatrischen Kliniken. Tatsachen, Ursachen, Prävention', *Sozial- und Präventivmedizin* 24: 34–7.

Farberow, N.L., Ganzler, S., Cutter, F., and Reynolds, D. (1971) 'An eight-year survey of hospital suicides', *Life-threatening Behaviour* 1(3): 184–202.

Foerster, K. and Gill, A. (1987) 'Suizid während stationärer psychiatrischer Behandlung – zur Frage der Häufigkeit und der Vorhersehbarkeit', *Nervenarzt* 58: 505–8.

Fujimori, H. and Sakaguchi, M. (1986) 'Der Suizid schizophrener Patienten in psychiatrischen Krankenhäusern', *Fortschritt in Neurologie und Psychiatrie* 54: 1–14.

Hessö, R. (1977) 'Suicide in Norwegian, Finnish and Swedish psychiatric hospitals', *Archiv für Psychiatrie und Nervenkrankheiten* 224: 119–27.

Hörte, L-G. (1983) 'Ovisshet – ett problem i suicidstatistiken', *Hygiea* 92: 251.

Langley, G.E. and Bayatti, N.N. (1984) 'Suicides in Exe Vale hospital, 1972–1981', *British Journal of Psychiatry* 145: 463–7.

Lönnqvist, J., Niskanen, P., Rinta-Mänty, R. *et al.* (1974) 'Suicides in psychiatric hospitals in different therapeutic eras: a review of literature and own study', *Psychiatria Fennica* 1974: 265–73.

Modestin, J. (1982) 'Suizid in der psychiatrischen Institution', *Nervenarzt* 53: 254–61.

Modestin, J. (1986) 'Three different types of clinical suicide', *European Archives of Psychiatry and Neurological Science* 236: 148–53.

Modestin, J. (1987) 'Suizid in der psychiatrischen Klinik', *Forum der Psychiatrie. Neue Folge 29*, Stuttgart: Enke.

Niskanen, P., Lönnqvist, J., Achté, K., and Rinta-Mänty, R. (1974) 'Suicides in Helsinki psychiatric hospitals in 1964–1972', *Psychiatria Fennica* 1974: 275–80.
Perris, C., Beskow, J., and Jacobsson, L. (1980) 'Some remarks on the incidence of successful suicide in psychiatric care', *Social Psychiatry* 15: 161–6.
Socialstyrelsen (1985–7) *Självmord inom den psykiatriska vården* (National Board of Health and Welfare: *Suicide in Psychiatric Care*, with a summary in English), Stockholm: Socialstyrelsen redovisar.
Waller, J.A. (1980) 'Injury as a public health problem', in J.M. Last (ed.) Maxcy-Rosenau. *Public Health and Preventive Medicine*, eleventh edition. New York: Appleton-Century-Crofts.

Chapter twenty

Prevention of long-term tranquillizer use

Paul Williams, Michael B. King,
and Edirimuni K. Rodrigo

Introduction

The prescription and consumption of benzodiazepines and other minor tranquillizers is a feature of the current health care scene which has engendered a great deal of public and professional debate (Gabe and Williams 1986a; Gabe and Bury 1987). The most important stimulus for this debate was the regular annual increase in the number of prescriptions for these drugs that occurred in many countries during the late 1960s and the early 1970s (e.g., Parish 1971; Trethowan 1975; Williams 1980; Marks 1983). The evidence clearly indicates that these increases in prescribing were largely due to an escalation in the extent of long-term benzodiazepine use (Williams 1983a); thus, it is not surprising that the extent of, and the alleged problems associated with, long-term use have been the major focus for critical comment, from both within and without the medical profession.

Most studies show that the prevalence of long-term (one year or more) tranquillizer use is between 1.5 per cent and 3 per cent of the population. Grossed up to the UK population, these estimates suggest that between 825,000 and 1,650,000 persons in the UK are long-term users of benzodiazepines and other minor tranquillizers.

Thus, it is undoubtedly a common problem; is it an important one? Tyrer (1984) observed that 'we should not assume that the long-term prescription of benzodiazepines and the consequent high risks of dependence are evils to be avoided at all costs'. He noted further that in spite of preliminary reports of possible neuroradiological changes after prolonged treatment (Lader et al. 1984) – not subsequently confirmed by other studies (Perera et al. 1987) – no permanent adverse consequences of long-term benzodiazepine use have as yet been described. However, since then, evidence has emerged of persisting cognitive deficit in long-term consumers of benzodiazepines (Lader 1987). Thus, as Tyrer pointed out in a later paper,

> when the benefits and risks of long-term treatment are compared, the
> balance tilts against benefit. The lessened efficacy of long-term dosage,

the increased risk of dependence, and the insidious cognitive effects can only be balanced against the relative safety of benzodiazepines compared with other (long-term) anti-anxiety drug treatments. (Tyrer 1987)

Indeed, current medical opinion is unequivocal: treatment with benzodiazepines should, wherever possible, be restricted to the short term (Tyrer and Murphy 1987). This, and the fact that the distribution of benzodiazepines is in many countries under the direct control of the medical profession, suggests that the prevention of long-term benzodiazepine use is an issue worthy of serious consideration.

Primary prevention

Clearly, there are two possible sites of preventive intervention in the chain { no benzodiazepine use → short-term use → long-term use }. Catalan and his colleagues (1984a, 1984b) conducted a controlled clinical trial in a group of British general practices. Patients entered into the trial were those who were judged by their general practitioners to require treatment with benzodiazepines, and they were randomly allocated to receive this treatment or not. Those not receiving benzodiazepines were to be 'counselled' by the general practitioners (although, in the event, the average duration of consultation was the same in both treatment groups, so that it is difficult to be sure what 'counselling' took place). The trial continued for six months, at the end of which there were no differences in clinical, social, or service use outcomes between the two groups.

While this study awaits replication, it certainly indicates the feasibility of primary prevention of long-term benzodiazepine use by means of decreasing initiation of benzodiazepine treatment. Indeed, there has in recent years been a levelling off and a subsequent decline in the prescribing of benzodiazepines in many countries (Marks 1983), and it has been suggested (Williams 1987) that this is the result of a decrease in incident prescribing, partly as a result of changes in the climate of medical and lay opinion about tranquillizer use.

The alternative approach to primary prevention of long-term use – that is, intervening to prevent short-term use becoming long term – also requires consideration. Since only a minority of benzodiazepine users become long-term users (Williams 1983b), the feasibility of this preventive strategy would be greatly increased by information about risk factors – that is, factors which can be identified at the beginning of benzodiazepine treatment, and which indicate an increased risk of chronicity.

To investigate such risk factors, we conducted a longitudinal prospective study of psychotropic drug use in a general practice setting (Williams et al. 1982; Murray et al. 1982; Williams 1983b). Six general practitioners in five south London practices were asked to identify and provide information about those patients to whom they supplied a new prescription for a psychotropic drug. 'New' was defined so as to include first-ever prescriptions as well as those written for the treatment of a new episode of illness. Subsequent prescribing was monitored for six months.

One hundred and fifty four patients were entered into the study, and follow-up prescribing information was available for 124 (81 per cent) of these. For each patient, the duration of continuous treatment was calculated, defined according to the method of Parish (1971) as the length of time elapsing between the initiation of treatment and the day on which medication would have been used up if it had been taken according to prescription (this is of course not necessarily the same as duration of consumption). Survival curves were then plotted using these data on duration of treatment.

Figure 20.1 shows the survival distributions according to the type of psychotropic drug prescribed at inception into the study. It can be seen that after six weeks, about one-third of the patients on tranquillizers (virtually all of which were benzodiazepines) were still receiving treatment. The

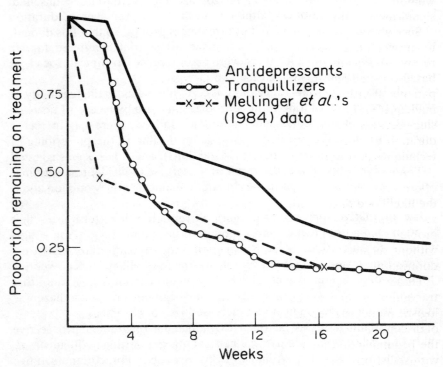

Figure 20.1 Survival distributions of duration of psychotropic drug use

figure also shows that just under 20 per cent of the tranquillizer recipients were prescribed drugs for the entire six-month period.

We then used survival analysis techniques to investigate factors which predicted the duration of treatment with psychotropic drugs (Williams 1983b). We studied the effects of two characteristics of the *patients* (sex; age), two aspects of their *health status* (GPs' assessment of severity of symptoms at inception of treatment; presence or absence of physical illness), a measure of *social functioning* (GPs' assessment of social problems), three aspects of the *treatment* (type of psychotropic drug prescribed; past psychotropic drug use; whether or not drugs were requested by the patient), and the *passage of time*.

The effects of these factors on the survival distribution of drug use were first examined one at a time. At this level of analysis, we found that symptom severity, type of psychotropic drug, and previous psychotropic drug use were each related to duration of treatment (severe symptoms, prescribing of antidepressants, and a previous history of psychotropic drug use each being associated with a more prolonged duration of treatment). We also found an association between increasing age and duration of tranquillizer, but not antidepressant, use and a longer duration of treatment in women than men, but only in those patients assessed by the GP as having significant social problems.

Such an analysis is sufficient for descriptive purposes; that is, it allows us to answer questions such as 'do patients with characteristic X tend to receive treatment for longer than those without it?' Indeed, a checklist based on such features might usefully be developed to help GPs identify patients at risk of becoming long-term users. However, this analysis is inadequate for explanatory purposes, since no account is taken of relationships between the predictor variables and possible interactive effects on the duration of drug use. We therefore applied multiple logistic regression techniques appropriate to the analysis of survival data.

Three significant prognostic factors were identified. These were a history of *previous psychotropic drug use* (the presence of such a history decreased the likelihood of discontinuing treatment), an interactive effect of *sex and social problems* (such that women in whom the GP identified social problems were less likely to discontinue treatment than were either women without such problems or men) and the *passage of time* – the longer the duration of treatment, the less the chance of stopping.

These findings applied equally to patients on antidepressants and tranquillizers, and an example of the state of affairs predicted by the logistic model is given in Table 20.1. This shows the estimated probability of discontinuing psychotropic drug treatment within the next two weeks, at the beginning and after four months of continuous treatment. A woman with social problems who has previously been treated with psychotropics has, compared with other women, little chance of early discontinuation of

Table 20.1 Probability of discontinuing psychotropic drug treatment within the next two weeks (women only: estimated from the logistic model in Williams (1983b))

	Social problems identified by GP	Previous psychotropic use	
		no	yes
At the beginning	none or one	0.34	0.21
of treatment	two or more	0.45	0.11
After 4 months	none or one	0.12	0.05
treatment	two or more	0.21	0.02

treatment at the start, and a negligible change after four months of drug treatment.

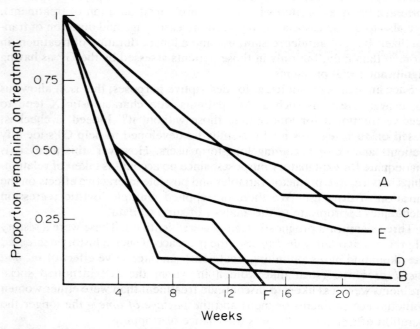

Figure 20.2 Survival distributions of duration of psychotropic drug use in patients of six general practitioners: between-doctor differences

A further analysis was conducted to explore the differences between the doctors with regard to their patients' use of psychotropics. Figure 20.2 demonstrates these differences very clearly: while all Dr F's patients had stopped treatment within four months, about one-third of Dr A's patients were still receiving prescriptions after six months. Survival analysis indicated that these disparities were due to differences neither between the practices with regard to the characteristics of their patients, nor between the patients' clinical status, nor between specific aspects of the treatment. However, the effect of the passage of time on the probability of discontinuing treatment did vary between doctors, suggesting that some doctors interact with their patients in such a way as to encourage, albeit not consciously, long-term use of benzodiazepines and other psychotropic drugs (for further details, see Williams (1983b)). These findings also suggest possibilities for interventions aimed at primary prevention of long-term tranquillizer use.

Recently, Mant *et al.* (1988) have reported a similar study conducted in Australia. They carried out a six-month prospective study of 104 general practice patients who started treatment with a benzodiazepine or an antidepressant drug. Again, survival analysis techniques were used, and the results were broadly similar to those reported above, except that no sex difference in duration of use was found.

Secondary and tertiary prevention

An important aspect of the knowledge base for secondary and tertiary prevention of long-term benzodiazepine use consists in information about the characteristics of long-term users. Who are they? In what way, if any, are they ill? What do they think about their drug treatment?

There is general agreement from cross-sectional studies that long-term tranquillizer users are predominantly middle-aged and elderly women (Woodcock 1970; Parish 1971; Cooperstock 1976, 1978; Mellinger *et al.* 1984; Rodrigo *et al.* 1988). Furthermore, long-term users of benzodiazepines and other tranquillizers report high levels of emotional distress. Mellinger *et al.* (1984) reported on sixty-eight respondents in a community survey who reported regular (daily for one year or more) use of anxiolytics. They found that half of these long-term users had high scores on their questionnaire measure of emotional distress, the Typology of Psychic Distress (PSYDIS – Mellinger *et al.* 1983), as compared with 20 per cent of the non-users. They noted, however, that in this respect 'the long-term users did not differ much from the other users', 45 per cent of whom were also high scorers.

In our study of long-term benzodiazepine users in a south London general practice (Rodrigo *et al.* 1988), we found that twenty-four (38 per cent) of an interview sample of sixty-four patients were rated by psychiatrists as cases on the Standardized Psychiatric Interview (Goldberg *et al.* 1970), a semi-structured interview designed to quantify psychiatric disorder in non-psychiatric settings. While in absolute terms this is a substantial level of psychiatric morbidity, it is not very different from that which would be found in an unselected series of general practice attenders. For example, Marks *et al.* (1979) obtained a psychiatric case rate of 39 per cent in their study of patients attending ninety-one general practitioners in Manchester, and Boardman (1987) recorded a level of 43 per cent in eighteen south London general practices, in both cases using the Standardized Psychiatric Interview as the case criterion.

In Rodrigo *et al.*'s (1988) study, the interviewing psychiatrists also assigned an ICD diagnosis to the twenty-four patients classified as cases. Table 20.2 shows that eighteen patients (75 per cent of the cases, or 28 per cent of the whole sample) were classified under the rubric neurotic depression (ICD 300.4),and that none were assigned a diagnosis related to anxiety. If this finding is replicated, it suggests that long-term benzodiazepine use might be used as a marker of hidden depression in general practice.

Table 20.2 Psychiatric morbidity in long-term benzodiazepine users in one general practice (Rodrigo *et al.* 1988)

Psychiatric cases, according to Standardized Psychiatric Interview	24
ICD diagnosis:	
300.4 neurotic depression	18
301.5 hysterical personality disorder	1
309.0 brief depressive reaction	1
309.1 prolonged depressive reaction	1
310.2 post-concussional syndrome	1
no ICD diagnosis	2
Not psychiatric cases, according to Standardized Psychiatric Interview	40
Not interviewed	18
Total long-term benzodiazepine recipients	82

There is evidence that *de novo* prescription of benzodiazepines and other psychotropic drugs frequently occurs in response to physical rather than psychological disorder (Solow 1975; Williams 1978). It is not surprising, therefore, that this has been investigated in the context of long-term drug use. Murray and her colleagues (1982) interviewed twenty-two patients who had been prescribed psychotropic drugs continuously for six months or more. She found that 'chronic physical complaints were common in the sample (diverticulitis, arthritis, hypertension, migraine) and 13 people were long-term users of non-psychotropic prescribed drugs'. Furthermore, in a questionnaire study of present and past long-term tranquillizer users (Murray 1981), only six out of 261 respondents were found to have no disability or physical symptoms as scored on the Belloc scale (Belloc *et al.* 1971). Mellinger *et al.* (1984), in the study of sixty-eight long-term consumers of anxiolytics referred to above, found that physical health distinguished between long-term users and other users more sharply than did any other factor they studied (including emotional distress). They noted that 'at least one-third of the long-term users reported four or more health problems – a rate twice that found among the other anxiolytic users and seven times that of the non-users'. These differences persisted when age was controlled for, and they observed further that much of the difference between the long-term users and the others could be accounted for by cardiovascular disorders and arthritis.

Rodrigo et al.'s (1987) study in south London confirmed Mellinger et al.'s findings, in that the patients showed evidence of substantial physical morbidity. For example, twenty-seven (42 per cent) had consulted their GP during the previous month for a physical illness (other than coughs, colds, and influenza), and twenty-two (34 per cent) had attended medical or surgical out-patient clinics in the previous year.

What do long-term users of benzodiazepines think about their drugs? Surprisingly, it is only recently that researchers have begun to concern themselves with this issue, and the impetus for such research has come primarily from social scientists rather than doctors. The methods used include postal survey (Murray 1981), structured interviews and question-naires (Rodrigo et al. 1987), in-depth semi-structured interviews (Helman 1981; Gabe and Lipshitz-Phillips 1982, 1984; Gabe and Thorogood 1986) and group discussion (Cooperstock and Lennard 1979). Two issues arising out of this research will be discussed here: long-term users' perceptions of the effects of the drugs; and their views as to their continued need for, and how they would cope without, their drugs.

Do long-term users regard their drugs as helpful? It appears that, in a general sense, most do (Murray 1981; Rodrigo et al. 1987). However, there is also evidence of considerable ambivalence: for example, 87 per cent of respondents in Murray's (1981) survey agreed with the statement 'I don't like taking the :e tablets but I could not manage without them'. Further-more, when Gabe and Thorogood (1986) asked women long-term users of benzodiazepines what they felt about taking the drugs, one-tenth of the sample emphasized the benefits and one-quarter the dangers, while the majority (about two-thirds) expressd mixed views. They also found that less ambivalence and fewer negative views were expressed by a sample of short-term users.

An important finding has been that, when asked to specify the ways in which benzodiazepines and other tranquillizers were helpful, long-term users frequently mention aspects of social functioning and performance. Table 20.3 shows the activities for which respondents expressed a need for drugs, as reported in Murray's (1981) questionnaire survey of long-term psychotropic drug consumers and in Rodrigo et al.'s (1987) interview study of long-term benzodiazepine consumers in a south London general practice. There are clearly marked differences between the two studies (which may well be accounted for by the nature of the samples and the methods used) but, taken together, they testify to the extent to which long-term users regard benzodiazepines and other psychotropic drugs as having a social as well as a purely clinical function. A similar finding emerged from Cooperstock and Lennard's (1979) series of group discussions with long-term benzodiazepine users, and over half of the long-term psychotropic drug users interviewed by Helman (1981) felt that withdrawal of the drugs would have a bad effect on their social relationships.

Table 20.3 Activities for which respondents felt a need for psychotropic drugs

	Current long-term users of psychotropic drugs (Murray 1981) n=183	Current long-term users of benzodiazepines (Rodrigo et al. 1988) n=68
	n %	n %
travelling	81 (44)	7 (11)
shopping	78 (43)	4 (6)
mixing with people	75 (41)	7 (11)
running the home	65 (36)	8 (13)
work	61 (33)	16 (25)
family problems	61 (33)	1 (2)
marriage	40 (22)	3 (5)
money matters	20 (11)	2 (3)
housing problems	13 (7)	1 (2)

Fifty-eight per cent of the current long-term users surveyed by Murray (1981) said that they would find it 'very difficult' to manage without their drugs, and a further 33 per cent claimed that they would not be able to manage at all. A similar picture emerges from Rodrigo *et al.*'s (1988) study: while a smaller proportion said that they could not 'do without' (17 per cent), more than half (54 per cent) of the long-term benzodiazepine consumers believed that they would need to take their drugs for 'years' or indefinitely.

In Rodrigo *et al.*'s (1988) study, long-term users were asked to suggest alternative strategies that they would use if the drugs were not available. Apart from distracting activities, the commonest strategy mentioned was the consumption of some alternative substance – other drugs, alcohol, and herbal remedies being the most frequently mentioned. Similarly, cigarette smoking was regarded as an alternative resource by the women inter-viewed by Gabe and Thorogood (1986).

Some of these various findings on users' perceptions and views can be integrated by using the concept of *meaning* – i.e., 'the interpretation a person gives to an object or event in his or her life' (Gabe and Williams 1986b). This approach has been taken by Helman (1981) and by Gabe and his colleagues (Gabe and Lipshitz-Phillips 1982; Gabe and Thorogood

1986). Gabe has developed the concepts 'lifeline' and 'standby' to describe the meaning of benzodiazepines to consumers. Those who viewed their drugs as a lifeline felt them to be 'something which they needed to take regularly and depended on simply to keep going in the face of chronic, unresolved problems'. Others viewed their drugs as a standby, to be kept in reserve and used occasionally to meet some short-lived crisis, while a minority of their respondents characterized their drug-taking behaviour in terms of both these meanings.

Helman (1981) conducted in-depth interviews with fifty long-term (six months or more) benzodiazepine users. He found, on the basis of their beliefs, attitudes, and expectations concerning the drugs, that 'long-term users of psychotropics can be classified into three main groups – called "tonic", "food" and "fuel"'.

Patients classified as 'tonic' (about one-third of the sample) were those who expressed maximum control over the drug, its dosage, and when it was to be used, tending to use the drugs on an occasional rather than a regular basis. They placed the site of action of the drug on themselves rather than on their relationships, and tended to have more anti-drug views than the other groups. Patients classified as 'fuel' (some two-fifths of those interviewed) expressed a variable degree of control over their medication but none the less felt that the drug played an important and constant part in their daily lives. Its maximum effect was thought to be on their relationships with others: in some cases, the drug was seen as an essential constituent of the patients' relationships. Helman used the concept of 'fuel', since, as he observed, without the drug 'the patient would not disintegrate but would just not function in conformity with familial and social expectations'.

The third group of patients (about one-fifth of the sample), for whom benzodiazepines were conceptualized as a 'food', expressed the least control over the drug and its ingestion, and over life generally. Helman noted that their psychological dependence appeared to be as much on the medical profession as on the drug. Furthermore, the drugs were seen by this group as acting both on the patient's emotional state and on social relationships: without it, both would disintegrate. Helman applied the concept of 'food' to these patients' drug use since without it they feared that they would not survive as independent, sane persons.

Conclusions

Despite dissenting opinions (e.g., Snaith 1984; Cohen 1987), short-term treatment with benzodiazepines and other tranquillizers continues to be accepted practice (Tyrer and Murphy 1987); in contrast, it is generally agreed that long-term use is to be avoided. Since only a minority of recipients become long-term users, the identification of risk factors for long-term use is of paramount importance for prevention. The work described here has identified a number of such factors, the relevance of which is enhanced by their being available at the beginning of treatment.

The extent to which steps should be taken to discontinue medication in an established long-term user is not so well established, although a number of studies testify that this is certainly possible (see Gabe and Williams 1987c). It is clear from the work described in this chapter that in such circumstances it is important to consider patients' own views on their drugs and drug treatment and the alternative resources available to them.

Even so, long-term use of benzodiazepines and other psychotropic drugs remains a major feature of medical practice. The phenomenon should not be conceptualized only within a pharmacological or even a strictly clinical context, and any approach to prevention, primary, secondary, or tertiary, must be grounded in recognition of the multifaceted nature of the problem.

Acknowledgements

This paper was written as part of a programme of research funded by the Department of Health and Social Security, and directed by Professor Michael Shepherd. Edirimuni K. Rodrigo was supported by a grant from Roche Products Ltd, and Paul Williams was in receipt of a grant from the Tregaskis Bequest fund of the University of London.

References

Belloc, N.B., Breslow, L., and Hochstim, J.R. (1971) 'Measurement of physical health in a general population survey', *American Journal of Epidemiology* 93: 328–36.

Boardman, A.P. (1987) 'The General Health Questionnaire and the detection of emotional disorder by general practitioners: a replicated study', *British Journal of Psychiatry* 151: 373–81.

Catalan, J., Gath, D., Edmonds, G., and Ennis, J. (1984a) 'The effects of non-prescribing of anxiolytics in general practice, I: controlled evaluation of psychiatric and social outcome', *British Journal of Psychiatry* 144: 593–602.

Catalan, J., Gath, D., Bond, A., and Martin, P. (1984b) 'The effects of non-prescribing of anxiolytics in general practice, II: factors associated with outcome', *British Journal of Psychiatry* 144: 603–10.

Cohen, S. (1987) 'Are benzodiazepines useful in anxiety?', *Lancet* ii: 1080.

Cooperstock, R. (1976) 'Psychotropic drug use among women', *Canadian Medical Association Journal* 115: 760–3.

Cooperstock, R. (1978) 'Sex differences in psychotropic drug use', *Social Science and Medicine* 12B: 179–86.

Cooperstock, R. and Lennard, H. (1979) 'Some social meanings of tranquillizer use', *Sociology of Health and Illness* 1: 331–47.

Gabe, J. and Bury, M. (1987) 'Tranquillizers as a social problem', *Sociological Review*, in press.

Gabe, J. and Lipshitz-Phillips, S. (1982) 'Evil necessity? The meaning of benzodiazepine use for women patients from one general practice', *Sociology of Health and Illness* 4: 201–9.

Gabe, J. and Lipshitz-Phillips, S. (1984) 'Tranquillizers as social control?' *Sociological Review* 32: 524–46.

Gabe, J. and Thorogood, N. (1986) 'Tranquillizers as a resource', In J. Gabe and P. Williams (eds) *Tranquillizers: Social, Psychological and Clinical Perspectives*, London: Tavistock, pp. 244–69.

Gabe, J. and Williams, P. (1986a) 'Tranquillizer use: a historical perspective', In J. Gabe and P. Williams (eds) *Tranquillizers: Social, Psychological and Clinical Perspectives*, London: Tavistock, pp. 3–17.

Gabe, J. and Williams, P. (1986b) 'The meaning of tranquillizer use: introduction', In J. Gabe and P. Williams (eds) *Tranquillizers: Social, Psychological and Clinical Perspectives*, London: Tavistock, pp. 197–8.

Gabe, J. and Williams, P. (1986c) 'Alternatives to tranquillizer use: introduction', in J. Gabe and P. Williams (eds) *Tranquillizers: Social, Psychological and Clinical Perspectives*, London: Tavistock, pp. 135–7.

Goldberg, D., Cooper, B., Eastwood, M.R., Kedward, H.B., and Shepherd, M. (1970) 'A standardized psychiatric interview for use in community surveys', *Journal of Preventive and Social Medicine* 24: 18–23.

Helman, C. (1981) 'Tonic, fuel and food: social and symbolic aspects of the long-term use of psychotropic drugs', *Social Science and Medicine* 15B: 521–33.

Lader, M.H. (1987) 'Long-term benzodiazepine use and psychological functioning', in H. Freeman and Y. Rue (eds) *The Benzodiazepines in Current Clinical Practice*, London: The Royal Society of Medicine International Congress and Symposium Series no. 114, pp. 55–69.

Lader, M.H., Ron, M., and Petursson, H. (1984) 'Computed axial brain tomography in long-term benzodiazepine users', *Psychological Medicine* 14: 203–6.

Mant, A., Duncan-Jones, P., Saltman, D., Bridges-Webb, C., Kehoe, L., Lansbury, G., and Chancellor, A.H.B. (1988) 'Development of long-term use of psychotropic drugs by general practice patients', *British Medical Journal* 296: 251–4.

Marks, J. (1983) 'The benzodiazepines: an international perspective', *Journal of Psychoactive Drugs* 15: 137–49.

Marks, J., Goldberg, D., and Hillier, V.E. (1979) 'Determinants of the ability of general practitioners to detect psychiatric disorder', *Psychological Medicine* 9: 337–53.

Mellinger, G.D., Balter, M.B., Uhlenhuth, E.H., Cisin, I.H., Manheimer, D.I., and Rickels, K. (1983) 'Evaluating a household survey measure of psychic distress', *Psychological Medicine* 13: 607–21.

Mellinger, G.D., Balter, M.B., and Uhlenhuth, E.H. (1984) 'Prevalence and correlates of long-term regular use of anxiolytics', *Journal of the American Medical Association* 251: 375–9.

Murray, J. (1981) 'Long-term psychotropic drug taking and the process of withdrawal', *Psychological Medicine* 11: 853–8.

Murray, J., Williams, P., and Clare, A.W. (1982) 'Health and social characteristics of long-term psychotropic drug takers', *Social Science and Medicine* 16: 1595–8.

Parish, P.A. (1971) 'The prescribing of psychotropic drugs in general practice', *Journal of the Royal College of General Practitioners*, 21, supplement 4: 1–77.

Perera, K.M.H., Powell, T., and Jenner, F.A. (1987) 'Computerized axial tomographic studies following long-term use of benzodiazepines', *Psychological Medicine* 17: 775–8.

Rodrigo, E.K., King, M., and Williams, P. (1988) 'The health of long-term tranquillizer users', *British Medical Journal*, 296: 603–6.

Snaith, R.P. (1984) 'Benzodiazepines on trial', *British Medical Journal* 288: 1379.
Solow, C. (1975) 'Psychotropic drugs in somatic disorder', *International Journal of Psychiatry in Medicine* 6: 267–82.
Trethowan, W.H. (1975) 'Pills for personal problems', *British Medical Journal* iii: 749–51.
Tyrer, P. (1984) 'Benzodiazepines on trial', *British Medical Journal* 288: 1101–2.
Tyrer, P. (1987) 'Benefits and risks of benzodiazepines', in H. Freeman and Y. Rue (eds) *The Benzodiazepines in Current Clinical Practice*, London: The Royal Society of Medicine International Congress and Symposium Series no. 114, pp. 3–11.
Tyrer, P. and Murphy, S. (1987) 'The place of benzodiazepines in psychiatric practice', *British Journal of Psychiatry* 151: 719–23.
Williams, P. (1978) 'Physical ill-health and psychotropic drug prescription: a review', *Psychological Medicine* 8: 683–93.
Williams, P. (1980) 'Recent trends in the prescribing of psychotropic drugs', *Health Trends* 12: 6–8.
Williams, P. (1983a) 'Patterns of psychotropic drug use', *Social Science and Medicine* 17: 845–51.
Williams, P. (1983b) 'Factors influencing the duration of treatment with psychotropic drugs in general practice: a survival-analysis approach', *Psychological Medicine* 13: 623–33.
Williams, P. (1987) 'Long-term benzodiazepine use in general practice', in H. Freeman and Y. Rue (eds) *The Benzodiazepines in Current Clinical Practice*, London: the Royal Society of Medicine International Congress and Symposium Series no. 114, pp. 19–32.
Williams, P., Murray, J., and Clare, A.W. (1982) 'A longitudinal study of psychotropic drug prescription', *Psychological Medicine* 12: 201–6.
Woodcock, J. (1970) 'Long-term consumers of psychotropic drugs', in M. Balint, M. Marinker, and J. Woodcock (eds) *Treatment or Diagnosis*, London: Tavistock, pp. 147–76.

Part six

Promoting healthier public policies

Chapter twenty-one

The World Health Organization's views on the prevention of mental disorders in developed and developing countries

Norman Sartorius

A high proportion of health and social welfare budgets in many countries is being spent on the care of individuals with mental disorders. Yet work in the field of mental health is not seen as a public-health effort and mental diseases are not considered a public-health problem. This is neither surprising nor a matter for a paranoid interpretation. It simply reflects the fact that until now mental disorders did not meet the three criteria which qualify a problem for public-health action. These are:

1. that the problem is severe enough, and occurs frequently enough, to significantly harm the well-being and productivity of the society;
2. that there are measures, acceptable to the individuals concerned, to their families and to the community, which are effective in preventing or reducing the problem and its consequences;
3. that all concerned – the community, the individual, and society as a whole – are convinced that both of the above criteria are fulfilled.

For most of the communicable diseases which have become a focus for public-health action, these three criteria are clearly met. These diseases are frequent; they cause damage to individuals and to society; there are measures which can be used to control them and most people in the community and also those in government know about this. For mental disorders this is not so. In most countries, most people are aware neither of the magnitude and nature of mental health problems, nor of the fact that preventive and curative action is possible.

WHO's work in this field over the past twenty years has concentrated on making mental disorders a focal point of public-health effort. Over the years, three phases in this work are discernible. First, in the early years of WHO, major emphasis was put on the development of instruments for the assessment of mental disorders, on a classification and nomenclature which would be acceptable to people in different parts of the world, and on other elements of a 'common language' which would permit scientists and public-health workers from different lands to understand each other and to communicate. A series of research projects have been undertaken, demonstrating the ubiquity of mental disorders and their seriousness. Among the WHO projects included in this first phase were studies of schizophrenia, depression, mental retardation, and suicide. These studies were complemented by an active effort to collate and transmit information obtained in research in different parts of the world, demonstrating the seriousness of mental disorders and their impact on society.

The second phase of WHO's work was characterized by efforts to demonstrate that treatment of the mentally ill is not only possible but also applicable in situations characterized by lack of resources and absence of highly trained personnel. Several studies exploring ways of providing mental health services in primary health care were conducted. These studies were carried out in Third World countries with few resources and even less acceptance of mental health problems. They had selected as targets mental and neurological problems of significant visibility, such as epilepsy and acute excitement, which were also characterized by their quick and full response to treatment. The demonstration that therapy can be provided under conditions prevailing in developing countries was also accompanied by convincing figures that such treatment is available at a price which even very poor countries could afford.

The third phase of WHO's work in the mental health field began relatively recently. It concentrates on directing public-health efforts towards the prevention of mental and neurological disorders. Although some publications on this topic were produced earlier, it was not until 1986 that a comprehensive document was presented to the World Health Assembly enumerating possibilities for intervention and giving estimates of public-health gain if preventive action in the mental health field were to be undertaken.

Three significant conceptual changes which have occurred over the past few years are incorporated in the document presented to the World Health Assembly. The first of these concerns the content of the term 'mental disorder'. In many countries until recently, these words referred only to functional disorders such as schizophrenia, affective disorders, and neurosis. In contrast, the document outlining possibilities for the prevention of mental and neurological disorders defined as legitimate targets for action by WHO not only functional disorders but also mental disorder due to organic damage of the central nervous system, mental retardation, certain forms of behavioural disorder and hazardous lifestyle, and psychosocial problems such as those related to the abuse of alcohol and drugs. While this expansion of the field makes the tasks for the mental health programme even more formidable, it also changes and enlarges the catalogue of activities that can be undertaken to prevent mental disorders and their consequences.

The second conceptual change concerns the assignment of principal responsibility for preventive programmes. While traditionally in the public-health field much of the responsibility for prevention of a disease has rested with the specialty or discipline which dealt with individuals suffering from that disease, recent years have seen a growing recognition that other public service sectors – for example, education, social welfare, and urban planning – have a crucial role in the prevention of mental disorder. Unless they assume it, programmes cannot be fully effective.

The third conceptual change concerns acceptable rates of success. In the prevention of many diseases a preventive measure is not considered useful unless it reduces the cases present in a community by, say, 70 or 80 per cent. This criterion has been applied to most communicable diseases, but it is doubtful whether it is useful in assessing success rates in the field of non-communicable diseases, and especially of disorders whose multiple causes are ubiquitous and frequent, and depend to a large extent on patterns of human behaviour.

Absolute numbers are usually shunned in assessing the effects of preventive measures; yet they are crucial in the instance of behavioural disorders. If, for example, simple advice to smokers, given during a medical encounter, causes 10 per cent of the smokers to quit smoking, this measure can be recommended for wide application: the intervention is cheap and without significant side effects, and although only one in ten will stop smoking, the total number of persons who smoke is such that if, for example, this measure were systematically applied in all medical encounters in the United States, approximately one million people would stop smoking. Furthermore, the role of peer pressure is of incomparably greater importance in the prevention of behavioural disorders than it is in the prevention of other diseases. If 5 per cent of the people in a community change their behaviour, they may in fact change standards of behaviour for the community as a whole. Ten years ago, in many settings non-smokers were a minority; today even though only 5 or 10 per cent of the population in these communities have stopped smoking, non-smokers have frequently become a majority: a majority which significantly reinforces further efforts to reduce smoking.

These three conceptual changes were of importance in deciding which measures to include in the proposals to the World Health Assembly. There is one additional conceptual shift which was not of major importance in our proposals, but may acquire importance as new methods of prevention become available. It concerns the definition of a mental disease. At present, a person who has had a single episode of a disease with symptoms usually described as schizophrenic will be considered by many as schizophrenic for the rest of his life, even though he may not have any further symptoms. If we were to consider each episode of schizophrenia as a new disease, the administration of chlorpromazine after a first attack of illness could be legitimately classed as another measure for the primary prevention of schizophrenia.

In the document presented to the World Health Assembly, we have estimated that approximately 50 per cent of all mental, neurological, and psychosocial problems could be prevented if there existed the political will to do so and if concerted action of all concerned could be brought about. The World Health Assembly is composed of representatives of different countries. Most of the delegates are public health administrators, and very few have any substantial knowledge of psychiatry. The challenge, therefore, was to find a way of presentation that would be acceptable, comprehensible, and convincing. Measures that were candidates for inclusion had to be cheap, without side effects, effective in producing a major reduction in the absolute size of the problem, and likely to be acceptable to the individuals and societies concerned. This proved difficult, and the material was therefore presented in three different ways.

First, a series of measures were presented according to the service sector which would have to take the primary responsibility for implementation (cf. Table 21.1).

Table 21.1 Proposals for an action plan for prevention of mental disorders

Health sector	Other sectors
Improvement of prenatal and perinatal care, including:	Improvement of day-care facilities for children
– advice on nutrition	Upgrading of long-term institutions
– prevention of smoking and drinking in pregnancy	Support of self-help groups
– prevention of tetanus	Optimization of schools
– iodine supply	Prevention of accidents
– recognition of high-risk pregnancy	Education through media
	Mobilization of social forces (religious bodies, cultural influences, etc.)
Programme of child nutrition	
Immunization programme	
Family planning	
Prevention of psychoactive substance abuse	
Crisis intervention facilities	
Prevention of iatrogenic damage	
Prevention or minimizing of specific impairments:	
– treatment of psychosis	
– treatment of depression	
– treatment of hypertension	
– treatment of febrile convulsions	
– correction of sensory impairment (e.g. provision of spectacles)	

Next, the measures were grouped in accordance with the level of responsibility, i.e., divided into those steps that can be taken at community level and by the people directly concerned themselves, and those that have to be taken by government with the sanction of the society as a whole, for example, new legislation. Then, to counter the argument that primary prevention of these conditions is impossible, the measures were presented as to whether they should be regarded as primary or secondary prevention.

Finally, a list of conditions was provided, indicating against each the measures which can be taken to prevent it (cf. Tables 21.2 and 21.3).

Table 21.2 Problems for which preventive measures were proposed

Mental retardation
Acquired lesions of the central nervous system
Peripheral neuropathy
Psychoses
Epilepsy
Emotional and conduct disorders
Substance abuse
Life styles that lead to disease
Excessive risk-taking behaviour among young people
Family breakdown

Table 21.3 Example of listing of preventive actions

Problem	Preventive actions
Mental retardation	Prenatal and perinatal care
	Immunization
	Family planning
	Epilepsy control
	Nutrition
	Day care
	Accident prevention
	Family support
	Teaching of parenting skills
	Upgrading of long-term care provision
	Recognition and correction of sensory and motor impairments

The reception of the document was enthusiastic. It was the first time, the delegates said, that a document presenting a list of specific measures had been presented. The multiple-entry organization of the document – by sector which should do the work, by condition which should be prevented, and so on – was not seen as a shortcoming: on the contrary, it was seen as making the use of the material easier.

The Assembly adopted a resolution urging member states and WHO to undertake the measures proposed; it also requested that each of the six regional committees of WHO discuss the topic in 1988, concentrating on conditions particularly prevalent in the respective region, and that the matter be put on the agenda of the World Health Assembly in 1989 to review progress and plan further work.

If prevention of mental and neurological disorders as a result of this action becomes an integral part of the countries' public-health programmes, the third phase of WHO's mental health programme will have been successfully completed, and the fourth – perhaps the most difficult of all – can commence. This will have to deal with the change of the abominably low place which mental life and health occupy on the scales of values of most societies. It is my conviction that this task is the most important. If we do not increase people's awareness of the value of mental health, and if mental health is not promoted on the scale of individual and societal values, all the achievements in the field of mental health will prove ephemeral and our programmes will remain fragile and vulnerable. It is in this promotive action that I see the main challenge for the mental health programmes of the future: the main challenge but also the greatest promise for lasting success.

Chapter twenty-two

Factors influencing the incidence of mental retardation, and their implications for prevention

Annalise Dupont

All efforts towards the primary prevention of mental retardation aim at a reduction of the incidence. Ever since it became possible in the study of mental disorders to differentiate between mental illness and mental retardation, the mental retardation research has aimed at new knowledge of causation in a consistent and systematic way. Especially during the last quarter of the century, progress in this field has been remarkable. Mental retardation has been called the Cinderella of mental health, and in many new psychiatric textbooks a chapter on mental retardation is searched for in vain. Yet in terms of research, and also of the prevention of new cases, successes have been outstanding. These successes have not been easy to achieve or to maintain. Throughout the many years of research it has been a constant pattern that as soon as one disease or group of diseases causing brain damage or dysfunction was controlled – as, for instance, certain sequelae of tuberculosis, syphilis, and rubella, and of diseases connected with incompatibility of blood groups – very quickly new aetiological factors came into play; for example, traffic accidents resulting in cranial trauma to the foetus, infant, or child, and followed by severe intellectual impairment for the rest of the person's life. Diminution in the incidence of a diagnostic group may not always be the result of scientists' and planners' preventive work, since in certain groups there is a considerable spontaneous fluctuation of prevalence at birth, as seen for instance for Down's Syndrome (Fryers 1984).

In mental retardation there is still no final solution with regard to definitions, classifications, and groupings within the total collective. Publication of the International Classification of Impairments, Disabilities, and Handicaps (WHO 1980) was a considerable step forward. In the following, the subdivision into severe and mild retardation is used (with IQ about 50 as the borderline). The new dynamic concept – especially of mild mental retardation – emphasizes the interaction of the person with a handicap and the social, educational, and other aspects of the community in which he lives.

Table 22.1 shows the many different aetiological factors for severe

Table 22.1 Distribution of severe and mild mental retardation by type of aetiology

Type of aetiology	Severe mental retardation (IQ ≤ 50)	Mild mental retardation (IQ ≥ 50)
	%	%
1. Prenatal	70:	40:
1.1 Hereditary:		
1.1.1 With chromosomal disorders	5	5
1.1.2 Without chromosomal disorders	15	5
1.1.2.1 Monogenic disorders (dominant, autosomal recessive, X-linked)		
1.1.2.2 Others (the hereditary pattern unknown)		
1.2 Chromosomal non-hereditary	35	15
1.3 Special syndromes	5	5
1.4 Acquired prenatally	5	5
1.5 Unknown how to group (but clinically prenatal)	5	5
2. Perinatal	8	2
3. Postnatal	2	15
4. Aetiology unknown (multifactorial; associated with psychosis, etc.)	20	43
	100	100

Sources: Gustavson *et al.* 1977a, 1977b; Hagberg *et al.* 1981;
       Rasmussen *et al.* 1982; Evans and Hamerton 1985.

mental retardation (SMR) and mild mental retardation (MMR). It is now possible, in a well-equipped diagnostic centre, to classify about 90 per cent of all cases of children with SMR according to aetiological factors. The largest group among the severely retarded is that of non-hereditary chromosomal disorders. Many numerical and structural abnormalities are now well recognized. However, the underlying – possibly environmental – causes of, for instance, non-disjunction (in Down's syndrome) are not yet clearly understood and the pathogenetic mechanisms which lead to mental and physical abnormalities in persons with abnormal karyotypic patterns are imperfectly understood (Annerén 1984). Nearly three-quarters of all the severely mentally retarded cases are prenatally determined. The mildly retarded cases include a much higher proportion with postnatal or unknown aetiology, and many of these are believed to be due to deprivation and under-stimulation during early development.

The rates of incidence of mental retardation in a defined population during a defined time period will depend upon the exposure to aetiological factors, but also the procedures for ascertainment. From a biomedical point of view, there may be a certain interest in the total inception rate. For the administrative planning of services it is necessary to know how many cases to subtract as abortions (spontaneous or induced) and the age-related mortality. McLaren and Bryson (1987) in a recent review found higher estimates in studies by investigators who included non-survivors in their counts, and concluded that lack of clear definitions makes cross-study comparisons difficult.

Some factors of importance in this context are:

– by definition all cases must commence before the age of 18 years;
– the majority of all cases have a prenatal aetiology;
– the mortality is high in infancy and childhood, especially for the severely retarded;
– the time of ascertainment varies greatly: that of SMR may today begin with a prenatal diagnosis, whereas the mild forms of retardation may not be ascertained until the child starts school.

Thus we have, in effect, a cumulative incidence of many different disorders associated with mental retardation in each cohort of conceptions (Fryers 1984). A high proportion of the cases are already abnormal at conception, some more arise early in foetal life, and others later on before birth. The perinatal period results in an increase in numbers, but thereafter the frequency of new cases decreases. Many impaired foetuses die early in foetal life, fewer later on. The perinatal period carries higher risks for the impaired foetuses, but after birth the mortality progressively diminishes. Ascertainment is progressively achieved.

In the western developed countries the incidence rate for all the different aetiologies combined, including also rare conditions, and all cases with IQ below 70, followed from birth to about 18 years, is about ten per 1,000 children up to the age of 18 (Rantakallio and von Went 1986). However, there is great variation, especially in some of the diseases; for example, the incidence of neural tube defects shows a substantial variation in time and place.

It is not possible to measure the result of preventive action unless the incidence of each aetiological group is known; however, as many cases are the cumulative or interactive effect of more than one factor, this may be difficult.

Preventive strategies in developing countries

Both the pattern of aetiology for mental retardation and the age-sex-specific prevalence ratios for a population are functions of the type of society under observation. A developing country with a high infant mortality and limited public-health facilities may very well be confronted by a new problem of increasing numbers of handicapped children once the infant mortality starts to decline. This development occurs as soon as the public-health services succeed in providing clean water, improving sewage disposal, combating malnutrition, and promoting immunization programmes.

With a limited budget, questions of priority will arise between specialist activities and general public-health measures. Unfortunately, few cost-effectiveness studies have been undertaken to guide the choice of programmes: for example, to decide whether it is more effective to establish units for genetic counselling or to concentrate on health education of groups at risk, to provide better primary health care systems, especially for pregnant women and newborn babies, or in some areas to use the available funds for training women and retraining staff personnel to avoid traditional harmful practices and achieve better recognition and diagnosis of birth complications such as asphyxia.

In the field of genetically determined diseases, first priority could be given to advisory service and counselling on general lines (for example, to avoid traditional family structures which will lead to consanguinity and intermarriage, with the risk for genetic diseases including mental retardation); or resources could be used to identify families with specific genetic anomalies and to spread knowledge of the genetic risks among certain ethnic groups, in order to reduce the incidence of metabolic diseases, malformations, and mental retardation. For the general population, awareness of the connection between high maternal age and increased risk for malformations and biological impairments is important. Here an appropriate training programme for primary health care workers is crucial.

Paradoxically, it has never been proved, and there is indeed no clear evidence, that poor infant nutrition will result directly in an increased frequency of brain damage among the survivors. An explanation for this fact has been suggested by Dobbing (1984) in the context of an industrial developed country. However, in considering the neuropathological basis of mental retardation, it is important to remember that the developing human brain has a very long period of special vulnerability compared with other organs. The aetiology of many cases of mental retardation and learning disability in developing countries may be explained by the following sequence: poor nutrition of the pregnant woman causes low birth-weight babies, whose poor postnatal growth and natural immunity leads to generalized and severe infections and a vicious circle of reduced capacity for learning and understimulation.

A major problem is the widespread occurrence of iodine deficiency.

It is estimated that some 800 million people are living in the iodine-deficient areas of the third world and are therefore at risk of developing iodine-deficiency disorders, including disorders with brain damage and mental retardation. The disorders include goitre and cretinism, but a much commoner manifestation is mental impairment due to the special sensitivity of both developing and adult brains to lowered blood levels of thyroxin. The prevention and control of iodine-deficiency disorders because of its dramatic impact on the quality of life, productivity and educability of millions would make a major contribution to the development of these countries and would contribute significantly to attaining the World Health Organization's goal of health for all by the year 2000.

This quotation is taken from a report by Hetzel (1987), which stresses the possibility, especially in some African countries, of using the relatively cheap measure of iodization of salt in order to prevent a high proportion of cases of intellectual impairment.

Another possibility of great importance in special population groups is the prevention of lead poisoning. There are many sources of lead encephalopathy in children. Lin-Fu (1982) showed that in countries where programmes to screen large numbers of children have been introduced, the incidence of lead encephalopathy with mental retardation has been reduced dramatically. One source of poisoning is the liberal use of 'Kohl', an eye cosmetic which is used in Arabian countries on infants and young children, as well as by pregnant women (Shaltout et al. 1986).

Preventive strategies in developed industrial countries

Epidemiological studies, especially of severe mental retardation, have shown that prevalence ratios have been fairly stable in recent decades. Although epidemiologists have stressed that both incidence and prevalence do vary considerably in time and place, for the severely mentally retarded rather stable figures were found in the western world from about 1925 to 1975 of around three to four per 1,000, as demonstrated by Fryers (1984).

This relatively constant prevalence is not an indication that preventive activities have been useless. In a 1982 publication, Alberman et al. examined trends in the prevalence at school age of cerebral palsy and severe educational subnormality in children of low birth-weight born in one region in Britain, and showed that the prevalence of both these defects was lower in the 1970 cohort than in cohorts born in the 1950s. This disparity was due both to a fall in the incidence of extreme gestational immaturity among children of low birth-weight and to a reduction in the risk of defects to the gestationally immature births that occurred. The decreased risk of these defects in children of low birth-weight was approximately counterbalanced by the increased likelihood of the children's survival. In many developed countries a steady decline of infant and maternal mortality has been recorded for as long as the statistics have been collected. Bloom (1984) has stressed that there are still important benefits to be gained by the improved application of modern medical technology in the perinatal period. However, the use of high technology to effect further reductions in perinatal damage means escalating medical care expenditures. Stahlman (1984) has posed the question concerning intensive care for the newborn: success or failure? His own longitudinal study of babies weighing less than 1,250 grams at birth showed that the number and severity of complications in this very low birth-weight group would give an IQ variation correlated to birth-weight and gestational age and complications. He also pointed out that at one time the lower limit of birth-weight for giving ventilatory support to infants was about 1,500 grams. Ten years ago the limit was 1,000 grams and today the limit is about 500 grams. The reason for this continued decline has been the successful survival in the low birth-weight group at which maximal effort had been used: enough normal babies had survived to encourage further development.

Although birth injury is still an important cause of mental retardation, perinatal causes for mental retardation have always been exaggerated by parents and non-obstetric professionals. With an improved knowledge of chromosomal disorders, inherited prenatal syndromes, metabolic diseases, and acquired prenatal aetiology for mental retardation, as well as of the damaged foetus and its difficulties during birth, it has become clear that cases in which a normal foetus is damaged during birth account for only about 15 per cent or fewer of the severely mentally retarded. Chaney *et al.* (1986) compared the final clinical diagnosis and the autopsy finding of a perinatal brain lesion in some 250 mentally retarded persons and found that only about one-third of clinical diagnoses of perinatal damage could be confirmed.

Mental retardation research has clearly demonstrated that it is not always necessary to know the aetiology of a disease in order to reduce its incidence. The classic example is Down's syndrome. A new chromosomal disorder, the fragile X syndrome, also offers a possibility of prevention without aetiological knowledge. Recent progress in genetic mapping makes the diagnosis more reliable both prenatally and in early life (Oberlé *et al.* 1987). Fragile X syndrome is said to be nearly as frequent a chromosome anomaly as Down's syndrome. By the finding of the fragile site at band q27 on the X chromosome it was found that some of the X-bound inherited cases of mental retardation, especially in males, were connected with this chromosomal anomaly. Affected males usually have a moderate degree of intellectual handicap, and some have autistic features or hyperactivity. The heterozygous females may be mildly handicapped intellectually in one-third of cases. Of the males with the mental handicap and fragile X syndrome, 80 per cent have a high forehead, big jaw, long ears, and enlarged testes. Visible expression of the chromosome anomaly is more variable and often absent in the females with carrier status.

Turner *et al.* (1986) have reported on a preventive screening programme for this syndrome. Their data indicate that cytogenetic screening of all mentally retarded persons in order to identify those with a fragile X syndrome is a potentially effective preventive measure because female carriers can then be identified in the course of the ensuing family studies. Moreover, a study of the costs of this survey showed that they compared favourably with those of other types of preventive programmes; thus, the cost of prevention of one case of fragile X was about the same as that of diagnosing one baby with phenylketonuria.

Causation related to environmental damage before or after birth has often been stressed in the individual case: for example, in connection with the exposure of pregnant women to chemical risk factors in industry. However, causal connections of this kind are hard to prove. The contemporary debate on possible teratogenic effects of such a well-known toxic risk factor as ethyl alcohol shows how many unsolved problems there are: how much alcohol? how often? Is it the substitution of alcohol for necessary protein, minerals, or vitamins that is responsible? In many countries the pattern of alcohol consumption has changed rapidly during the last decades: for instance, it is well documented that abuse of alcohol has become increasingly common among young adults in many countries, as girls and young women adopt the heavy drinking habits and drinking patterns earlier reserved by tradition for men. In Sweden active anti-alcohol drives have been initiated by the school health, child health, and maternal health authorities. The establishment of special maternal health teams to trace and actively support women at risk very early in pregnancy or before pregnancy has proved to be a promising approach (Hagberg and Kyllerman 1983).

With the rapid development of molecular biological techniques, many new possibilities of prevention are being opened. In tuberous sclerosis, for example, a single gene locus has been identified on chromosome 9 at band q34 and the specific DNA probes are now being used to facilitate first trimester prenatal diagnosis and genetic counselling (Connor et al. 1987). Automatic equipment for chromosome analysis is being developed and tested in many centres. The result may be such a reduction in costs that it will become possible to test all pregnant women who wish it. The measure of acceptance in the population will of course depend upon religious and sociocultural factors.

Special strategies of prevention and amelioration for Mild Mental Retardation

Many of the biomedical factors of significant importance for the aetiology of severe cases of mental retardation also play an important role for the cases of MMR. However, syndromes based on clinical symptoms, without specific biochemical or chromosomal disorders, are very difficult to diagnose in *forme fruste* cases. Preventive strategies aimed at SMR may also reduce the numbers of MMR (Gustavson *et al.* 1987).

Prevention of a reduced function in education and in social competence of persons with MMR and the possibilities of facilitating their integration into the community have been studied intensively during recent decades (Clarke and Clarke 1985). In this secondary prevention, early intervention and stimulation, special training of language and communication, improvement of behavioural competence, and promotion of social interaction and vocational skills have been stressed.

Our scientific knowledge of the scope for prevention of all degrees of mental retardation is now far ahead of what is being practised today, either in developed or in developing countries. Even in Europe, for example, few countries have developed national screening programmes for inborn errors of metabolism, as recommended by the Council of Europe (1981). Such programmes are still beyond the reach of many developing countries, yet effective prevention could still be possible by means of other, quite simple efforts. For all communities there is a link between the social conditions of the population and the occurrence of mental retardation, since mild mental retardation always has a higher prevalence in the groups of low social status, and in some populations the same may hold good also for the severely retarded (Cooper and Lackus 1984).

Economic aspects

Kramer (1980) has drawn attention to the rising pandemic of mental retardation and mental illness. If the mentally retarded survive the first years of life, they may now live nearly as long as other persons in the population (Dupont *et al.* 1987).

Leaving aside for a moment the emotional and psychological implications for the family of having a handicapped child, let us look at the hard economic facts. Braddock and Hemp (1986) have shown that the USA is spending a rapidly growing amount of money on mental retardation, and that federal, state, and combined spending for both community services and institutional care for mental retardation and developmental disabilities increased by 23 per cent (nearly two billion dollars) during the period of the fiscal years 1977 to 1984 (measured in 1977 dollars).

The increasing survival rates for the mentally retarded also present a challenge to psychiatrists. Lund (1985) has demonstrated that attempts to integrate the mentally retarded into the community may in fact serve to increase the numbers of admissions to psychiatric beds. It is therefore not only a question of a reduction of the incidence of new cases, but also of making preventive efforts in order to avoid a prohibitive increase in care costs.

Conclusion

Research into the aetiological factors of all types of mental retardation has brought important new knowledge, so that it is now possible to identify such factors in about 80 per cent of cases of severe mental retardation and 60 per cent of cases of mild retardation. Since many of the possibilities for prevention are linked to a knowledge of aetiology, this has meant significant progress concerning the potential scope for preventive action. In countries where such measures are not ruled out on religious, cultural, or ethical grounds, it has proved possible to make prenatal diagnoses and then, in accordance with the mothers' and the families' wishes, to perform abortions, thus limiting the numbers of both hereditary and non-hereditary chromosomal disorders. In cases of monogenic disorders and in some special syndromes, the development of DNA probes has also opened up new possibilities for prenatal diagnosis. In many industrialized countries there has been an improvement in the environmental conditions for pregnant women, especially with regard to the exposure to infection, trauma, radiation, and chemical risk factors in industry, as well as in the facilities for counselling (e.g., on the intake of medicines, drugs, and alcohol) and for supervision of the pregnant woman's health and nutrition. Improvements in the obstetrical services and in neonatal care have resulted in a better prognosis, especially for low birth-weight babies. In some developing countries also there has been an amelioration of the conditions of women, infants, and children, while specific preventive measures are being promoted with respect, for example, to the control of iodine-deficiency disorders and exposure to lead-containing substances.

The decline in early mortality now observed for all grades of mental retardation represents a challenge to the planners of health and social welfare services in all parts of the world. The growing demand for care provision for the mentally retarded and the increasing financial costs that this entails make it doubly imperative to apply the possibilities for prevention that now exist in order to contain and reduce the burden of mental retardation.

References

Alberman, E., Benson, J., and McDonald, A. (1982) 'Cerebral palsy and severe educational subnormality in low-birth-weight children: a comparison of births in 1951–53 and 1970–73', *Lancet* 13 March 1982: 606–8.

Anneren, G. (1984) 'Down's syndrome: a metabolic and endocrinological study', *Acta Universitatis Upsaliensis* 384.

Bloom, B.S. (1984) 'Changing infant mortality: the need to spend more while getting less', *Pediatrics* 73: 862–6.

Braddock, D. and Hemp, R. (1986) 'Governmental spending for mental retardation and developmental disabilities, 1977–1984', *Hospital and Community Psychiatry* 37: 702–7.

Chaney, R.H., Givens, C.A., Watkins, G.P., and Eyman, R.K. (1986) 'Birth injury as the cause of mental retardation', *Obstetrics and Gynecology* 67: 771–5.

Clarke, A.M., Clarke, A.D.B., and Berg, J.M. (1985) 'Lifespan development and psychosocial intervention', in A.M. Clarke and A.D.B. Clarke (eds) *Mental Deficiency: The Changing Outlook*, fourth edition, London: Methuen, pp. 440–64.

Connor, J.M., Pirrit, L.A., Yates, J.R.W., and Fryer, A.E. (1987) 'Linkage of the tuberous sclerosis locus to a DNA polymorphism detected by v-*abl*', *Journal of Medical Genetics* 24: 544–6.

Cooper, B. and Lackus, B. (1984) 'The social-class background of mentally retarded children: a study in Mannheim', *Social Psychiatry* 19: 3–12.

Council of Europe (1981) *Neonatal Mass Screening for Metabolic Disorders*, Strasbourg: Council of Europe.

Dobbing, J. (1984) 'Pathology and vulnerability of the developing brain', in J. Dobbing, A.D.B. Clarke, J.A. Corbett, J. Hogg, and R.O. Robinson (eds) *Scientific Studies in Mental Retardation*, London: The Royal Society of Medicine, pp. 89–101.

Dupont, A., Vaeth, M., and Videbech, P. (1987) 'Mortality, life expectancy and causes of death of mildly mentally retarded in Denmark', *Upsala Journal of Medical Science*, supplement 44: 76–82.

Evans, J.A. and Hamerton, J.L. (1985) 'Chromosomal anomalies', in A.M. Clarke, A.D.B. Clarke, and J.M. Berg (eds) *Mental Deficiency: The Changing Outlook*, fourth edition, London: Methuen, 213–66.

Fryers, T. (1984) *The Epidemiology of Severe Intellectual Impairment: The Dynamics of Prevalence*, London: Academic Press.

Fryers, T. (1987) 'Epidemiological issues in mental retardation', *Journal of Mental Deficiency Research* 31: 365–84.

Gustavson, K.-H.,Hagberg, B., Hagberg, G., and Sars, K., (1977a) 'Severe mental retardation in a Swedish county, II: etiologic and pathogenetic aspects of children born 1959–1970', *Neuropädiatrie* 8: 293–304.

Gustavson, K.-H., Holmgren, G., Jonsell, R., and Blomquist, H.K:son (1977b) 'Severe mental retardation in children in a northern Swedish county', *Journal of Mental Deficiency Research* 21: 161–81.

Gustavson, K.-H., Holmgren, G., and Blomquist, H.K:son (1987) 'Chromosomal aberrations in mild mental retardation', in K.H. Gustavson, B. Hagberg, L. Kebbon, and S.A. Richardson (eds) 'Scientific studies in mild mental retardation: epidemiology, origin and prevention', *Upsala Journal of Medical Science*, supplement 44: 165–8.

Hagberg, B. and Kyllerman, M. (1983) 'Epidemiology of mental retardation – a Swedish survey', *Brain Development* 5: 441–9.

Hagberg, B., Hagberg, G., Lewerth, A., and Lindberg, U. (1981) 'Mild mental retardation in Swedish school children, II: etiologic and pathogenetic aspects', *Acta Paediatrica Scandinavica* 70: 445–52.

Hetzel, B.S. (1987) 'Progress in the prevention and control of iodine-deficiency disorders', *Lancet* 1 August 87: 266.

Kramer, M. (1980) 'The rising pandemic of mental disorders and associated chronic diseases and disabilities', in E. Strömgren, A. Dupont and J.A. Nielsen (eds) 'Epidemiological research as basis for the organization of extramural psychiatry', *Acta Psychiatrica Scandinavica* 62, supplement 285: 382–96.

Lin-Fu, J. (1982) 'The evolution of childhood lead poisoning as a public health problem', in J.J. Chisolm and D.M. O'Hara (eds) *Lead Absorption in Children*, Baltimore, MD: Urban and Schwarzenberg.

Lund, J. (1985) 'Mentally retarded admitted to psychiatric hospitals in Denmark', *Acta Psychiatrica Scandinavica* 72: 202–5.

336

McLaren, J. and Bryson, S.E. (1987) 'Review of recent epidemiological studies of mental retardation: prevalence, associated disorders, and etiology', *American Journal of Mental Retardation* 92: 243–53.

Oberlé, I., Camerino, G., Wrogemann, K., Arveiler, B., Hanauer, A., Raimondi, E., and Mandel, J.L. (1987) 'Multipoint genetic mapping of the Xq26–q28 region in families with fragile X mental retardation and in normal families reveals tight linkage of markers in q26–q27', *Human Genetics* 77: 60–5.

Rantakallio, P. and von Wendt, L. (1986) 'Mental retardation and subnormality in a birth cohort of 12,000 children in Northern Finland', *American Journal of Mental Deficiency* 90: 380–7.

Rasmussen, K., Nielsen, J., and Dahl, G. (1982) 'The prevalence of chromosome abnormalities among mentally retarded persons in a geographically delimited area of Denmark', *Clinical Genetics* 22: 244–55.

Shaltout, A.A., Ghawaby, M.M., Hunt, M.C.M., and Guthrie, R. (1986) 'High incidence of lead poisoning detected by free erythrocyte protoporphyrin screening in Arabian children', in J.M. Berg (ed.) *Science and Service in Mental Retardation*, London and New York: Methuen, pp. 429–35.

Stahlman, M.T. (1984) 'Newborn intensive care: success or failure?' *Journal of Pediatrics* 105: 162–7.

Turner, G., Robinson, H., Laing, S., and Purvis-Smith, S. (1986) 'Preventive screening for the fragile X syndrome', *New England Journal of Medicine* 315: 607–9.

World Health Organization (1980) *International Classification of Impairments, Disabilities, and Handicaps*, Geneva: WHO.

Chapter twenty-three

Increase of suicide due to imitation of fictional suicide on television

H. Häfner and A. Schmidtke

Introduction

Effects of fictional suicidal behaviour

For more than 200 years the imitation of fictional suicide models has been known as the 'Werther effect'. In 1774 Johann Wolfgang von Goethe published his novel *The Sorrows of Young Werther*, whose hero finally shot himself after a sentimental, hopeless love-affair, and which in Goethe's own words had 'a great, indeed, an immense impact'. The imitation hypothesis was supported at another level in an impressive way: Werther's clothing (blue tailcoat with brass buttons, yellow vest, yellow breeches, brown turndown boots, felt hat, and loose, unpowdered hair), which Goethe had described so vividly, became the gentlemen's fashion of the last quarter of the eighteenth century and was known as the 'Werther dress'.

The term 'Werther effect', however, is derived not from gentlemen's fashions, but the, in those days widespread, impression that Goethe's novel led to an increase in suicides of the same type, i.e., shooting with a pistol. This impression was so strong that authorities in Denmark (Copenhagen), Saxony (Leipzig), and Milan banned the book. Thereafter, the unproven assumption that fictional suicide models might trigger suicides through imitation effects fell largely into oblivion, whereas the issue of whether press reports on real suicides had comparable effects continued to be of interest (Unus Multorum 1910; Hemenway 1911).

Television as a mass medium has made the Werther effect of topical interest again. In this medium, attractive models of suicidal behaviour, portrayed in a realistic manner but mostly avoiding the deterrent impressions of suffering and dying, are transmitted to a great number of individuals in the privacy of their own homes.

The conceptual framework: learning by modelling

Learning by modelling refers to the acquisition of new patterns of behaviour by observation without a necessary reinforcement (Bandura

1976). In experiments the effect of modelling depends on the characteristics of the model, such as age, sex, and social status, and the corresponding characteristics of the observer. Similarity between certain characteristics of the model and those of the observer increases the effects of learning from symbolic models (Bandura 1977). Applied to the imitation of fictional models this means that the dependency of the size of the effect upon the degree of similarity between the characteristics of the model and those of the observer must be examined.

Background of the present study

A six-episode television film, broadcast twice by one of the two nation-wide television networks in the Federal Republic of Germany (ZDF) in 1981 and 1982 gave us a unique opportunity of fulfilling all the above-mentioned methodological requirements (Schmidtke and Häfner 1986, 1988a; Häfner and Schmidtke 1988). At the beginning of each episode a train is shown slowing down, the dead body of a schoolboy is found, and the police investigations begin. The episodes two to six also showed the 18- or 19-year-old schoolboy on his way to the railway line in a mood of resignation, determined to let himself be run over by a train. Each episode described, partly mirrored by the police investigations, one particular aspect of the schoolboy's life leading up to the suicide, as seen by the student himself, his parents, classmates, teachers, and girl-friend. The film has received several awards because of its outstanding aesthetic quality.

The programme was rebroadcast eighteen months later, in 1982. By using this natural experiment we were able to test repeated imitation effects, especially in relation to the size and characteristics of both viewing audiences.

Material and methods

Research design

The programme was first broadcast in January and February 1981 on six successive Sunday evenings (18, 25 January, 1, 8, 15, 22 February; each time at 8.15 p.m.). The second broadcast took place in October and November 1982 (24, 31 October, 7, 14, 17, 21 November; Sundays at 4 p.m.). To obtain a natural 'ABABA-design' (A = baseline phase; B = intervening phase) we selected time periods before and after the transmission from 1 January 1976 to 31 December 1984 with an A-phase of about one-and-a-half years between the two broadcasts (Figure 23.1). In order not to miss any effects persisting over a longer time period, we studied time periods of differing length following the broadcasts, including the five weeks between the first and the last episode. The results presented here are

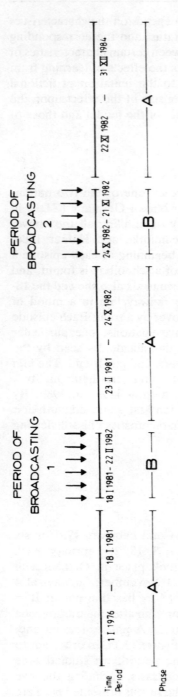

Figure 23.1 Design: ABABA
Source: Schmidtke and Häfner 1986

based on a time period beginning two hours after the broadcasting of the first episode and ending seventy days later (including 29 March 1981). Thus, the period studied after the last of the six episodes was five weeks or thirty-five days for each broadcast. To control for long-term trends, seasonal and other covariations, we included analogous time periods in the years 1976–1984. We also used the periods immediately before the first episode of each broadcast.

Model variables

The model variables were the method of suicide (being run over by a train), age (18/19 years), and sex (male). We were not able to assess the influence of socio-economic status because of the strict data protection regulations in the Federal Republic of Germany. We collected information on all suicidal events that had occurred on the entire West-German railway network (the Deutsche Bundesbahn) over the nine-year period 1 January 1976 – 31 December 1984, each of which was recorded exactly by the date and the hour. Problems of assessing attempted suicides and dating suicidal acts precisely, one of the major difficulties in studies based on official mortality statistics, did not arise, because all such events on the railways were recorded precisely, and 92 per cent of all the suicide attempts in the nine-year period under study ended lethally.

Research findings

When 15- to 29-year-old males were taken as the first group similar to the model in age, in order to use an age grouping comparable with that used for the audience figures, sixty-two suicides were obtained for the observation period of seventy days from the first broadcasting of the film (see Figure 23.2). The mean value for the remaining years studied was 33.25 (σ= 6.50), which corresponded to an increase over the expected number of twenty-nine suicides (86 per cent). Among females of the same age fourteen suicides occurred, compared with eight expected (σ= 4.07), thus amounting to an increase over the expected number of six suicides (75 per cent).

When smaller age groups were examined, the effect was observed to be strongest among males 15–19 years of age, i.e., the group most similar to the model. Twenty-one suicides (σ= 2.92) occurred in the seventy days during the first broadcasting of the suicide model, corresponding to an increase of 175 per cent, compared with a mean of 7.63 for the same time periods in the remaining years. Among girls 15–19 years of age, six suicides occurred, amounting to an increase of 167 per cent, when compared with the expected number of 2.25 (σ= 1.98).

In age groups less similar to that of the model the effect levelled off.

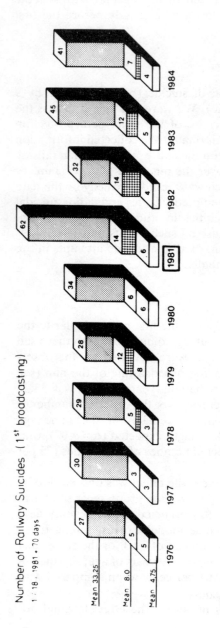

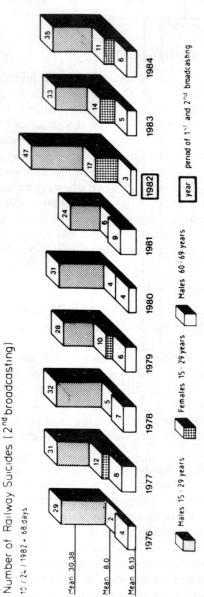

Number of Railway Suicides (1st broadcasting)
1 / 18 . 1981 + 70 days

Mean 33.25
Mean 8.0
Mean 4.75

1976 1977 1978 1979 1980 1981 1982 1983 1984

Number of Railway Suicides (2nd broadcasting)
10 / 24 / 1982 + 68 days

Mean 30.38
Mean 8.0
Mean 6.13

1976 1977 1978 1979 1980 1981 1982 1983 1984

Males 15 - 29 years
Females 15 - 29 years
Males 60 - 69 years
period of 1st and 2nd broadcasting
year

Figure 23.2 Number of railway suicides (first broadcasting) 18.1.1981 + 70 days
Source: Häfner and Schmidtke 1988

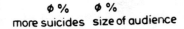

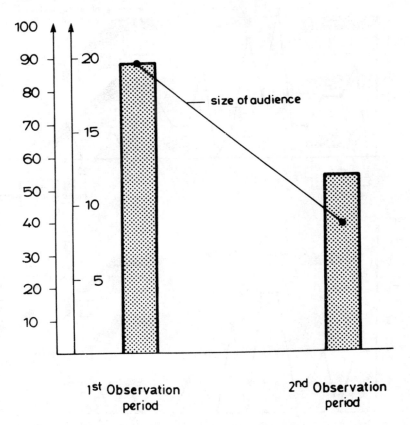

Figure 23.3 Ratios of the increases in railway suicides among 15- to 29-year-olds in the observation periods at the first and the second broadcasting and ratios of the sizes of audience (14- to 29-year-olds)
Source: Schmidtke and Häfner 1986

Among males aged 30–39, suicides increased by six only, when compared with the mean of the remaining years, and by ten, when compared with the preceding and following years. Among 40- to 49-year-old males, the small increase of suicides did not exceed the standard deviation of the expected figure. Among females no increase could be observed in the age group 30 to 39 years (seven suicides observed against 7.5 expected). In higher age groups of both sexes, especially in that of 60- to 69-year-olds, which we

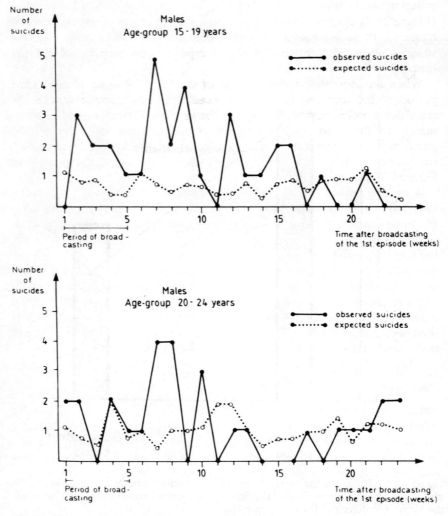

Figure 23.4 Suicides per week after broadcasting the first episode
Source: Schmidtke and Häfner 1988b

have included in Figure 23.2 for comparison, we did not observe any increase related to the showing of the suicide film.

The effects of the repeat broadcasting were weaker than those of the first, but there was again a significant increase in suicide numbers above the expected figures. The number of suicides for males 15–29 years of age showed an increase of 54 per cent (forty-seven suicides observed as against

30.38 expected). Compared with the time periods immediately before and after the broadcast the increase was 61 per cent. Females of the same age group showed a similar trend, with a relatively high increase of 113 per cent (Figure 23.2). As with the first broadcast, the effect was strongest in young males 15–19 years of age, the group most similar to the model: eighteen suicides observed, compared with 8.4 expected, an increase of 115 per cent.

When the increases in the suicides of males 15–29 years of age in the period of the first and the second broadcasts were compared with the television viewing figures, the ratio of the increases corresponded approximately to the ratio of the numbers of viewers accounted for by the comparable age group of 14–29 years in the two periods of broadcasting (on average 19 per cent and 8.9 per cent respectively of this age group; see Figure 23.3).

A striking finding was that the frequency of suicide remained raised for a longer period of time after the broadcasting of the model than indicated in Phillips's studies (Phillips 1978, 1980, 1982), and longest in the group most similar to the model. When the number of suicides each week after the first broadcasting of the film was examined for the group most similar to the model and the group next most similar (Figure 23.4), suicides in the group of 15- to 19-year-old males remained above the expected number, with slight fluctuations, for sixteen weeks. In the group of 20- to 24-year-old males suicides ceased to show any excess after the tenth week. After the second broadcasting the increased suicide rate of the 15- to 29-year-old males declined slowly over the entire following year.

Discussion

Before any conclusions can be drawn, alternative explanations have to be ruled out. All the usual alternative explanations, such as secular trends, economic, seasonal or other variations, or increased sensitivity to un-natural causes of death, can be ruled out on the basis of the design used and the time-series analysis performed over experimental and control periods; or simply because they were of no relevance in our study.

There are two really relevant alternative explanations:

1) Durkheim's assumption (1897) that imitation only precipitates suicides that are already intended, can be refuted, as already demonstrated by Phillips (1974) and Phillips and Carstensen (1986), and also on the evidence of our data. The decrease in suicides that should occur after a certain period of time, if the timing of suicides had been 'brought forward', was not observed. On the contrary, a slow reversion to the mean after the second broadcast, lasting well into the following year, could be observed.

2) The model may have simply determined the method of suicide for those individuals who already intended to commit suicide by one method or

another. To forestall this objection, we examined the frequencies of suicides by other 'hard' methods (hanging: ICD E 953; jumping from a high place: ICD E 957) in the relevant age groups. The results did not support the alternative hypothesis. Suicides by the other two 'hard' methods did not decrease when railway suicides increased in the two periods of broadcasting; on the contrary they increased slightly, though not significantly, in the relevant age groups. Had the model in fact only suggested the means of suicide to persons who would otherwise have chosen a 'soft' method – which is very unlikely – the overall frequency of suicidal behaviour would have remained unchanged. The increased use of a highly lethal method, however, would have caused the number of deaths from suicide to rise, even if the number of attempted suicides had remained unchanged.

The repeated nation-wide broadcasting of a clearly defined suicide model with well-identifiable model characteristics, and the collection of complete and precise nation-wide data on the modelling effect over a period of sufficient length, enabled us to assess the imitation effect of a televised suicide model with some experimental rigour. The findings show that the maximum increase in suicides occurred in the same age and sex group as that of the model. The increase in frequency was less the greater the difference from the model in terms of age and sex. The results thus confirm the results of laboratory research showing that imitation effects depend on the similarity of the characteristics of the model to those of the imitator.

In contrast to the findings of previously published studies (Phillips 1978, 1980, 1982; Gould and Shaffer 1986; Phillips and Carstensen 1986), our findings seem to suggest that the imitation effect probably persists for more than just a few days after the perception of a model.

Some important questions still remain unanswered; for example, what makes suicide models so attractive to persons at risk that they overcome the instinct of self-preservation and lead to suicide; and what characteristics, besides age and sex, make individuals susceptible to the provocation of suicidal acts by suicide models.

A more immediate preventive issue also arises, namely, could the increase in suicide rates in the younger age groups, which has been observed for some decades now in several industrial countries – the trend has been confirmed for the USA (Murphy and Wetzel 1980), Canada (Solomon and Hellon 1980), Australia (Goldney and Katsikitis 1983), the FRG (Häfner and Schmidtke 1985), and Switzerland (Häfner and Schmidtke 1985) from about 1950–60 onwards – have something to do with the expansion during this period of the mass media and their increasing tolerance of attractive models of destructive and autodestructive behaviour?

References

Bandura, A. (1976) *Lernen am Modell*, Stuttgart: Klett.

Bandura, A. (1977) 'Self-efficacy: towards a unifying theory of behavioural change', *Psychological Review* 84: 191–215.

Durkheim, E. (1897) *Le suicide: Etude de sociologie*, Paris: Alcan. (German edition: Durkheim, E. (1973) *Der Selbstmord*, Neuwied: Luchterhand).

Goldney, R.D. and Katsikitis, M. (1983) 'Cohort analysis of suicide rates in Australia', *Archives of General Psychiatry* 40: 71–4.

Gould, M.S., and Shaffer, D. (1986) 'The impact of suicide in television movies', *New England Journal of Medicine* 315: 690–4.

Häfner, H. and Schmidtke, A. (1985) 'Do cohort effects influence suicide rates?', *Archives of General Psychiatry* 42: 926–7.

Häfner, H. and Schmidtke, A. (1988) 'Do televised fictional suicide models produce suicides?', in C.R. Pfeffer (ed.) *Suicide among Youth: Perspectives on Risk and Prevention*, Washington, DC: American Psychiatric Press.

Hemenway, H. (1911) 'To what extent are suicide and other crimes against the person due to suggestion from the press?', *Bulletin of the American Academy of Medicine* 12: 253–63.

Murphy, G.E. and Wetzel, R.D. (1980) 'Suicide risk by birth cohort in the United States, 1949 to 1974', *Archives of General Psychiatry* 37: 519–23.

Phillips, D.P. (1974) 'The influence of suggestion on suicide: substantive and theoretical implications of the Werther effect', *American Sociological Review* 39: 340–54.

Phillips, D.P. (1978) 'Airplane accident fatalities increase just after newspaper stories about murder and suicide', *Science* 201: 748–9.

Phillips, D.P. (1980) 'Airplane accidents, murder, and the mass media: towards a theory of imitation and suggestion', *Social Forces* 58: 1001–24.

Phillips, D.P. (1982) 'The impact of fictional television stories on U.S. adult fatalities: new evidence on the effect of the mass media on violence', *American Journal of Sociology* 87: 1340–59.

Phillips, D.P. and Carstensen, L.L. (1986) 'Clustering of teenage suicides after television news stories about suicide', *New England Journal of Medicine* 315: 685–9.

Schmidtke, A. and Häfner, H. (1986) 'Die Vermittlung von Selbstmordmotivation und Selbstmordhandlung durch fiktive Modelle. Die Folgen der Fernsehserie "Tod eines Schülers"', *Nervenarzt* 57: 502–10.

Schmidtke, A. and Häfner, H. (1988a) 'The Werther effect after television films: evidence for an old hypothesis', *Psychological Medicine* 18: 665–76.

Schmidtke, A. and Häfner, H. (1988b) 'Are there differential effects in the imitation of suicidal behavior?', paper presented at the First Combined Meeting 'Suicide and Cultural Values: National and International Aspects' of the American Association of Suicidology and the International Association for Suicide Prevention, San Francisco, 1987: 460–1.

Solomon, M.I. and Hellon, C.P. (1980) 'Suicide and age in Alberta, Canada, 1951 to 1971', *Archives of General Psychiatry* 37: 511–13.

Unus.Multorum (1910) 'Kapitel I', in Vereinsleitung des Wiener psychoanalytischen Vereins (ed.) *Über den Selbstmord, insbesondere den Schülerselbstmord*, Wiesbaden: Bergmann, pp. 5–18.

Chapter twenty-four

Preventive interventions in the workplace

Evelyn J. Bromet and David K. Parkinson

Introduction

The aims of this review are to describe (a) the empirical evidence supporting the establishment of mental health intervention programmes in the workplace and (b) the basic elements of an occupational psychiatry programme with a major preventive intervention component. On a conceptual level, occupational psychiatry may be considered a branch of occupational medicine which has as its primary goals the identification, treatment, and *prevention* of occupationally related diseases. Implicit in the interventionist approach of occupational medicine is the acceptance of three sets of hypotheses to be developed more fully in this chapter.

1. The first hypothesis is that some health problems, including psychiatric problems, are caused or triggered by workplace conditions. Psychiatric manifestations may result directly from environmental exposures which at high levels are extremely pathogenic, such as carbon disulphide (Mancuso and Locke 1972), lead (Cantarow and Trumper 1944), organic solvents (Baker and Fine 1986; Cavanagh 1985), and mercury (Hunter 1978). Although the evidence for effects at lower levels is less consistent, Ashford (1976) hypothesized that the combination of such exposure and stress in the workplace may be particularly harmful. It is thus surprising that over the last twenty to thirty years, although most adult study participants in psychiatric epidemiological research are employed full-time, workplace exposures have not routinely been assessed, even in studies focused specifically on identifying causal factors in the environment (e.g., Aneshensel and Stone 1982; Dohrenwend *et al.* 1978) or on explaining the inverse relationship between social class and mental illness (Link *et al.* 1986). Rather, the vast majority of community studies have drawn inferences from job title or assessed such environmental risk factors as general life event stressors or chronic strains (Dohrenwend and Dohrenwend 1982). Although life event checklists contain items pertaining to work difficulties or changes in work status, their scope is typically limited in nature. Only environmental studies using non-checklist forms of

data collection have obtained detailed information on the work setting (e.g., Brown and Harris 1978; Bromet *et al.* 1988). On the other hand, just as community studies pay insufficient attention to the work environment, research on the relationship of occupational stress to mental health has tended to ignore potential effects of non-work sources of stress, making little attempt to integrate non-occupational risk factors when modelling the effects of stress on psychological well-being (e.g., Caplan *et al.* 1975; Glowinkowski and Cooper 1985; Karasek 1979; Kasl 1978).

2. The second hypothesis is that psychiatric problems in the workplace contribute to low productivity and high costs of medical insurance (White 1983). As early as 1916, the medical director of a US silk company acknowledged that 'the psychoneuroses and emotional attitudes of the employees toward their employment, their foremen and fellow workers and the machines were responsible for a greater loss in dollars and cents than accidents or contagion' (Rennie *et al.* 1947: 67). The Hawthorne experiments of the 1930s underscored the relationship between positive social relationships at work and high productivity (Rothlisberger and Dickson 1939). Thus, improving mental health and morale is viewed as economically sound because of the potential for increasing productivity and decreasing absenteeism and turnover (Levi 1981). With respect to the effects of mental health on health care costs, a recent study of a large corporation found that, in 1984, the cost of medical care for 14,162 insured employees and their families was \$29.4 million, with psychiatric treatment accounting for 8 per cent of this total but representing 3 per cent of the claims (Tsai *et al.* 1987). Because the average psychiatric hospital stay was significantly longer than that for other illnesses (20 days vs. 6.1 days), the average total expenditure per admission was three times higher. Direct mental health care costs, of course, represent only a small fraction of the total impact of psychological and substance-related morbidity on total health care expenditure since individuals with diagnosable mental disorders more frequently utilize general medical services than their well peers (Shapiro *et al.* 1984). Many large corporations have established health promotion programmes and Employee Assistance Programmes (Roman 1983; Walsh 1982) which offer a variety of services ranging from comprehensive health assessments to stress management. These programmes are viewed as a means of improving productivity and reducing health costs (Warner *et al.* 1988) and reflect a belief that reduction in morbidity and disease prevention are in the best interest of both the employer and the employee.

3. Presuming the validity of these two hypotheses, the third hypothesis is that mental health conditions which are work-environment related are preventable by eliminating the exposure from the work setting. That is, just as asbestosis can be prevented by removing asbestos dust from the environment, so can some mental health problems be prevented. For

example, toxic encephalopathy can result from solvent exposure at high levels (Gregersen *et al.* 1987) and can be prevented by modification of the work setting, such as by improved ventilation.

Given these three hypotheses, we first discuss the links between workplace conditions and mental health, and then describe the basic elements of a mental health prevention programme in the workplace.

Mental health and the work environment

Prevalence

Surprisingly few epidemiologic studies have documented the extent of psychiatric mortality and morbidity in the workplace. Perhaps the earliest descriptive data were reported by two French physicians regarding symptoms of exposure to carbon disulphide which included excess suicide and psychosis, termed 'sulphide of carbon neurosis' (Hunter 1978). The increased rate of suicide due to carbon disulphide exposure was subsequently quantified by Mancuso and Locke (1972) in an American cohort of viscose rayon workers. The age-sex-adjusted rate for suicide among these workers was 22.7/100,000 compared to 15.1/100,000 for the total US population.

The first large-scale prevalence study of the rate of psychiatric morbidity in a workforce was conducted in New York City in the 1920s at Macy's Department Store (Anderson 1929). Although details on the sampling technique were sketchy, psychiatrists and trained social workers conducted psychiatric evaluations on 1,200 employees of various departments of the store. Twenty per cent of the employees were categorized as 'problem individuals', i.e., were diagnosed as having neurotic disorders. It was suggested that 'a sufficiently large number of problem cases will improve under psychiatric treatment to make the application of such measures profitable – not only in terms of human salvage – but in terms of dollars and cents' (Anderson 1929: 9). This study and the recommendations deriving from it served as the basis for Macy's decision to employ psychiatrists in its personnel department and to conduct psychiatric assessments on all job applications and workers seeking transfers. However, the Great Depression led to a curtailment of most aspects of the programme.

Interest in establishing the prevalence of psychiatric disorders among workforces appears to have waned after the Macy's study. This was undoubtedly due in part to recognition of the limitations in the measurement of psychiatric disorders, which affected psychiatric epidemiology more generally, and to the shifts in focus among psychiatric researchers during the Depression and two world wars. Thus, our recent research on power-plant workers from two nuclear and two coal-fired power-plants was the first occupational psychiatry study in the United States to administer structured diagnostic interviews (the Schedule for Affective Disorders and Schizophrenia – Lifetime Version, Endicott and Spitzer 1978) to a well-defined occupational group (Bromet *et al.* 1982; Bromet *et al.* 1988). The one-year prevalence rate of affective disorders was 16 per cent, and a similar proportion had diagnosable alcohol problems. In a subsequent study addressing effects of low-level lead exposure in the workplace, we administered the Diagnostic Interview Schedule (DIS, Robins *et al.* 1981) to 288 lead-exposed workers from three lead battery plants and 181 non-exposed controls (Parkinson *et al.* 1986). Lifetime rates of depression were considerably lower than those noted above, ranging from 4.3 per cent to 5.3 per cent, whereas alcohol abuse rates were somewhat higher, ranging from 10.6 per cent to 24 per cent. Whether these differences reflect true variations in morbidity rates between these populations is difficult to determine since the instruments used for ascertaining psychiatric history differed. In addition, the lead-exposed workers were older and had worked in the plants for a longer period of time compared to the power-plant workers, and, according to the Epidemiologic Catchment Area findings of a decreased prevalence of depression with increasing age (Robins *et al.* 1984), these demographic differences may also have contributed to the lower rate of depression observed among the lead workers. We are currently conducting a prevalence study of depression and alcohol abuse/ dependence in a sample of 2,000 male and female managers and professionals of a large multinational corporation, and for the first time will have data on the lifetime and recent prevalence rates for these segments of the workforce.

Thus, there is a need at present for more descriptive epidemiological studies of the prevalence of psychiatric disorders in different occupational groups. Prospective studies of the incidence of psychiatric disorders in cohorts of new employees, which are virtually non-existent, would be even more valuable in establishing the extent to which the work environment is implicated in the development of new cases of psychiatric disorders. Although a sizeable literature on occupational mental health exists, most such studies examined non-specific psychological symptoms and drinking behaviour, often employing unstandardized inventories (Kasl 1978). Estimates of the prevalence of clinical disorders, which are more informative with respect to the planning of intervention programmes, cannot adequately be determined from such data. However, findings from community studies have repeatedly shown an inverse relationship between social class and mental illness (Dohrenwend and Dohrenwend 1969). Similarly, workers in less skilled occupations report higher levels of symptomatology than workers in jobs with more prestige and responsibility (Kahn 1981). Findings from treated populations have produced similar results. For example, Ødegaard (1956) analyzed 34,457 psychotic patients admitted to all psychiatric hospitals in Norway and demonstrated that the highest admission rates were in occupations requiring the least skill and social prestige. Thus, although we do not have specific prevalence estimates at present, there are sources of data which would suggest where the greatest needs for psychiatric intervention might be located.

Work-related correlates

In contrast to the dearth of information on the incidence and prevalence of clinical disorders in the workplace, considerable knowledge has accumulated about the work-related correlates of psychiatric symptoms and problem drinking. One variable of particular relevance to blue-collar workers is chemical exposure. As noted above, high levels of toxic substances that affect the nervous system, such as lead, cyanide, carbon monoxide, carbon disulphide, and mercury have been known for years to precipitate symptoms such as depression, anxiety, euphoria, giddiness, short-term memory dysfunction, disorientation, convulsions, and loss of appetite (Collier 1939; Hunter 1978). Collier's description of symptoms resulting from carbon monoxide (an exposure found in workers in blast furnaces, fire fighters, and workers, such as fork-lift truck operators, exposed to exhaust gas from internal combustion engines) also emphasized the following personality disturbances resulting from exposure to high levels of this toxic substance:

> the inability of the sufferer . . . to criticize his own actions or to maintain a clear insight into his own condition. . . . Irresponsible actions, the taking of foolish risks, the inability to realize danger, are characteristic effects and may account perhaps for some of the 'catastrophes of rashness' that are observed during rescue work. (Collier 1939: 92)

Some effects of exposure were so well known that they have been incorporated into the English language. The phrase 'mad as a hatter' stems from observations of clinical syndromes among workers in the hatting industry in Europe during the nineteenth century who were exposed to high levels of mercuric nitrate. Similar conditions were described over a century later in the hatting industry in Danbury, Connecticut, and the associated syndrome became known as 'the Danbury shakes'.

These historical descriptions were associated with high-level exposures where it was easy to identify a single substance responsible for the symptoms. With the lower levels of exposure and the increase in the variety and multiplicity of chemicals used in the workplace today, it is difficult to isolate specific effects except under experimental research conditions. Furthermore, current exposure levels are regulated in most western countries by government standards, and exposures at these lower levels have not consistently been shown to produce psychiatric effects. For example, in our research on occupational lead exposure conducted after the 1978 US occupational lead exposure standard which resulted in major environmental modifications, we found little evidence to support the hypothesis that low-level lead exposure was associated with psychiatric, psychosocial, or neuropsychological performance (Parkinson *et al.* 1986). Furthermore, even workers with previous high exposures did not differ on the measures applied from non-exposed controls, suggesting that if effects had occurred in the past, either they had been reversed, or our sample of long-term employees did not include affected workers who had left the battery plants when exposures were high.

Epidemiological research on effects of low-level exposure to other substances, such as arsenic, mercury, and organic solvents, is needed to determine whether such exposures adversely affect the central nervous system in male and female employees. Our current work on effects of solvent exposure suggests that lower-level exposures may indeed trigger a variety of physical and psychological symptoms in female blue-collar workers, a group who have long been neglected in occupational exposure research (Dew *et al.* in press). Interviews were conducted with more than 160 female assembly-line workers from a light manufacturing plant. After controlling for relevant demographic risk factors, as well as for work stress, increased exposure to solvents at work was significantly associated with psychosomatic, cardiovascular, and respiratory symptoms. We have confirmed these findings in subsequent analyses of 567 female workers from a second light manufacturing plant, a large percentage of whom experienced multiple chemical exposures on their work sites (Bromet *et al.* submitted). The findings from the two plants are noteworthy because a series of case studies was published purporting to describe episodes of 'mass psychogenic illness' in workplaces with predominantly female employees; in each case, solvent exposure was present but was dismissed as a causal agent because the level was below the government-prescribed threshhold. However, these values were determined from human studies of male workers and were based on crude outcomes (e.g., dizziness, mucous membrane irritation) that did not include psychological or neuropsychological measures. They may therefore not be clinically meaningful, particularly for female employees.

The environmental focus of occupational research on white-collar workers has been on the psychosocial milieu, and little attempt has been made to examine the physical environment (Moss 1981). A variety of workplace stressors have been delineated, including status level of the job, monotony, overload, under-utilization of abilities, job ambiguity, inadequate decision latitude, problems with supervisor, and 'person-environment fit' (Baker 1985; Brook 1981). In Kasl's (1978) review of epidemiological studies, the correlations between such workplace factors and various mental health symptoms were typically less than .30. In addition, recent evidence suggests that particular combinations of these stressors, such as high demands coupled with low decision latitude, may have more deleterious effects than single stressors (Karasek 1979).

From a methodological viewpoint, most occupational mental health research has several important shortcomings. Such research is typically cross-sectional, limited to male workers, focused on symptoms that are at times confounded with the measurement of occupational stress, directed exclusively at psychosocial exposure, and (with the exception of our own work) has failed to consider the role of other known risk factors as well as other non-work sources of stress that may affect the outcomes under investigation. (For example, workers with a history of psychiatric problems predating employment might be more vulnerable to the effects of chemical or social stresses.) There are also no prospective studies of healthy workers entering their first jobs and followed over time; such a design would permit an understanding of the unique contribution of the work environment to the onset of newly diagnosed psychiatric disorders. In spite of these limitations, it is still reasonable to conclude that psychiatric disorders, such as depression, which have an environmental component to their aetiology, may at times be precipitated by factors in the work environment. Because adult populations spend at least half of their waking hours at work, these settings provide ideal sites in which to offer intervention and prevention programmes.

Elements of an occupational psychiatry programme

Occupational psychiatry programmes are concerned with two classes of workers: (1) those who develop a mental disorder as a direct result of workplace exposures; (2) workers who develop mental health problems for reasons unrelated to the work environment but which affect work performance. It is often impossible to differentiate between these two groups. Thus, as in general occupational medicine, a comprehensive programme must contain both clinical and preventive components; it should be directed by physicians who are knowledgeable about psychiatry in general and of the workplace specifically. It is important to emphasize that, in practice, most occupational psychiatry problems will be seen initially by a primary care physician whose training in both psychiatry and occupational medicine is not just limited but more often than not absent.

As in other medical care programmes, the clinical service component must address three issues: diagnosis, treatment, and referral. It is the special knowledge of workplace exposures as potential triggers of psychiatric problems that distinguishes occupational psychiatry from other forms of community psychiatry. This 'case management' aspect of occupational psychiatry (Task Force on Psychiatry and Industry 1984) requires that workers have access to competent medical and psychiatric care under conditions that guarantee confidentiality. There must also be a policy in the workplace that such consultation will be offered in cases where deterioration of job performance has triggered the possibility of termination.

With respect to prevention, which is the focus of this chapter, four interrelated components can be identified:

1. identification and measurement of exposures;
2. screening of persons working in high-risk settings;
3. health promotion/stress management;
4. educational programmes for:
   – supervisors,
   – union health and safety officials,
   – primary care physicians or company physicians.

The identification of workplace exposures which may lead to disease is the most fundamental and important part of a prevention programme. Traditionally, walk-through inspections to identify potential exposures, review workplace processes, and identify specific chemical or biologic substances from material safety data sheets are carried out before designing a sampling programme for specific toxic elements in the environment. The measurements are obtained by an industrial hygienist. Exposures which are potentially neurotoxic should be reviewed by a psychiatrist, in consultation with the industrial hygienist. The identification of a toxic exposure should lead to the implementation of engineering and ventilation modifications to reduce the exposure to levels at which no health risk exists.

There is, however, an additional problem that until now has defied proper definition and measurement, namely, the issue of stress in the workplace. Thus, another methodology of particular relevance for identifying non-chemical exposures in the workplace is a screening programme that can identify high-risk settings within an organization. Such a programme may be based on information from current and former employees in those settings as well as periodic analyses of the plant location of individuals utilizing mental health services. Data which may provide indications of stressful situations might also be obtained from grievance actions, records of labour-management difficulties, or sickness absence. Even without a formal occupational stress study, these data would permit a mental health specialist to locate potential high-risk settings and to investigate changes in the work environment which might prevent the onset of new cases in the future. In the Macy's study noted earlier, departmental conditions believed to affect workers unfavourably were modified in an attempt to reduce the level of psychological morbidity. If modifications are introduced using an experimental protocol, effects can be formally evaluated. Unfortunately, as Fielding stated:

355

> Few employers are enthusiastic about long-term studies ... which require serial data collection over many years. ... The cost of data cleaning, collection, and merging of the health and economic data bases, even when logistically possible, can be as expensive or more expensive than the intervention being assessed. (Fielding 1988: 113)

Health promotion and stress management programmes are designed to prevent the onset of mental and physical disorder in workers. Given the relatively high rates of participation in programmes such as Johnson and Johnson's 'Live for Life' (Bly *et al.* 1986) and the lack of stigma (compared to mental health services, such as Employee Assistance Programmes), the expansion of such comprehensive programmes may well be beneficial to employees. It should be noted that no economic analyses of stress management programmes in the workplace and only a little evidence on the benefits of health promotion programmes are currently available (Warner *et al.* 1988). It would be useful if a needs assessment preceded the establishment of such programmes (Roman 1983) so that they could be tailored to the specific needs of a workforce. Programme evaluation studies are needed to determine in what ways and for which workers these programmes are effective in reducing morbidity levels.

Finally, a major pillar of any prevention programme is education. An excellent model for such an educational programme is the National Institute of Mental Health's Depression/Awareness, Recognition and Treatment (D/ART) programme. With respect to occupational mental health, the three groups most likely to encounter psychiatrically disturbed employees are supervisors, union health and safety officials, and primary care physicians. Each of these groups has a different baseline understanding of mental health, and individualized educational programmes should be developed.

Our own team has experience in designing and implementing prevention programmes collaboratively with industry and unions. One such effort, although not a mental health intervention, nevertheless serves as a useful model of a collaboration between union workers (the United Steel Workers of America) and a university team which together designed, delivered, and evaluated a health education programme. Specifically, we initiated an educational programme for coke-oven workers aimed at altering workplace behaviours believed to put these workers at increased exposure to coke-oven emissions and thus at increased risk for lung cancer (Parkinson *et al.* 1989). Seven randomly selected coke-oven plants were given an educational programme, and seven coke-oven plants matched for location and size served as controls. The educational programme, delivered on four occasions over a two-year period, entailed (a) a formal set of lectures on workplace behaviours mandated by the coke-oven standard and the health effects of coke-oven emissions, (b) meetings with local health and safety officials to determine special local problems in the coke-oven batteries, and (c) plant inspections of the coke-oven batteries. To evaluate the effectiveness of the programme, we collected baseline questionnaires prior to the start of the lecture, and one- and six-month telephone follow-up interviews conducted by laid-off coke-oven workers.

Workers from the control plants were divided into two groups: those randomly selected at the time of each educational programme, and those randomly selected at the time of the first educational programme and followed up by telephone contacts throughout the two years in which the educational programme was delivered. The latter group was followed up because we hypothesized that continually asking workers about their workplace behaviours and their knowledge of the coke-oven standard and health risks might remind them about the dangers entailed by their jobs and thus engender the same level of behavioural change as might occur among workers attending the programme. The results showed that workers attending the educational programme changed their workplace behaviours and knew more about the coke-oven standard and potential physical health effects than did those in either control groups.

Conclusion

The work setting has the potential to produce mental health problems because of the presence of chemical, physical, and stress-related exposures, or interactions among these exposure elements. If an environmental factor is the source of the health problems, then reduction of exposure to it must be the primary goal of a prevention programme. This may involve engineering or ventilation changes, or, in the case of stress, reduction of the psychosocial factors believed to have produced the increase in psychiatric symptoms. It is inevitable that prevention programmes will incur considerable cost to be born primarily by companies, and they in turn will support such efforts because improvements in mental health are presumed to increase productivity and decrease health care costs. Thus, senior company officials play a critical role in both prevention programmes and changes to be implemented in the work setting. As noted earlier, ideally, formal evaluations of the effectiveness of prevention programmes and environmental modifications should be implemented from their inception.

Historically, occupational psychiatry has been a component of occupational medical care. For example, the study at Macy's was conducted under the auspices of the company's medical director. In most large companies in the US, the corporate medical department refers workers with psychiatric and substance abuse problems to consultants with whom a formal relationship has been established. Recently, the development of Employee Assistance Programmes (EAPs) has led to a partial removal of responsibility for alcohol, drug abuse, and psychological problems from the purview of the medical department. This development came about at least in part because of concerns about the confidentiality of information regarding drug and alcohol abuse. We suspect that another related reason was a concern among employees that the physician's first loyalty was to the company rather than to the employee. This, however, is certainly not the case in companies where the medical director is a board-certified occupational physician. The American Occupational Medical Association's code of ethics specifically delineates the priorities of occupational physicians and emphasizes that an industrial physician's priorities are first and foremost the health problems of the employee.

Organizationally, occupational psychiatry and EAPs might interact more effectively if they were both under the direction of the corporate medical department. Furthermore, since physical and mental health problems often co-exist, a unified approach can be more easily applied and the relationship of the work environment to such problems, which is an integral component of general occupational medicine, can be more easily investigated.

In closing, we return to our central theme, namely, that there is strong evidence demonstrating a causal relationship between workplace exposure and mental health. Since positive mental health within a workforce is in the best interest of both management and employees, work settings provide ideal places in which to launch and evaluate intervention and prevention programmes.

References

Anderson, V.V. (1929) *Psychiatry in Industry*, New York: Harper & Brothers.

Aneshensel, C. and Stone, J. (1982) 'Stress and depression: a test of the buffering model of social support', *Archives of General Psychiatry* 39: 1392–6.

Ashford, N. (1976) *Crisis in the Workplace: Occupational Disease and Injury*, Cambridge, Mass: MIT Press.

Baker, D. (1985) 'The study of stress at work', *Annual Review of Public Health*, 6: 367–81.

Baker, E. and Fine, L. (1986) 'Solvent neurotoxicity: the current evidence', *Journal of Occupational Medicine*, 28: 126–9.

Bly, J., Jones, R., and Richardson, J. (1986) 'Impact of worksite health promotion on health care costs and utilization: evaluation of Johnson & Johnson's Live for Life Program', *Journal of the American Medical Association* 256: 3235–40.

Bromet, E., Dew, M.A., Parkinson, D.K., and Schulberg, H.C. (1988) 'Predictive effects of occupational and marital stress on the mental health of a male workforce', *Journal of Organizational Behaviour* 9: 1–13.

Bromet, E., Parkinson, D., Schulberg, H., *et al.* (1982) 'Mental health of residents near the Three Mile Island reactor: a comparative study of selected groups', *Journal of Preventive Psychiatry* 1: 225–75.

Bromet, E., Parkinson, D., Cohen, S. *et al.* (1989) 'Health effects of solvent exposure in a female blue-collar cohort', (submitted for publication).

Brook, A. (1981) 'Mental health of people at work', in R. Schilling (ed.) *Occupational Health Practice*, second edition, London: Butterworth.

Brown, G. and Harris, T. (1978) *Social Origins of Depression*, New York: Free Press.

Cantarow, A. and Trumper, M. (1944) *Lead Poisoning*, Baltimore, MD: Williams & Wilkins.

Caplan, R., Cobb, S., French, J., *et al.* (1975) *Job Demands and Worker Health*, Washington, DC: HEW Pub. No. (NIOSH) 75–160.

Cavanagh, J. (1985) 'Solvent neurotoxicity', *British Journal of Industrial Medicine* 42: 433–4.

Collier, H.E. (1939) 'The mental manifestations of some industrial illnesses', *Occupational Psychology* 13: 89–97.

Colligan, M. and Murphy, L. (1979) 'Mass psychogenic illness in organizations: an overview', *Journal of Occupational Psychology* 52: 77–90.

Colligan, M., Pennebaker, J., and Murphy, L. (1982) *Mass Psychogenic Illness: A Social Psychological Analysis*, Hillsdale, NJ: Erlbaum.

Dew, M.A., Bromet, E.J., Parkinson, D.K., *et al.* (in press) 'Effects of solvent exposure and occupational stress on the health of blue collar women', in K. Ratcliff (ed.) *Women, Health and Technology*, Ann Arbor, Mich: University of Michigan Press.

Dohrenwend, B.P. and Dohrenwend, B.S. (1969) *Social Status and Psychological Disorder*, New York: Wiley.

Dohrenwend, B.P. and Dohrenwend, B.S. (1982) 'Perspectives on the past and future of psychiatric epidemiology', *American Journal of Public Health* 72: 1271–9.

Dohrenwend, B.S., Krasnoff, L., Askenasy, A.R., and Dohrenwend, B.P. (1978) 'Exemplification of a method for scaling life events: the PERI Life Events Scale', *Journal of Health and Social Behavior* 19: 205–29.

Endicott, J. and Spitzer, R. (1978) 'A diagnostic interview: The Schedule for Affective Disorders and Schizophrenia', *Archives of General Psychiatry* 35: 837–44.

Fielding J. (1988) 'Editorial: the proof of the health promotion pudding is ... ', *Journal of Occupational Medicine* 30: 113–15.

Glowinkowski, S. and Cooper, C. (1985) 'Current issues in organizational stress research', *Bulletin of the British Psychological Society* 38: 212–16.

Gregerson, P., Klausen, H., and Elsnab, C. (1987) 'Chronic toxic encephalopathy in solvent-exposed painters in Denmark 1976–1980: clinical cases and social consequences after a 5-year follow-up', *American Journal of Industrial Medicine* 11: 399–417.

Hunter, D. (1978) *The Diseases of Occupations*, sixth edition, London: Hodder & Stoughton.

Kahn, R. (1981) *Work and Health*, New York: Wiley.

Karasek, R. (1979) 'Job demands, job decision latitude, and mental strain: implications for job redesign', *Administration Science Quarterly* 24: 285–306.

Kasl, S.V. (1978) 'Epidemiological contributions to the study of work stress', in C. Cooper and R. Payne (eds) *Stress at Work*, New York: Wiley.

Levi, L. (1981) *Preventing Work Stress*, Reading, Mass: Addison-Wesley Publishing Co.

Link, B., Dohrenwend, B., and Skodol, A. (1986) 'Socioeconomic status and schizophrenia: noisome occupational characteristics as a risk factor', *American Social Review* 51: 242–58.

Mancuso, T. and Locke, B. (1972) 'Carbon disulphide as a cause of suicide', *Journal of Occupational Medicine* 14: 595–606.

Moss, L. (1981) *Management Stress*, Reading, Mass: Addison-Wesley Publishing Co.

Ødegaard, Ø. (1956) 'The incidence of psychoses in various occupations', *International Journal of Social Psychiatry* 2: 85–104.

Parkinson, D.K., Bromet, E.J., Dew, M.A., *et al.* (1989) 'Impact of a health programme for coke-oven workers', *Journal of Occupational Medicine* (in press).

Parkinson, D.K., Ryan, C., Bromet, E.J., and Connell, M.M. (1986) 'A psychiatric epidemiologic study of occupational lead exposure', *American Journal of Epidemiology* 123: 261–9.

Rennie, T.A.C., Swackhamer, G., and Woodward, L.E. (1947) 'Toward industrial mental health: an historical review', *Mental Hygiene* 31: 66–88.

Robins, L., Helzer, J., Croughan, J., and Ratcliff, K. (1981) 'National Institute of Mental Health Diagnostic Interview Schedule: its history, characteristics and validity', *Archives of General Psychiatry* 38: 381–9.

Robins, L., Helzer, J., Weissman, M., *et al.* (1984) 'Lifetime prevalence of specific psychiatric disorders in three sites', *Archives of General Psychiatry* 41: 949–58.

Roman, P. (1983) 'Employee Assistance Programs in Australia and the United States: comparisons of origin, structure and the role of behavioral science research', *Journal of Applied Behavioral Science* 19: 367–9.

Rothlisberger, R. and Dickson, W. (1939) *Management and the Worker*, Cambridge, Mass: Harvard University Press.

Shapiro, S., Skinner, E., Kessler, L., *et al.* (1984) 'Utilization of health and mental health services: three Epidemiologic Catchment Area sites', *Archives of General Psychiatry* 41: 971–8.

Task Force on Psychiatry and Industry (1984) 'Report of the Task Force on Psychiatry and Industry', *American Journal of Psychiatry* 141: 1139–44.

Tsai, S., Bernacki, E., and Reedy, S. (1987) 'Mental health care utilization and costs in a corporate setting', *Journal of Occupational Medicine* 29: 812–16.

Walsh, D. (1982) 'Employee Assistance Programs', *Milbank Memorial Fund Quarterly/Health and Society* 60: 492–517.

Warner, K., Wickizer, T., Wolfe, R., *et al.* (1988) 'Economic implications of workplace health promotion programs: review of the literature', *Journal of Occupational Medicine* 30: 106–12.

White, S. (1983) 'Recent trends in occupational mental health: an overview', in S. White (ed.) *Advances in Occupational Mental Health*, San Francisco: Jossey-Bass.

Index

Müller's fibers, 56, 249, 353, 356-358, 378-379
neurobiones, 385
optic nerve fibers, 353, 358-360
plexiform (external molecular) layer, 353
rods, 353, 361, 364-370, 387-388
Rods, *see* Retina
Round column of His (dorsal funiculus), 48, 104 (*See also* Spinal cord)

S

Schwann cells, *see* Lemmoblasts
Scientific drawings and photomicrographs, 72-73, 98
Sensory ganglia, 32-41
Sensory pathways, 44-58
  medula and midbrain, 49-51
  retina, 51-58
  spinal cord, 44-49
Spider cells, *see* Neuroglia
Spinal cord, 217-249
  collateral fibers of, 225, 226, 228, 233-236, 238
  commissural cells of, 224-225, 228-229, 240-242
  dorsal root fibers, 33-34, 103-106, 221-222, 236-240
  ependymal cells of, 246-248
  funicular cells of, 242-243
  secondary sensory pathways, 44-49
  spinal ganglia, 32-35
  ventral root fibers, 15ff., 236, 243
Spiral ganglion, 174, 176. *See also* Cochlea.

Stellate cells of cerebellum
  large, 258-259, 263, 268, 270, 280-281, 292-295
  small, 266, 267, 297-301
Stereotropism, 123-124, 125-126, 127, 134-135, 159-160, 187, 397 (*See also* Mechanism of nerve outgrowth and orientation)
Superficial granular zone of cerebellum, 263-267, 272-274, 276, 290-292, 305, 311, 313
Sympathetic nervous system
  development of cells of, 58-61, 106-110
  nucleus of origin of, 25
  relation to motor plaque, 207, 210
  visceral component of, 60, 80-81
Symphonocyte, 123 (*See also* Lemmoblast)

T

Tactile hairs, 166-173
Tongue
  development of glossopharyngeal nerve terminations, 195-196
  development of gustatory nerve terminations, 188-196
  development of lingual nerve terminations, 185-188
  development of nerve terminations, 185-196
  motor nerve terminations of, 206-214

V

Vestibular nerve, 39-40, 178-184